Organization and Management of IVF Units

Steven D. Fleming • Alex C. Varghese
Editors

Organization and Management of IVF Units

A Practical Guide for the Clinician

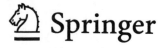 Springer

Editors
Steven D. Fleming, BSc, MSc, PhD
School of Medicine
University of Sydney
Sydney, NSW, Australia

Alex C. Varghese, PhD
ASTRA Fertility Group
Mississauga, ON, Canada

ISBN 978-3-319-80555-9   ISBN 978-3-319-29373-8   (eBook)
DOI 10.1007/978-3-319-29373-8

Printed on acid-free paper

This Springer imprint is published by Springer Nature
The registered company is Springer Science+Business Media LLC New York

Preface

A number of books have been published on the scientific aspects of assisted reproduction. However, they have been mainly aimed at the experienced practitioner alone, with limited benefit to those working in ancillary areas relevant to the IVF unit in its entirety. In contrast, the primary objective of this book is to provide an easy to read, comprehensive guide to establishing and managing an IVF unit from its very inception, with an emphasis on quality control. Therefore, an attempt has been made to direct the material at a broad readership, including those in the clinic, the laboratory, marketing, and IT.

While every effort has been made to ensure that the information contained in this book is as up to date as possible, it should be noted that manufacturers and distributors reserve the right to change product specifications and discontinue product lines without prior notice. New products will invariably be introduced in the future, and it is hoped that future editions of this book will address such innovations. The editors welcome feedback and further discussion regarding any of this book's content.

Sydney, NSW, Australia　　　　　　　　　　　　　　　　　Steven D. Fleming
Mississauga, ON, Canada　　　　　　　　　　　　　　　　　Alex C. Varghese

Contents

Contributors

Baiju P. Ahemmed, MBBS, DGO, DNB Reproductive Medicine, NCARE IVF CENTRE, Balram Memorial Building, Kannur, Kerala, India

Charles L. Bormann, PhD, HCLD Department of Obstetrics, Gynecology, and Reproductive Biology, Brigham and Women's Hospital, Harvard Medical School, Boston, MA, USA

Stuart Campbell, DSc, FRCPEd, FRCOG Create Fertility, London, UK

James Catt, PhD Optimal IVF, Melbourne, VC, Australia

Anne Melton Clark, MPS, MBCHB, FRCOG, FRANZCOG, CREI Fertility First, Hurstville, NSW, Australia

Ian D. Cooke, FRCOG, F Med Sci, FRANZCOG (Hon) Academic Unit of Reproductive and Developmental Medicine, The University of Sheffield, Sheffield, UK

Simon Cooke, BSc Agr, PhD (Med) IVF Australia, Greenwich, NSW, Australia

Denise Donati, RN, CM, BAppSc(Nsg), MN Fertility Solutions, Sunshine Coast Clinic, Buderim, QLD, Australia

Jane Fleming, BSc, MSc, PhD Master of Genetic Counselling Program, Royal North Shore Hospital, Sydney, NSW, Australia

Steven D. Fleming, BSc (Hons), MSc, PhD Discipline of Anatomy and Histology, School of Medical Sciences, University of Sydney, Sydney, NSW, Australia

Joyce Harper, BSc, PhD Embryology, IVF and Reproductive Genetics Group, Institute for Women's Health, University College London, London, UK

Shahryar K. Kavoussi, MD, MPH Austin Fertility and Reproductive Medicine/ Westlake IVF, Austin, TX, USA

Mara Kotrotsou, MUDr Create Fertility, West Wimbledon, UK

Erin I. Lewis, MD Department of Obstetrics, Gynecology, and Reproductive Biology, Brigham and Women's Hospital, Harvard Medical School, Boston, MA, USA

Veronica Montgomery Department of Marketing, Barbados Fertility Centre, Hastings, Barbados

Geeta Nargund, FRCOG Create Fertility, West Wimbledon, UK

John Peek, PhD Fertility Associates, Auckland, New Zealand

Jonathan Pollinger Intranet Future – Social Media Consultancy, Cheltenham, UK

Thomas B. Pool, PhD, HCLD Austin Fertility & Reproductive Medicine/Westlake IVF, Austin, TX, USA

Fertility Center of San Antonio, San Antonio, TX, USA

Amparo Ruiz, MD, PhD IVI-Valencia, Valencia, Spain

John P. Ryan, BSc Agr, MSc Agr, PhD Fertility Specialists of Western Australia and School of Women's and Infants' Health, University of Western Australia, Claremont, WA, Australia

Luis Saurat, MD (Economics), MD (Law) IVI Group, Valencia, Spain

Jason Spittle, BSc Reproductive Health, Cook Medical, Eight Mile Plains, QLD, Australia

James D. Stanger, PhD FertAid Pty Ltd, Newcastle, NSW, Australia

Alex Steinleitner, MD Department of Obstetrics and Gynecology, Sierra Vista Medical Center, San Luis Obispo, CA, USA

John P.P. Tyler, PhD Next Generation Fertility, Parramatta, NSW, Australia Castle Hill, NSW, Australia

Alex C. Varghese, PhD Astra Fertility Group, Mississauga, ON, Canada

Part I
IVF Unit Establishment and Organization

Chapter 1
IVF Unit Location, Design, and Construction

Jason Spittle

Primary Considerations During Planning

Purpose of Clinic

Firstly define what work will be conducted in the clinic. Will it be a full-service clinic offering everything from diagnostic services to IUI, IVF, and PGD? Will it be a boutique clinic offering personalized treatment by a small team or a large clinic offering efficient service to a large patient population? A clear vision of what services are intended will help define the space required and lead to effective planning.

It is also important to consider how the clinic will grow and expand over the next decade and beyond. Try to create some flexibility in the design to allow for changing the room configuration. Assisted reproduction is rapidly evolving and is quick to adopt new technologies. Space requirements will change as the science of IVF evolves. It is very challenging to renovate in an operational clinic. Similarly, it is hard to shut down a busy clinic, so time spent now on planning for the future will save a lot of problems later.

Patient Pathway Review: What Will Be Done in the Clinic?

Viewed simplistically, the process of diagnosing the cause of infertility followed by appropriate treatment represents the basis of care for patients and is universal. How this is implemented in practice varies widely around the world based on factors such as private versus public clinic operations, government and private insurance

J. Spittle, BSc (✉)
Reproductive Health, Cook Medical, 95 Brandl St, Eight Mile Plains, QLD 4113, Australia
e-mail: jason.spittle@cookmedical.com

© Springer Science+Business Media New York 2016   3
S.D. Fleming, A.C. Varghese (eds.), *Organization and Management of IVF Units*, DOI 10.1007/978-3-319-29373-8_1

reimbursement, local legislative directives as to what techniques can be performed, relative affordability of treatment in a country, location, proximity of associated medical services, and the vision of the clinicians/owners/managers.

Careful consideration of the patient treatment pathway (Fig. 1.1) will indicate possible services the clinic can provide.

Many clinics, particularly those competing in a crowded marketplace, look to differentiate themselves by expanding their range of services and taking a more holistic approach to patient care.

Such ancilliary services includes: diagnostic services such as pelvic ultrasound examinations eg., sonohysterography (SHG) or hysterocontrastsonography (HyCoSy), hysterosalpingography (HSG), or testicular ultrasound (increasingly used to assist in diagnosis of male infertility); hormone analysis; andrology; and gamete cryo-banking.

With improvements to the size of instrumentation, hysteroscopy can now be performed in-office with minimal anesthesia requirements. This reduces the cost to the patient of performing hysteroscopy and might assist in improving patient outcomes [1].

Given the proven benefits to reproductive performance of weight reduction [2] and improving patient health prior to undergoing IVF treatment, many clinics now offer dietary advice and management, stress management classes that cover modalities such as meditation, tai chi, and yoga. Psychological counseling is also mandatory in some countries, such as Australia, and routinely offered in many others.

Pre-implantation genetic diagnosis (PGD) is an area of ART that has undergone rapid technological change over the last decade. The advent of next generation sequencing (NGS) of the entire genome promises to simplify the process of PGD, making it more cost effective, easier and faster to perform and more accurate in

PATIENT PATHWAY

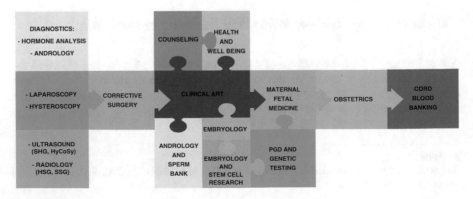

Fig 1.1 Patient treatment pathway

detecting a wider range of genetic abnormalities [3]. Accordingly, provision for performing embryo biopsy and NGS testing and accompanying genetic counseling for the patients may be warranted.

Following successful treatment, pregnancy management including high-risk pregnancies, maternal fetal medicine procedures such as fetal karyotyping from maternal blood, chorion villus biopsy, amniocentesis, and ultrasound might also be offered alongside obstetric services. Finally clinics might also wish to offer cord blood banking to parents.

Although private research is diminishing as ART treatment protocols and outcomes are optimized, some clinics may wish to pursue research. This can be entirely self-funded or performed in conjunction with universities or commercial partners. Depending on the local tax laws in each country, clinics might be able to claim a tax rebate on medical research or attract grant funding from bodies such as the National Health and Medical Research Council or similar.

Determining what will be done in the clinic both now and with a view to future expansion is vital. This vision will be used to create a description of space needed, services required and ultimately the business model to describe how the clinic will be funded. It might not be possible to offer all services initially; however, these can be added later as the clinic expands if allowance (and space) is made during planning.

Outsourcing Versus Insourcing

Determining what services can be offered within your clinic coupled with financial modeling and possibly space restrictions are likely to determine what services might need to be outsourced. This in turn gives indications as to potential locations for basing the clinic; as for patient efficiency, having facilities nearby that can offer the needed services is important. If they are within easy walking distance or have readily accessible parking, so much the better.

Location

Patient Population Demographics

Establishing a new clinic requires significant financial input, so careful estimation of expected cycle numbers is necessary to determine the size and scope of what the clinic can offer. As revenue is driven by patient throughput, if available, population demographics may assist to identify areas within a city or region populated by people of childbearing age (20s to early 40s). Identification of areas populated by potential patients and not well serviced by existing clinics may provide a better opportunity to found a successful clinic rather than opening up across the road from a well-established clinic.

Zoning

Having identified potential locations for the clinic, check the relevant zoning requirements for that location along with any building restrictions likely to impact on the design and construction of the building. It is essential to first clarify what permits/permissions, etc., the local council or government requires as these might restrict what can be done on any chosen site. Always obtain permissions in writing before commencement.

Patient Access

In today's society everyone, it seems, is time-conscious and patients are no different; they are keen to minimize the inconvenience of infertility treatment in their lives. If they have a choice they may opt for clinics that offer the simplest access and most rapid turnaround. It is therefore important to consider how easy it is for patients to access the clinic. Is it close to public transport such as train stations and bus stops? Is there sufficient car parking available for patients—and staff? Are there bicycle racks where nearby residents wishing to ride can secure their bicycles? If in a multistory building, are the lifts efficient so that waiting time is minimal? These might seem like small issues, but to patients attending regularly for injections, ultrasound, and blood tests they can be a major annoyance and add to the stress they experience.

Another consideration is wheelchair access for patients with mobility restrictions as well as for emergency access for ambulance services, should any patient require this.

External Pollution

It is well established that volatile organic compounds (VOCs) are commonly found inside IVF laboratories [4] and can significantly affect the performance of an IVF lab. It is possible to remove these from the lab environment, but it is better to try to minimize those entering the lab if possible. For this reason when choosing a site for a new lab be aware of what VOCs might be emitted upwind of your clinic from local industry, particularly in heavily industrialized cities where environmental controls on emissions might not be rigidly enforced. On a more local level also take note of major roads, as they can be a large source of VOCs, particularly from diesel vehicles and particulates. This necessitates finding a balance between providing easy access for patients and sufficient distance to minimize external pollution. Obviously it may not be possible to avoid exposure to external VOCs in which case focus can be put into removing these from the internal air inside the clinic and this is discussed below.

Another good reason for maintaining a sufficient distance from major roads is that the exposure to traffic pollution has been well studied and linked to respiratory disease and generally poor health of individuals exposed. External pollution tends to concentrate inside buildings, particularly in winter, and combined with seasonal viruses can contribute to health issues in those working in the building. As no clinic can afford to have staff absent a case can be made to consider using HEPA and carbon filters to purify all the internal air fed into the clinic.

External vibration and ICSI do not mix. Anti-vibration tables will assist; however, if external sources of noise and vibration such as trains, subways, and roads carrying heavy vehicles, plant and equipment can be avoided, do so. ICSI is stressful enough to perform without being challenged by vibrating pipettes!

Electromagnetic Fields

The question, do electromagnetic fields (EMFs) have the potential to negatively impact embryos in culture is one that has not been adequately answered and it could be said that research in this area is still in its infancy. Luo et al. found that EMFs could cause DNA damage in pre-implantation embryos in vitro; however, the electromagnetic field was directly applied close to the culture dishes inside an incubator [5]. It is possible that the metal walls of an incubator could act as a Faraday cage to insulate the contents from EMFs thereby protecting embryos in culture. At the moment this is a topic with more questions than answers, however as laboratories have significant electrical wiring and electronic equipment, and we move to greater use of computers communicating wirelessly to equipment via wireless routers, it is apparent that we work in a "sea" of electromagnetic radiation. Electrical equipment particularly that accredited for use in operating theaters is required to meet regulatory standards for EMFs to avoid interference with other electronic equipment. Nonetheless, it may be advisable to consider what has the potential to emit radiation and to consider its location relevant to where embryos are cultured. The health of staff working in the laboratory should also be considered from this perspective, as there is increasing evidence that some individuals can be sensitive to electromagnetic radiation [6].

Design

The principles discussed apply to both building a new clinic from the ground up and adapting an existing building or space. If renovating an existing space, it is worthwhile considering stripping back the space provided to an empty "shell" as then you can identify what materials and piping are in that space and have complete control over what you then place into that space. This also aids the design process as it is then constrained only by the floor area available, ceiling height and any load bearing walls or piers.

The Planning Process

Starting with a blank sheet of paper can be a daunting task, so the following may assist to provide a starting point and aid logical decision making as part of the planning process.

How Much Space Is Required?

Create a list of the functions that will be performed in the clinic and assign a room or rooms to each. Nominate who will work in that room and assign a floor area to it. Equipment and furnishings can also be listed, and this will help determine floor area.

Spheres of Influence

The heart of an IVF lab is the embryo culture area. Consider viewing this as the central point in a series of concentric circles comprising the other areas of the clinic. These will impact what happens in the embryo culture lab to a greater or lesser extent, so mapping the areas of influence may help provide a visual map of interacting functions and factors. Locating related areas close to one another creates efficiency, while separating high traffic areas such as waiting rooms from vibration sensitive areas such as the intracytoplasmic sperm injection (ICSI) workstation just makes sense. The same applies to separating areas sensitive to VOCs such as the culture laboratory from the more dirty areas in the clinic such as the cleaner's room. Using this method and the rooms listed in the section above, create a layout for the clinic. Common sense dictates that areas with similar functions will be grouped together. For example, the egg collection room/operating theater and culture lab will be side by side. The patient reception, waiting room, consulting and accounting areas will similarly be located in close proximity, etc. (Fig. 1.2).

Process Mapping

This is an old concept that can be incredibly useful when designing a clinic. Basically it involves mapping on paper (or using one of many available computer programs) the processes that will occur in the clinic. Maps provide direction. They indicate dangerous ground as well as safe paths, highways versus tracks. Committing ideas to paper allows the design team to break down processes into critical steps, to objectively examine these and identify issues. This allows potential difficulties to be avoided early in the design process. The clarity that comes with process maps should aid in creating efficient systems and reduce risk.

Process mapping can be used to map patient flow through the clinic, and include who comes into contact with the patient, what interactions occur, what resources are required, what time who spends where, what risks are involved, where bottlenecks are likely to occur, etc. Similar maps can be undertaken for almost every activity or procedure. Examples for consideration include, sample

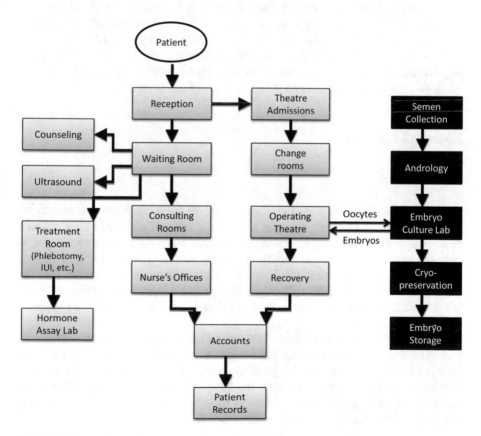

Fig 1.2 Patient and sample flow through the clinic guides proximity of functional areas

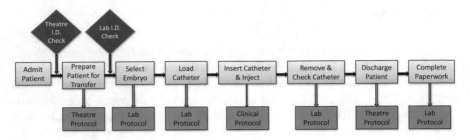

Fig 1.3 Example of a flowchart for an embryo transfer procedure. Each process will have a separate, more detailed protocol assigned to it

collection (e.g., blood or semen), the ovum aspiration process, handling of oocytes, ICSI, embryo culture, IUI, cryopreservation, embryo transfer (Fig. 1.3), data entry, billing, and giving patients disappointing news.

If you are new to process mapping, it is easier to start with the big picture processes and keep them simple. Each of the steps mapped can be the basis of another layer of process mapping and these can be built up until all the key processes in the clinic are described. Once the basics have been outlined they can then be used as the basis for more detailed examination, particularly those related to risk management, creation of standard operating procedures (SOPs), designing training requirements, and a myriad of other uses.

Essential Services

Power

All the critical functions of an IVF theater and lab are dependent upon electricity. Not only is failure of supply a major issue, the quality of electricity supplied to a clinic is also important. Spikes and surges otherwise known as brown outs and white-outs and other fluctuations of supply can cause problems for sensitive electronic equipment. These can occur in the short term resulting in shorts or failure, or over the long term having a cumulative effect, gradually weakening the equipment until failure occurs. This commonly occurs in many developing countries, where the power supply is inconsistent.

Backup in case of power failures is essential and options can include generators and uninterruptable power supply (UPS) systems. Many backup systems also provide power filtering to remove the problems associated with spikes and surges. It is worthwhile in any country to consider the benefits of additional power filtration. It can assist protecting vital lab systems, computers, databases, and the increasing number of electronic devices being employed in medicine.

Generators are usually located external to the building in a secure room, which is readily accessible for servicing, often near to the car park. Generators usually run on diesel or petrol, which is stored in a tank near the generator. Fuel is a potential source of VOCs so should be placed as far away from the air-conditioning air intake as possible.

Gas

The IVF lab requires special mix gas or N_2 and CO_2 for its incubators and clinics with an operating theater will require anesthetic gasses. Gas cylinders are both heavy and dirty and are difficult to move around. The ideal location for cylinders is next to the car park or in a location where fresh cylinders can be collected and empties removed without the need to transport cylinders far from the delivery vehicle. If the clinic is located within a multistory building, ensure that access is available to a service elevator to separate deliveries of gas, liquid nitrogen, and supplies from patient access elevators.

Assigning a small room or caged area to store cylinders and the regulators for each of the gasses used is the ideal solution. Keep gas cylinders out of the culture lab wherever possible. Appropriate storage racks for securing the cylinders from accidentally falling over will reduce the risk to property and staff. Appropriate fittings can be obtained from a local gas supply company.

Any gasses supplied to the laboratory or operating theater should be connected via an automatic changeover regulator system, to ensure that the gas supply does not run out. These are usually supplied and installed by an anesthetic gas supply company. Investigate the quality of the regulators used in the changeover units as these can vary in quality. Some can contain neoprene diaphragms, which have the potential to release VOCs into the gas stream. Regulators with stainless steel diaphragms avoid this issue.

During installation of the gas supply system plumbing will be installed to supply gas into the laboratory. Gas piping is usually made from copper or stainless steel and much debate has occurred over what is the best material for use in an IVF setting.

Another option is to use polytetrafluoroethylene (PTFE) tubing for plumbing gas. This is an inert, non-embryo-toxic material that is ideal for special mix gases as it is not permeable to CO_2. Of the many types of plastic available, even those recommended as food or medical grade, PTFE is the most inert and has less extractable elements such as plasticizers (e.g., phthalate) that can cause embryo toxicity. Silicone is another inert plastic but is permeable to CO_2, so not suitable for premixed gases as the CO_2 concentration will drop proportionately with the length of the tubing, leading to wrong gas concentrations entering the incubator. PTFE tubing has the added advantage that being flexible it can be easily rerouted in the event that the lab requires reconfiguration. It can be purchased as plain tubing or covered in braided stainless steel for protection. It is available from companies like Swagelok®. The addition of Swagelok® fittings allow it to be readily attached to regulators, gas taps and other gas supply fittings.

Liquid Nitrogen (LN₂)

Liquid nitrogen is an important consumable used in cryopreservation and storage of gametes and embryos. It is also hazardous and requires care in handling. If cryo-storage will be performed in the lab a regular supply of LN_2 will be required. The volume of cryopreservation performed and quantity of samples stored will determine delivery and storage methodology. Small and startup units usually use standard dewars containing from 6 to 10 canisters; larger units may choose to use liquid or vapor phase storage vats. Large cryobanks are better served by having a large on-site storage vessel, preferably sited directly outside the lab and in a room that can be easily accessed by delivery personnel. Piping can then deliver LN_2 to the cryolab where it can be used to top up dewars, feed directly to storage vats via an automated top-up system, and provide a source of LN_2 for filling vitrification vessels. Keep piping as short as possible and insulate to minimize loss of LN_2 during delivery. Depending on the volumes used, LN_2 is either delivered in the form of several small tanks or for high volume users the external tank of LN_2 is filled from a delivery truck. In either event external access by delivery vehicles and a transport path needs to be planned.

The cryolab or room where LN_2 will be dispensed and used requires careful design. Some spillage of LN_2 from dewars is inevitable, so floor coverings need to be able to resist the sudden change in temperate and contraction that accompanies this without cracking. Proper ventilation is critical to ensure that LN_2 vapor is rapidly removed and replaced with fresh air, and an oxygen meter installed to warn staff if nitrogen gas has displaced all the oxygen in the room. As this can cause staff to fall unconscious and asphyxiate the investment is warranted.

Air-Conditioning and Air Quality

The relationship between air quality and environmental health is a global issue, although worse in some cities than others. IVF laboratories require pure air to ensure that culture systems remain uncontaminated with pollutants such as VOCs, particulates, and infectious agents such as bacteria and fungi. After ensuring the stability and rapid recovery of temperature and pH of the embryo culture system, VOCs present the next major risk factor to be controlled. As VOCs are ubiquitous it is safe to assume that they will be present in and around any building, although those close to heavy industry and freeways are likely to be more challenged by high concentrations. The first need is to understand where the air is sourced from and potentially what is in it that will need to be removed. VOC meters are available for hire or purchase and can be very useful in this respect, although they do vary in sensitivity. Parts per billion (PPB) meters are by far the better choice as many VOCs can be deleterious to embryos at a PPB level and will of course not be detected by a parts per million (PPM) meter. If VOCs are detected, having the air analyzed to determine what chemicals are present can assist in determining what is the potential risk of toxicity, as not all VOCs are embryo toxic.

Apart from the general quality of air in the environment around your chosen site, consider where the air inlets will be placed to feed air into the air-conditioning and supply system. Conventional wisdom dictates that the air-conditioning system be placed next to the car park to make it easy for the service agent to drive their vehicle close to the machinery for easy servicing. Unfortunately this results in car exhaust fumes being routinely sucked into the air-conditioning and fed into the lab, particularly if the car park is enclosed. Ideally the air intake should be on the top of the building or as far away from car exhaust fumes as possible.

The second consideration is design of air recirculation pathways within the building. It is common for internal air to be recirculated to reduce the expense of heating or cooling external air. Air exhaust vents carry the room air back into the conditioning system where it is mixed with a percentage of external air and then fed back into the building, the key point being that air from "dirty" areas that may contain VOCs might be piped back into the lab. As VOCs are concentrated inside buildings and many are emitted from furnishings, finishes and construction materials, it is wise to view internal air as potentially toxic. One solution is to keep the culture lab's air-conditioning on a completely separate circuit, to more closely control the air quality entering.

While it is possible to remove VOCs from within a lab by use of Coda® Towers or similar filtration systems, it is preferable to remove the contaminants before they enter the lab in the first instance. While HEPA filters will remove particulates, they will not remove VOCs so consideration should be given to installing appropriate filtration systems designed specifically to remove VOCs. They usually comprise filtration systems consisting of activated carbon and an activated alumina substrate impregnated with potassium permanganate. More recently photocatalytic systems that work with titanium oxide have become available. These are designed to fit industry standard air-conditioning ducts and can be retrofitted into existing buildings. Polarized media filtration devices that function using electrostatic attraction may also be useful to filter submicron particles.

Clinics that operate in particularly humid environments should also consider means of controlling the relative humidity in a laboratory. This is due to the correlation between relative humidity and the growth of molds. The presence of mold in an incubator can be disastrous to the embryos in culture and once colonized an incubator can be very difficult to completely sterilize. In addition, high humidity levels can saturate the carbon being used in carbon filters to remove VOCs rendering them ineffective and releasing the VOCs trapped by the carbon.

The ambient temperature in both the theater used for oocyte pickups and transfers and the culture lab is best run as warm as bearable, preferably above 24 °C, to reduce thermal shock to oocytes and embryos exposed to room air, unless environmental chambers are used for all embryo handling, ICSI, and manipulation procedures. It is therefore preferable to have these rooms on a separate circuit whereby their temperature can be controlled without affecting other areas in the building.

Lifts

Lifts are a source of vibration and VOCs so while they may be essential to assist patient access, consideration should be given to the siting of the lift in relation to the culture and ICSI laboratory. Ideally there should be separate lifts for patients and for moving deliveries of consumables such as gas and liquid nitrogen.

Emergency Access

Consideration should be given in the planning phase to emergency access for services such as the ambulance and fire brigade.

Paramedics may require access to the operating theater or collection room in the event that a patient suffers a mishap that is not treatable with the facilities available in the clinic. Passages and doorways should be wide enough to permit easy passage of a gurney to remove patients.

Similar thought should be given to the access that may be required for fire brigade personnel to enter the building in case of fire. This will accompany thought on how to rapidly remove tanks of stored embryos and patient records should the integrity of the building be in jeopardy.

The Floor Plan and Room Design

Clinic: The Doctor, Nurse, and Patient Interface

Ambiance and Stress Reduction

As attending an infertility clinic brings attendant stress for patients, the creation of a welcoming, relaxed ambiance can do much to help put patients at ease. This can be achieved in many ways, limited only by imagination. Plants, fish tanks, external views of a natural environment, paintings, music, lighting, and specific wall colors can all assist in relaxing patients. Other examples (that have been tried) extend to having a grand piano in the foyer playing relaxing music to patients attending for morning blood tests, having four or five small separate waiting rooms, so that patients have complete privacy and rarely see other patients, having tea, coffee, and refreshments on hand, a library of relevant books on infertility for patients to read, Internet stations, TVs for entertainment, etc.

Depending on cultural background, patients often like to mix with other patients and share the highs and lows of the journey. This can be beneficial as a means of mutual support. In this instance creating a space where patients can socialize with

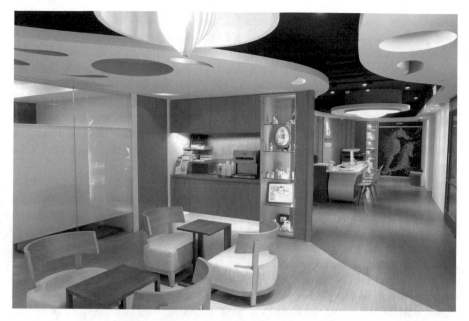

Fig 1.4 A relaxing waiting room where patients can socialize

each other before or after treatment can help create a supportive environment. Figure 1.4 shows a relaxing waiting room where patients can socialize over coffee.

Patients are often in a rush to return to their regular employment, so efficiency in checking in patients in and then seeing them for blood tests, ultrasound, and consultations is appreciated and can help mitigate stress.

A clinic does not need to be "clinical" in appearance, particularly the patient consultation areas. With appropriate design clinics can operate in old, renovated homes, with antique furniture, that feel more like visiting a friend's house than attending a medical practice. There is no right or wrong in styling, only efficiency in how the patient flow works and what suits the cultural temperament of the patients. Advice from a qualified interior designer can be beneficial and as they are used to working with architects, and they can be a useful part of the design team.

Privacy and Confidentiality

Maintaining patient confidentiality, if not a law, is a significant expectation in most countries. In an infertility clinic, this is hard to maintain as patients usually see one another while attending for appointments or tests. Patient files can be left on desks, or patient lists posted where patients can see. Some of this is unavoidable, however beyond seeing a face in the waiting room, it is imperative that patient data and treatment records are kept strictly confidential and access is controlled to those who have a legitimate need to work with it. Commonsense is the cornerstone of building processes that maintain confidentiality. Methods for controlling access to different sections of the clinic should be decided during the planning phase. Numerical keypads or key cards that electronically open doors to admit staff can help control who can access particular areas such as the lab or record storage/filing rooms. Patient files should be kept in a locked room, or locked filing cabinet. Files should not be left unattended on desks; they should be secured when not being worked on.

As many clinics are becoming paperless or at least moving to patient management software and databases, regulations and training for staff on how maintain confidentiality in terms of what can be accidentally viewed on a screen, can assist to maintain what is becoming an important issue for clinics. Similarly, maintaining log-in passwords and changing them regularly is also key to maintaining the integrity of patient data, as is restricting access to areas where computers are kept.

Many countries now have strict privacy laws and take a dim view if patient data is stolen so systems need to be put into place to secure any data put into laptops and taken outside the clinic, as well as access protocols to virtual private networks (VPN'S) used to allow external access to the clinic's data.

When designing the consulting rooms consider the use of soundproofing materials so that the people in the next room cannot hear what is being said. Plasterboard used for building walls comes in a soundproof grade and insulation installed inside wall cavities can also assist.

Semen Collection Rooms

Providing a semen sample is a part of undergoing infertility treatment, but this can be embarrassing for men. While the option of producing at home is one possibility each clinic usually has one or more rooms for semen collection. Discreet placement of these rooms so that they can be accessed without walking in front of a waiting room full of other patients is desirable. So too is having a system that clearly indicates which room is occupied as this can save much embarrassment and additional stress to the patient. Consideration should also be given to using soundproofing materials to reduce extraneous noise entering these rooms.

Treatment Rooms

As most patient examinations and treatments involve at least a partial disrobing, give attention to ensuring privacy for patients in treatment rooms. Pay particular attention to possible lines of sight through open doors, to avoid inadvertently exposing patients when clinic staff enter and leave rooms.

Counseling Rooms

As psychological counseling is mandatory in many countries and commonly offered to assist patients cope with their treatment these rooms should be soundproofed and designed to present a comfortable and safe environment. Even in clinics with high pregnancy rates, many patients do not become pregnant, so both patients and staff appreciate having a private space to deliver disappointing news.

Patient Traffic and Ergonomics

Creating an efficient environment to receive and see patients can make a huge difference to how a clinic functions, especially at the busiest times. Think about the most common patient pathway within the clinic and consider how the clinic layout can best facilitate this. For example patients tend to flow from the main entrance, to reception, the waiting room, Doctor's office, nurses' office, back to reception and out the main entrance again. Designing a floor plan to allow patients to move through the clinic with minimal crossing of paths or backtracking, can make the clinic function much more efficiently and avoid bottlenecks, confusion, and patient mix-ups. Spending time with a good architect and discussing patient flow and the different services offered will be of great assistance in finalizing a design that works well.

Information Technology

IVF clinics run on data, much of it based around patient records. A paper-free record system is a possibility that can add efficiency to a clinic's operation. The advent of tablet computers means that data collection can be portable and adaptable to a clinic's needs. Whether designing a new system or purchasing a commercial system consideration needs to be given as to how the computer system that runs the clinic will operate. The reason for this is that a computerized clinic will require considerable wiring of consulting and examination rooms, the accounting department, nursing and reception, and each workstation in the IVF lab. Even if wireless is used, wiring of routers is also a consideration. In addition, the scope of computerization required to run the clinics of the future will require a central server to operate the system and this will require a temperature controlled room with secure access and a UPS, so this needs to be added to the floor plan.

In addition, as clinics become more computer-dependent and as clinical and patient data is mined for information, office space for information technology (IT) personnel will also be required.

Laboratory

The IVF laboratory forms the heart of an IVF clinic and has a major role to play in creating pregnancies. Given its importance, significant planning time should be allocated to optimizing the design of this space.

Modern assisted reproduction requires several functional areas such as the andrology lab, embryology/culture lab, cryopreservation area, and perhaps a research lab. While it may be tempting to place all these into one big lab for efficiency the negatives outweigh the benefits and it is better to keep these as separate, though closely related rooms.

Planning should be done with risk management principles in mind. These principles form the cornerstone of thought processes, design and operation of the lab and are intended to manage and reduce the risk of adverse events happening to patients, staff and the gametes and embryos in the lab. There are a number of good texts published on the subject, for example Mortimer and Mortimer [7], and an understanding of the principles of quality assurance and risk management will be a great help in designing any new clinic.

Security: Stored Embryos, Patient Data, and Staff

Controlled Access

Given the irreplaceable value of gametes and embryos, both stored and in culture, the embryo lab and environs is not a place for through traffic or persons who do not have a legitimate reason for being there. For this reason securing access to this part of the facility is a simple measure that can help avoid many problems. This can be achieved through the use of security doors operated with key cards or keypads with a numeric access code. The benefit of key cards is that the door locks can be connected to a central computer and staff movements traced if required. This can be particularly useful as units commonly operate seven days a week and after-hours access by staff is both common and necessary.

Ergonomics and Efficiency

IVF laboratories can be extremely busy places with a lot of traffic through the lab. This creates the risk of embryologists bumping into each other and the possibility of dropped dishes containing patient's embryos. Planning the layout giving consideration to the movement of gametes and embryos through the culture processes will help avoid excessive and unneeded staff movement and crossing of pathways. Manufacturing companies aim to have a one-way flow of the product during manufacturing with no crossing or backtracking of this pathway. This minimizes the risk of mixing batches or raw materials. The same considerations apply to IVF labs. Consider that the journey begins in the operating theater or room used for egg pickups. From there the follicular aspirates go to a workstation for oocyte identification. The oocytes are then placed in an incubator waiting insemination. If ICSI is being performed the oocytes will then move to the ICSI stations and then back to incubators for culture. From there embryos are then graded and prepared for transfer and finally excess embryos are moved to a cryopreservation area where they are frozen or vitrified.

Aim to keep this path unidirectional with zones defined by the work performed in them. ICSI is a task that requires intense concentration, so aim to keep the ICSI area segregated from the rest of the lab to avoid the distractions caused by staff moving behind the ICSI embryologist. Accidental bumping and the added vibration caused by movement make performing ICSI harder, so if these risks can be removed it makes the process more efficient. For example consider having an alcove off the main area of the lab set aside for ICSI, or place the ICSI area at the end of a room where there is no through traffic.

Most embryology involves moving eggs or embryos from an incubator to a microscope and back again. The closer that incubators are to the microscope the less movement involved, which reduces the risk of accidents, reduces the time out of the incubator and increases efficiency. The advent of small benchtop incubators means that these can be easily sited next to microscopes and workstations, reducing the need to stand up and move embryos across a lab to a bank of large "box style" incubators. As it is well known that temperature and pH fluctuation is undesirable for embryo culture, another advantage of having benchtop incubators close to the microscopes is that it helps to minimize the duration of exposure of the embryos to ambient conditions and the faster recovery times of benchtop incubators return the culture conditions to the desired state quicker, thereby reducing stress [8].

Airflow

Hospital theater complexes operate as a series of cleanrooms, where the most critical area, usually the operating theater, is the cleanest and kept at a higher pressure than surrounding rooms to ensure air flows out from this room and in doing so prevent contaminants entering the room.

If the embryology lab is adjacent to the operating theater, consideration should be given to running the lab on a separate circuit and trying to minimize the ingress of air from the theater into the lab. The reason for this is that anesthetic gases, sterilizing and cleaning solutions used between cases, and disinfecting solutions are all potentially embryo toxic compounds and should be excluded from the lab environment. This is particularly true if the theater is used for purposes other than ovum aspiration and embryo transfer as a wider range of chemical substances may be used.

Careful consideration also needs to be given to the location of air-conditioning outlets with respect to placement of incubators. As the physical mass of benchtop style incubators is smaller than that of conventional big box incubators, they are more sensitive to being cooled by drafts of cold air exiting the air-conditioning vents. Transient cooling can sometimes trigger their alarm systems, which is an annoyance, particularly after hours. Therefore ensure that cool air does not blow directly onto the benches where incubators will be sited.

Windows and Sunlight

A similar problem to that caused by cool air from air-conditioning vents can be caused by direct exposure to sunlight. If there are windows in the lab, sunlight shining directly onto incubators can cause transient heating and alarming. In general most labs aim for a low level of light to minimize light exposure to embryos while out of the incubator, so would usually shade windows to reduce the amount of ambient light entering the lab.

Andrology and Diagnostic Labs

These labs commonly work with a wide range of potentially toxic chemicals (e.g., PAP stains) as well as pathogens. These areas should be separated physically and be served by separate air-conditioning systems to ensure no crossover of toxins from the diagnostic lab into the culture areas. The use of biosafety cabinets should be considered.

Computerization and Wiring for Quality Management

Modern IVF laboratories should run a comprehensive quality assurance program to ensure consistent outcomes and rapid identification of nonconformance. To this end most items of lab equipment should be independently monitored to ensure they are functioning correctly. Examples are remote temperature and CO_2 monitoring of incubators, fridge and freezer temperatures, liquid nitrogen levels in dewars, ambient temperature sensors, etc. Monitoring devices can be hard wired to a central monitoring database, so plan to incorporate wiring channels for monitoring equipment to the planned location for all capital equipment in the lab.

As some level of computerization is required within any lab, space needs to be allowed for computer access for data entry and review. Depending on the type of patient management system used, the lab could be paperless in which case touch screens for data entry may be located next to each work station and connected by hardwiring or wireless communication to the central server.

The growth of wireless technology means that hardwiring may be replaced by wireless in the near future, so this will require consideration particularly around "future proofing" the design. If the lab is large, several wireless routers may be required, which will require wiring to the server room. Different systems exist for routing wiring and maintaining access to the wiring for maintenance and reconfiguration. These can be sited under the floor, in the roof space or in ducting mounted in or on the walls. Reviewing what systems are available with consideration to future expansion or changes to room layout and function will help considerably as change is inevitable.

Safety

Ensuring the safety of the staff that work within the lab is an obvious expectation so once the initial floor plan has been decided upon, give consideration to the space required for hazardous biological waste disposal bins near the ovum pick up stations, sharps bins for disposal of pipettes and ICSI and holding pipettes. External rubbish disposal areas where hazardous waste from the labs can be safely stored until the waste disposal company can collect also need to be planned.

Safety extends to hand washing areas, eye baths, and potentially safety showers that need to be located in close proximity to the IVF and diagnostic laboratories.

Process mapping of the tasks being performed in the laboratory and a physical map of personnel movement though the lab will also help to minimize crossing over of movements, particularly those that could result in accidents, spillages or disruption to staff performing delicate tasks such as ICSI.

Storage

The operating theater and IVF lab utilize many different consumables; these require storage space and should not be stored in the lab or theater. Firstly, cardboard packaging is a source of dust, bacterial contamination, and most cardboard is saturated with VOCs. Consumables should be removed from cardboard packaging outside the lab complex and transferred to plastic storage tubs for storage close to the lab. As the plastic packaging surrounding the consumables (e.g., plasticware) can also be a source of VOCs it is preferable to keep consumables in a storeroom area outside the lab and only transfer into the lab a small quantity of what is required for use.

Construction

Construction methods will vary according to whether the clinic is being built new from the ground up or installed into an existing space in a hospital or commercial building. One of the added challenges of using an existing space is that floors and ceilings are often cast concrete and it may not be possible to create holes for plumb-ing, piping and wiring, so this may create some constraints over what can be put where.

Minimizing the use of solid, loadbearing walls in the building design means that walls can be constructed in a way that allows them to be readily moved. There are now many demountable or modular styles of wall construction available. These give future flexibility in the use of the space and simplify the process of remodeling the floor-plan, minimizing construction time. Pay close attention to the composition of materials suggested.

Any clinic performing embryo culture should be extremely aware of potential sources of irritant and toxic gases and aim to exclude these sources wherever possible. Laboratories in particular should be airtight spaces in order to prevent the uncon-trolled entry of external containments. Careful consideration as to the materials used for floors, walls, wall insulation, ceiling and ceiling insulation materials is required. Formaldehyde and other VOCs are commonplace and will outgas from sources including linoleum and synthetic carpet floor coverings, the glues used to install these, particleboards, wall coverings, furniture, paints and plastics.

Floor Coverings

Given the impact that VOCs can have on culture outcomes, the types of materials used in constructing and furnishing the culture lab are critical. The less outgassing that occurs, the less VOC removal systems will have to deal with. Beginning with the floor, a lab requires a surface that is non-slip, nonpermeable to fluids, easy to clean, and does not outgas. This reduces the options considerably.

Tiles are one possibility, however should be large to minimize the usage of grout and ideally the grout should be sealed to prevent trapping bacteria or fungi. A more common floor covering is commercial linoleum supplied specifically for laborato-ries and resistant to chemicals, LN2, and other spillages. When installed it should extend up the walls so that no right angle corners are formed which can trap bacteria and fungi and can be difficult to clean.

Walls

Laboratory and operating theater walls should be sealed and have a nonpermeable surface that can be easily cleaned, or fully decontaminated if required. Wall con-struction can be of aluminum, coated steel, plastered brick or plasterboard sealed with paint. Most paints are a potent source of VOCs and can continue to outgas for months. Major paint manufacturers often sell low VOC paints, but this does not remove the problem, it just decreases it slightly. There are now specialist manufac-turers that make zero VOC paints so it is worthwhile making an effort to find these if they are present in your region.

A trap to be wary of is that although one can specify to the architect and builder the need to avoid glues, solvents and the many building products that contain VOCs, they are not embryologists and have no idea that even tiny concentrations of VOCs can have a significant effect on embryo culture. The builder might subcontract out work; particularly painting, meaning the painters are removed from the education provided to the builder about the need to avoid toxic products. Despite specifying the brand of paint, painters may ignore this and use their preferred brand. The message is that extreme vigilance is required to ensure that every member of the construction team is aware of toxicity issues and held responsible for only using the products specified. Regular, frequent site visits during construction are recommended as uncovering problems at this stage can save much time and money later in the commissioning process.

If there are windows inserted into the walls ensure that there are no flat windowsills to trap dust. Windowsills should be angled so that particulates are shed downwards onto the floor or the glass placed flush with the wall.

Ceilings

Ceilings should be sealed to prevent the ingress of particles and similarly constructed of a material that can be completely cleaned. Coated steel or painted plasterboard are the main options and the same considerations apply to paint as mentioned above. Suspended ceiling tiles should not be used as they are not impermeable to dust, particles and the air circulating within the space between the suspending ceiling and the roof.

Lighting for the Culture Lab

As the interior of the fallopian tube is not exposed to visible light concern about the exposure of embryos to light has existed since the beginning of IVF. Many labs did and still do work with low ambient light levels, preferring incandescent lighting over fluorescent lighting due to concerns about the wavelengths emitted. Ottosen et al. performed an informative evaluation of light exposure to oocytes and pre-implantation embryos and concluded that subdued yet comfortable ambient light presents no threat to embryos [9]. They do however suggest that the damaging effect of visible light results from wavelengths of 400 to 500 nm and this primarily comes from tungsten halogen incandescent light supplied by microscope light sources. They recommend reducing the light intensity as much as possible during embryo observation and using filters to exclude radiation energy in this range.

Whatever lighting is chosen, the light fitting should be enclosed to avoid contaminants from the ceiling space entering the room.

Lab Benches and Cupboards

A very common building material for cupboards and bench-tops is medium density fiberboard (MDF) covered with a plastic laminate. MDF is essentially made from wood particles bonded together with a variety of resins. These can outgas for extended periods of time (several months or more), releasing formaldehyde, classified by the WHO International Agency for Research on Cancer as a known carcinogen, and other potentially embryo toxic VOCs. Particleboard is another commonly used material with the same issues as MDF. If either of these is present it is suggested to paint the raw surface to help to seal in the VOCs and inhibit their outgassing.

Materials that do not outgas such as stainless steel or stone or engineered stone surfaces may therefore be a better choice for bench-tops.

Lab Furnishings

Chairs or stools are commonly used in IVF labs and it is generally accepted that one needs to be seated to work on microscopes. Chairs move on their castors however and can present a hazard to moving around the lab when holding embryo dishes. By adjusting the heights of bench-tops and microscopes it is possible to work standing up, which has the side benefit of improved ergonomics for the staff, no outgassing from the plastics used in chair construction and less clutter in the lab.

Conclusion

This chapter only briefly touches on many of the topics involved in building or renovating an ART clinic. The intention is to provide the reader with ideas for further research as they formulate plans for their clinic. Time spent thinking about current and future needs, planning the layout and reviewing designs before commencing building is critical to achieving a functional, pleasant, and efficient place to treat patients and work. A healthy building creates a pleasant working environment and in a business where stress minimization leads to better patient's outcomes, careful planning and attention to detail will reap rewards for both the clinic staff and the patients undergoing treatment.

References

1. Pundir J, Pundir V, Omanwa K, Khalaf Y, El-Toukhy T. Hysteroscopy prior to the first IVF cycle: a systematic review and meta-analysis. Reprod BioMed Online. 2014;28(2):151–61.
2. Norman RJ, Noakes M, Wu R, Davies MJ, Moran L, Wang JX. Improving reproductive performance in overweight/obese women with effective weight management. Hum Reprod Update. 2004;10(3):267–80.

3. Martin J, Cervero A, Mir P, Martinez JAC, Pellicer A, Simón C. The impact of next-generation sequencing technology on preimplantation genetic diagnosis and screening. Fertil Steril. 2013;99(4):1054–61.

4. Cohen J, Gilligan A, Esposito W, Schimmel T, Dale B. Ambient air and its potential effects on conception *in vitro*. Hum Reprod. 1997;12(8):1742–9.

5. Luo Q, Yang J, Zeng Q, Zhu X, Qian Y, Huang H. 50-Hertz electromagnetic fields induce gammaH2AX foci formation in mouse preimplantation embryos in vitro. Biol Reprod. 2006;75:673–80.

6. Genuis SJ, Lipp CT. Electromagnetic hypersensitivity: fact or fiction? Sci Total Environ. 2012;414:103–12.

7. Mortimer S. Quality and risk management in the IVF laboratory. Cambridge: Cambridge University Press; 2005.

8. Cooke S, Tyler JPP, Driscoll G. Objective assessments of temperature maintenance using in vitro culture techniques. J Assist Reprod Genet. 2002;19(8):368–75.

9. Ottosen LDM, Hindkjaer J, Ingerslev J. Light exposure of the ovum and preimplantation embryo during ART procedures. J Assist Reprod Genet. 2007;24:99–103.

Chapter 2
Batch IVF Programme in ART: Practical Considerations

Baiju P. Ahemmed and Alex C. Varghese

Batch IVF Programme

Batch IVF programme may be defined as a planned process of recruitment and synchronisation of menstrual cycles and ovarian stimulation in a cohort of woman seeking IVF/ICSI to facilitate the completion of the process of assisted reproduction treatment (ART: oocyte retrieval, IVF/ICSI, embryo transfer (ET) and cryopreservation) within a designated time period [1]. Batch IVF may or may not be directly or indirectly influenced by limited resources (financial and otherwise) or number of patients. It may or may not also be associated with a certain degree of conciliation to get the embryologist and at times a trained fertility specialist on board. Essentially batch IVF is a cusp of science and logistics. The crux of batch IVF is how to implement the programme within that stipulated time without compromising the quality in ART on clinical as well as on the embryology side.

Background of Batch IVF Programme

IVF therapy costs 2–3 times more for the couple when they have to travel to distant cities when we consider the lost working days and the financial burden of IVF that may necessitate batching of cases in the peripheral centres. In some settings batching may be practised because it is cost beneficial to the programme and/or the

B.P. Ahemmed, MBBS, DGO, DNB
Reproductive Medicine, NCARE IVF CENTRE,
Balram Memorial Building, Rajiv Gandhi Road, Kannur 670 001, Kerala, India
e-mail: baijupookilath@hotmail.com

A.C. Varghese, PhD (✉)
Astra Fertility Group, 4303 Village Centre, Mississauga, ON, Canada, L4Z 1S2
e-mail: alexcv2008@gmail.com

© Springer Science+Business Media New York 2016
S.D. Fleming, A.C. Varghese (eds.), *Organization and Management of IVF Units*, DOI 10.1007/978-3-319-29373-8_2

patient. Some centres with high volumes of patients may also need to batch their cases to facilitate co-ordination of work and individualise treatment and cycle management according to logistics. It is important that the fertility specialist is well versed with the specifics of embryology as well so as to facilitate cover in the absence of an embryologist. Arrangements should be in place to make sure services of an alternative embryologist are available in case of need. While the practice of batch IVF may be a controversial issue with both proponents and opponents of this practice, one cannot underestimate the necessity of batching in some settings. Strategies to prevent market pressure constraints from affecting clinical management, and methods to deal with these constraints are important. Formulating a set of standard guidelines to facilitate transparent and smooth running of the process of batching may ensure increased success without compromising patient care. In an era of individualisation and tailored management, patient selection is very important to optimise the results of batch IVF [1].

Types of Settings of Batch IVF

Well organised and well equipped set-ups with in-house embryologist and infertility specialist may choose to batch to optimise resources such as drugs, media, consumables, incubator and availability of the fertility specialist and hospital facilities such as operating theatre (OT), anaesthetist, beds, ancillary staff, etc. These settings do not have time constraints. By batching, they are able to allow time for the lab to recover and also time for the audit process. Media, consumables and other logistics can be economised to make IVF more cost effective to the patient and the centre. Many of the drugs and media used have short shelf life and batching would help reduce costs. For example, rFSH can be shared, if only a small dose of it is needed in a step down protocol. Resources in the centres, particularly those where other gynaecological specialties are also practised, can be streamlined. Consumables and media are better utilised, team is geared up better and quality control can be assessed better.

Set-ups with in-house fertility specialist and a visiting embryologist may do batching based on the availability of the freelancing embryologist. This setting may also give optimal results and resource utilisation provided there is ample flexibility in time period given by the embryologist or a back-up provided and proper planning of the entire batch.

General set up (usually run by a general gynaecologist) with visiting fertility specialists and embryologists coming in for the designated days may do batching out of sheer necessity and with rigid constraints. The gynaecologist recruits a batch of patients and starts stimulation as per remote instructions given by a fertility specialist. This may lead to suboptimal stimulation. The fertility specialist joins at the time of oocyte retrieval and/or ET and may not be aware of the full clinical details of the patients. Laboratory may lack optimal working conditions and availability of necessary logistics in absence of trained in-house staff or an embryologist. Such a setting functions more as a recruitment centre and may lead to serious compromises in key issues of patient management. Such settings are also more prone to inconsistent results and inappropriate utilisation of the available resources. This might lead to overall sub-standard care.

Shortage of well trained, skilled and experienced embryologists and lab technicians may be one of the main reasons for programmes to resort to batching. Arrangements should be in place to make sure there is availability of additional embryologists and ancillary staff to allow effective, uncompromised and undisturbed functioning of the entire process. This may mean having additional junior embryologists and lab technicians to handle the workload with the visiting senior embryologist supervising. Advantages and disadvantages depend on the setting and the organisation of batching. Specialists practising batch IVF should be aware of their limitations and be able to refer couples with complex issues (e.g. poor responders or hyper-responders, and recurrent implantation failures) to better-suited fertility centres as and when necessary. Seropositive and immunocompromised patients should be diagnosed early and should be referred to an IVF unit which handles those cases and has the facility to do such cases separately, including cryopreservation. Strategies to identify such couples beforehand are one of the key factors to ensure proper success while batching [2].

Batch IVF Preparation

Preparation of Patients

Complete the pre-IVF investigations of the couple—haematological, endocrinological and imaging studies should be completed and patients should be reassessed before enrolling onto a batch IVF programme.

Consents forms of all couples should be signed and completed.

Also complete pre-IVF procedures before starting a batch IVF programme—hysteroscopy, mock ET, coring (endometrial scratch), etc.

Verify all records including the completed consent forms just before commencement of batch IVF.

Determine the number of patients included in a particular batch IVF programme and adjust and confirm the available dates of embryologists according to the number of recruited patients.

Ensure individual couple counselling and explain the procedural details of batch IVF to the individual couples participating in the programme.

Plan the treatment protocol suiting each couple based on the individual characteristics; e.g. type of protocol for stimulation, type and dose of gonadotropins, freezing strategy, sperm retrieval and sperm freezing, IVF/ICSI/IMSI, luteal support, etc.

The choice of the protocol should be based on the women's ovarian reserve and the experience of the fertility units and specialists. If the unit is depending on the visiting reproductive medicine specialists to perform the cycles, it is good practice to be in constant touch with the visiting experts right from the start of the treatment cycle.

Keep back-up frozen semen samples depending on the requirement based on the quality of each person's sample.

Keep always a frozen TESA/PESA sample in cases of non-obstructive azoospermia/obstructive azoospermia.

Ordering for Gonadotropins

Determine the initial starting dose for each patient and multiply it by 10 to get the total amount of gonadotropins needed for that particular batch.

Decision over the choice of gonadotropins is purely on personal preferences.

Keep 5–10 % of the calculated total dose of gonadotropins extra for back-up use to meet additional requirements in case of emergency.

Ensure the availability of gonadotropins 1 week prior to the commencement of a batch.

A dedicated, designated staff member responsible for gonadotropin injections should be posted in the IVF unit.

Keep a separate refrigerator with uninterrupted power supply (UPS) back-up exclusively for gonadotropins and maintain a strict cold chain in the IVF unit.

Getting the Lab Ready for Batch IVF

Make a list of all things to do in consultation with the visiting embryologist and proceed accordingly without any flaws.

Make sure all disposables are available in sufficient amount and quantity at least 1 week prior to the commencement of the programme. All disposables should be kept and stored in an air-conditioned separate area near to the laboratory in an orderly manner (see Tables 2.1 and 2.2).

Make sure and verify all equipment and confirm that they are in good working condition at least a few days before commencement of the programme.

Arrange for any additional equipment and disposables, if needed, according to the number of patients in that particular batch.

Check all UPS connections and verify their status at time of preparation for the batch IVF programme.

Calculate the media needed for a particular batch and make it available at least 5 days before starting the programme, and they should be kept in a separate fridge with UPS back-up at reachable distance from the laboratory (see Table 2.2).

It is advisable to do a sperm survival test with all lots of new media prior to each batch.

Table 2.1 Disposables required for one patient (NCARE IVF, India)

Disposable item	Quantity in number
Semen collection container	1
Sterile probe cover	1
Oocyte aspiration needle	1
Hand care gloves	5
Sterile powder free latex gloves	5
Round bottom tube 14.0 ml	20
Round bottom tube 6.0 ml	2
Screening dish 3034	10
Serological pipette 10.0 ml	2
Serological pipette 5.0 ml	2
Pasteur pipette 5.0 in.	3
Falcon centrifuge tube 15.0 ml	2
BD 7575 pipette 3.0 ml	10
Denuding pipette 170 μm	2
Denuding pipette 140 μm	2
Diamond microtip	2
Disposable BD syringe 1.0 ml	7
ICSI dish	1
Holding pipette	1
Injection needle	1
Nunc four well dish	4
Nunc culture dish	1
Embryo transfer catheter	1
Embryo transfer stylet	1
Goblet	1
Cryolock	2
Aluminium cane	1

Table 2.2 Amount of media required for one patient (NCARE IVF, India)

Type of media	Amount
Cleavage media	2.5 ml
Extended culture media	1.5 ml
Fertilisation media	5.0 ml
Sperm rinse	5.0 ml
Flushing media—MOPS	15.0 ml
Hyaluronidase 0.1 ml	0.05 ml
ICSI PVP 0.1 ml	0.03 ml
Double density gradient	1.0 ml
Paraffin oil	12.0 ml
Vitrification kit (SAGE)	4.0 ml for nine patients
Warming kit (SAGE)	4.0 ml for eight patients

Calibration of Instruments

Calibration of instruments should be done before commencing each batch. Temperature and CO_2 control of all incubators and consistency of temperature of all heated stages should be verified and adjusted accordingly.

Cleaning and Air Quality

In spite of the fact that batch IVF units perform only intermittent cycles unlike regular programmes, cleaning and sterilisation of laboratory and adjacent rooms needs to be undertaken as part of clean room discipline. Embryosafe cleaning solutions need to be used such as Oosafe or Fertisafe. Excessive use of any alcohols can have a deleterious consequence on preimplantation embryo development. Hence it is better to avoid use of any alcohols in the vicinity. It is observed that many laboratory areas where batch IVF is performed is shut down completely once the batch is over. This may not be good practice. Regular inspection of equipment performance and lab cleaning ensures good laboratory practice. Since many batch IVF units are in low resource settings, a compromise is made by many units when it comes to installing the air handling units. Since much evidence indicates that air quality, especially the volatile organic compound (VOC) level, can have a negative impact on embryo culture systems, at least minimal investment should be made to procure air handling systems in laboratory areas which can reduce the particulate matter and VOC level. An external validation of the facility by quality control (QC) experts might be a good idea to evaluate laboratory conditions.

Laboratory Cleaning Procedure [3–5]

The laboratory and OT areas should be cleaned on a regular basis with the intention of minimising particle and microbial contaminants. The cleaning materials should not introduce any kind of volatile chemicals and/or organic compounds into the laboratory or OT.

Cleaning Solutions Used

1. Oosafe (OODIH 1000)—For cleaning laminar airflow cabinets (LAF's), CO_2 incubators and bench tops.
2. Oosafe (OODSF 02000)—For IVF and andrology laboratory, OT—Cleaning walls and floor.
3. Tissue culture (TC) grade water.

Materials Used for Cleaning

Designated mops, autoclaved gauze, sterile water in separate utensils for laboratory, OT and normal areas.

Method of Cleaning

Day 1—Cleaning the laboratory and OT area
Day 2—Incubator cleaning
Day 3—Incubator decontamination

Cleaning of Laboratory Equipment, Laboratory Areas and Surroundings

This has to be done by authorised personnel. Use OODSF—Disinfectant Oosafe in 1:100 dilution (10 ml of OODSF in 1000 ml of distilled water) for IVF laboratory walls, ceiling, floor and its premises. Use separate mops exclusively for each area and these should be marked accordingly. Use separate cleaning utensils for OT and IVF laboratory.

All cleaning movements should be in a single unidirectional way. This will prevent the spread of contaminants and dust in the area which has been cleaned. Also keep a pattern for cleaning of surfaces and do not move from area to area randomly. Follow the principle: The area that has to be completely sterile has to be cleaned last. So in an IVF laboratory, the inner surfaces of the incubators should be the last area to be cleaned.

Use cotton gauze for cleaning the ceiling, walls and floor of the OT. Routinely this should be regularly and frequently changed during the procedure. First clean ceiling, then walls and lastly floors using diluted Oosafe solution and this should be followed by distilled water. Keep changing the gauze wrapped around the mop. This precaution is done to prevent carry-over of dirt from place to place. Clean the laminar flow outer surface (not the working area) with the gauze.

Then start cleaning the lab benches and equipment with distilled water and then with Oosafe solution (OODIH 1000). Use autoclaved gauze for this purpose. Carefully clean the microscopes and outer surface of incubators taking enough time. The door gaps of incubators should be cleaned carefully. Working area in the laminar flow should be cleaned thoroughly and cautiously from the top followed by the sides and lastly the bench. Used only TC grade water inside the laminar flow. This should be followed by thorough cleaning with Oosafe solution (ODIH 1000). Oosafe solution should be applied evenly on surfaces and allowed 15 min to dry out for the best results, and cleaned with a sterile gauze impregnated with sterile water.

Incubator cleaning should be done exclusively on a separate day. But on that day, again the LAF should be cleaned as mentioned previously and the surface of the LAF should be used to store the incubator racks while cleaning the incubators.

Incubator Cleaning

The person cleaning incubators should be in sterile attire and gloves. They should use sterile gloves and have to take care not to touch any outside surfaces. Racks should be taken out and kept in the cleaned LAF. One person should be available to assist the person cleaning the incubators. For cleaning one should use autoclaved cotton gauze and cleaning should be unidirectional with smooth movements from inside to outside. Start from the top and then go to the sides and finally to the floor spaces. Cleaning has to be started using TC grade water followed by OODIH 1000. After OODIH 1000 washing wait for 15–20 min to dry out the surfaces. While using OODIH 1000, do not flood the surfaces inside; instead make the cotton wet and then clean the surfaces. Later cleaning should be repeated with sterile gauze impregnated with TC grade water. The cleaning process should be repeated twice and gauze and gloves should be changed in between. After cleaning, incubator doors should be kept open and allowed to dry.

Once inner surfaces are cleaned, close the incubator doors and start cleaning the racks that are placed on the laminar flow. Racks are also cleaned in a similar way that inner surfaces are cleaned and allowed to dry. Make sure that only one incubator is cleaned at a time and after completion of that, change over to the next one.

Next day, incubator decontamination and start-up is done as mentioned in the operating manual. It is not mandatory that every month incubator decontamination is done. The decontamination process can be repeated once in every 3 months. If the microbial culture report is negative after mechanical cleaning, decontamination can be done once in every 6 months also. Any further manipulations inside the incubator, like adding sterile water, etc., should be under strict aseptic conditions.

Laboratory Maintenance Schedule

Weekly—Laboratory and OT wall, roof and ceiling areas
Fortnightly—Changing water in incubators, taking swabs for culture, LN_2 dewar filling
Monthly—Incubator cleaning, calibration of incubators, instruments and heated stages
3–4 Monthly—Charcoal in-line filter replacement, LAF pre-filter changing [6]

Work Co-ordination in Batch IVF

Optimum Number of Patients

Decide on the number of couples to be included in a given batch depending on the availability of the embryologist and keeping in mind the capacity of the laboratory. Most recommend a maximum of 4–5 patients per incubator (Standard CO_2 Incubator) per day, however this also depends on the number of oocytes harvested and the number of embryos from each patient. Practically speaking, it is ideal to restrict activity to around five oocyte pick-ups (OPU's; a maximum of 5–6 OPU's) while seeing to it that the aimed average targeted yield is around 10 (maximum of 15) oocytes per patient. This would require individualised targeted ovarian stimulation. While estimating the work load the time needed for ET's should also be accounted for, since fresh transfers would start from day 2 onwards. As an example, if one is scheduling about five women in one batch it would make it necessary for the embryologist to remain onsite for Day −1 to confirm readiness of the laboratory; Day 0 would be for oocyte retrieval and an additional 2 days to ensure Day 2 ET's. Additional time, staff and laboratory equipment may become inevitably necessary and needs to be arranged if planning for complex procedures such as TESE in that batch, for vitrification and if any blastocyst transfers are required.

Optimum Number of Incubators

The number of incubators will play a crucial role in the success of an IVF programme. It is more important in a batch IVF setting. This is because crowding of cases in a limited duration of time will definitely lead to compromised culture conditions if not managed properly with an adequate number of incubators. In a set-up where we are planning to do five cases per month should have two incubators. During a batch IVF programme, one incubator should be completely dedicated to store culture media, oil, dishes and consumables. This incubator can also be used for keeping the oocytes after OPU, before denudation/co-incubation. The second incubator should be exclusively used for culture. In a standard CO_2 incubator, ideally 4–5 cases should be kept at a time. If the number of cases increases, it increases the frequency of door opening and a crowded incubator will compromise the quality of culture conditions. So if a centre is doing 15–20 cases per batch, they should be ideally having 4–5 standard CO_2 incubators to avoid compromising culture conditions [6].

IVF Batching: A Practical Approach to Make It Possible (See Table 2.3)

If the days when the embryologist is available on site are considered as Day 0, Day 1 and so on, this would be a general framework for planning the whole cycle. All scheduling is done based on these dates and going back from these available days.

Day 0 minus 2 days (36 h earlier) will be the day of trigger. Day of trigger minus 10 days will be the day of starting stimulation if an antagonist cycle and minus 11 days will be the day of starting stimulation if a long agonist down-regulation cycle. That means day of starting stimulation has to be Day 2 or 3 of menses. So we have to stop the oral contraceptive pill (OCP) 7–8 days prior to starting stimulation.

Sample BATCH Calendar for 4-5 Patients with D2 Transfers						
Sun	Mon	Tue	Wed	Thu	Fri	Sat
		1	2	3	4 GnRHa Depot	5
6	7	8 Start GnRHa	9	10	11 Stop OCP	12
13	14	15	16	17 Start Gonadotropin	18	19
20	21	22 Start Antagonist	23	24	25	26
27 Trigger	28	29 Availability of embryologist	30 Availability of embryologist	31 Availability of embryologist		

Table 2.3 Sample calendar

Again day of trigger minus 17 days will be the day for stopping of OCP and day of trigger minus 21 days will be the day for starting GnRHa if going for daily GnRHa. By that we expect to achieve 10–14 days of down-regulation with 4–5 days of over-lap of the OCP with GnRHa to prevent cyst formation due to the flare effect of GnRHa. Another way of achieving down-regulation is to give a single dose of Depot GnRHa, 7 days prior to stopping the OCP's which will ensure complete down-regulation for the next 28 days.

In antagonist cycles, usually in batch IVF one keeps the stimulation days as 10. For practical purposes and convenience, it is better to adhere to a fixed day antago-nist start policy of Day 6 of stimulation in batch IVF. A fixed day antagonist proto-col will reduce the number of visits of patients to the clinic and will make the scheduling easy. Studies have proved beyond doubt that a fixed day antagonist will not compromise the results of an IVF cycle [30].

Fundamentals of Stimulation in Batch IVF

1. Minimum number of days of OCP required is 12 days [7].
2. Majority of the patients will bleed on 3.5 ± 1 day after stopping OCP [8].
3. In a long agonist cycle 3–4 days of OCP−GnRHa overlap is needed [9].
4. Number of days of GnRHa required to achieve down-regulation is 10–14 days [10].
5. Single dose of Depot GnRHa will ensure complete down-regulation after 14 days of its administration and patient can be stimulated with any other interven-tion for the next 14 days [10].
6. Average duration of stimulation in a long agonist cycle is 11 days.
7. Average duration of stimulation in an antagonist cycle is 10 days.

Cycle Programming

Cycle Pretreatment with Combined OCP (COCP)

Pretreatment of the batch of women with oral contraceptives helps synchronise cycles (Fig. 2.1). While the main advantage of the pill includes cycle programming, it also helps avoid cyst formation and has a role in preventing premature LH surge and maintaining persistently decreased LH levels till the trigger and P_4 suppression. Pill pretreatment causes sensitisation of receptors to FSH. Also it ensures the complete endometrial shedding/thinning effect may last until the early follicular phase [11].

However pill pretreatment does not improve oocyte yield due to excessive suppression of the pituitary gland and may even exert a negative effect on outcome by causing impaired endometrial receptivity executed through the gestagen component in the pill. It also increases the duration of stimulation required and the dose of the gonadotrophins required for stimulation. Pretreatment with pills and a short washout period may lead to profound LH suppression and may increase miscarriage and decrease pregnancy rates by impairing oocyte quality. The endometrial thinning effect may persist until the late stimulation phase and there may be an impact of the gestagen component on the endometrium. The most recent Cochrane Review and other meta-analyses are not in favour of pill pretreatment in antagonist cycles [12]. But in long agonist protocols, the COCP can be used effectively for cycle programming, which is called the dual suppression strategy. Here also, instead of COCP's, combination of oestrogen and 19 nor progesterone or 19 nor progesterone alone can be used to induce bleeding, and also for cycle programming [13].

If we go through the recent literature there is lack of evidence for and against pill pretreatment [15, 16]. But when patients received the pill only for 12–16 days, and had a wash-out period of 5 days, no difference could be found in live birth rates between the groups. In a further randomised controlled trial, cycle outcome was compared in women who planned their cycles with the pill versus cycle planning with only oestrogen, as previously described. Again, no differences could be found in live birth rates. Therefore, it could be concluded that the benefits of cycle scheduling with the pill (equal distribution of work load in large busy units and staff distribution, avoiding weekend retrievals in small units, synchronisation of follicular cohort, avoiding excessive incubator openings) must be weighed against the

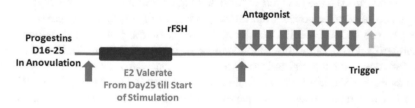

Fig. 2.1 Cycle programming with estradiol valerate pretreatment

drawbacks (i.e. higher FSH consumption and longer duration of the stimulation). When given for a minimum number of days, and if ovarian stimulation is started after a wash out period that resembles the natural cycle, OCP pretreatment might not have a negative effect on endometrial receptivity and IVF outcome might be comparable to women undergoing a classical long protocol or who were pretreated only with oestrogen [14].

Other Strategies for Cycle Programming

Cycle Pretreatment with Estradiol Valerate in Antagonist Cycles [17]

Estradiol (E_2) programming of the cycle is started during the preceding cycle. Usually in anovulatory women it can be started on D25 of the previous cycle and can be continued beyond the menses, till the day of starting stimulation. E_2 pre treatment can be safely extended up to 8 days beyond menses before starting stimulation without compromising cycle outcome. The wash-out time for E_2 pretreatment is just 1 day whereas this period for the COCP is 5 days. The endocrinological milieu and follicular cohort size are much similar to that of a natural cycle immediately the next day after stopping the E_2 tablets. Usual recommended dose of E_2 valerate is 2 mg twice daily orally.

In cases of women with irregular periods/anovulation, cycle scheduling is done by adding progestogens (MPA or NET) from D16 to D25 and then starting E_2 valerate orally 2 mg twice daily from D25 onwards till the day of starting stimulation. Progestogens will ensure proper withdrawal and timely menses with complete shedding of endometrium.

Ovarian Stimulation in Batch IVF

Individualising the FSH Dose

Selecting the initial starting dose of gonadotropin is vital to prevent ovarian hyperstimulation syndrome (OHSS) as well as for obtaining optimum numbers of oocytes. Many suggest decreasing the gonadotropin starting dose, but merely decreasing the dose is not enough. The CONSORT (CONsistency in r-FSH Starting dOses for individualized tReatmenT) dosing algorithm individualises recombinant human follicle-stimulating hormone doses in ART, and assigns 37.5-IU increments based on simple characteristics such as basal FSH, BMI, age and antral follicle count (AFC). Using this CONSORT algorithm may help achieve an adequate oocyte yield and better pregnancy rates. Of late there are another few algorithms (PIVEt alGORITHM, LA MARCA ALGORITHM) also available for selecting the individual initial starting dose [18–20].

Addition of LH Activity [21, 22]

Most normogonadotrophic women have adequate endogenous LH for steroidogenesis and oocyte maturation. However in about 20 % of women there could be a poor response to FSH, otherwise known as steady response, which may be due to low bioactive LH or due to an FSH receptor polymorphism. Addition of LH may help in these women. In women with hypogonadotrophic hypogonadism addition of LH adds to the success of assisted reproduction treatment (ART). Poor responders and patients >35 years of age and older may benefit from exogenous LH.

Table 2.4 is an example of individualising gonadotropin doses based on patient characteristics and selection of protocol based on the ovarian response using the most robust ovarian reserve assessment tools, anti-mullerian hormone (AMH) and AFC.

Optimum Number of Oocytes for Best Outcome

The key is to aim for an optimal number of oocytes to avoid overburdening resources, embryologists, and to avoid OHSS. This can be achieved by individualising the protocols based on patient characteristics and standardising them for use in a batch programme. Determining ovarian reserve using valid indicators such as age, AFC and AMH is extremely useful. Careful monitoring will help with following strategies to control progesterone elevation and timing the trigger. If oocyte recovery rates were restricted to <12 eggs, OHSS would almost cease to exist as a risk factor of IVF. This type of targeted stimulation aims to marginally elevate the basal FSH such that only the most responsive follicles are recruited, potentially leading to more chromosomally competent oocytes and embryos and OHSS-free clinics. This would also facilitate better endometrial receptivity and endocrine milieu, and maximises the chances of fresh transfer cycles and minimises the need for "freeze all" cycles, thereby improving overall outcomes in a batch programme. Excess embryos are frozen so that patients can have a repeated cryo-cycle in case of failure and will help us to improve the cumulative pregnancy rates also [19].

Table 2.4 Ovarian stimulation strategy—choosing a protocol (NCARE IVF, India)

	Hyper-responder	Normo-responder	Poor-responder
	AMH >3.0	AMH 1.2–3.0	AMH <1.2
	AFC >15	AFC 5–15	AFC <5
GnRHa	Antagonist	Agonist	Antagonist/micro dose flare
Gonadotropin[a]	rFSH	rFSH	rFSH ± rLH
Starting dose	75–150 IU	150–262.5 IU	300–375 IU
Trigger	rhCG/GnRHa	rhCG	rhCG

[a]Type of gonadotropins used can be according to clinician's personal choices

Monitoring of Ovarian Stimulation (NCARE IVF, India)

One of the most important requirements in ensuring smooth progress in a batch programme is a standardised and individualised mechanism to monitor controlled ovarian hyperstimulation. Correlation of three components is important. These include the ultrasound and/or hormonal monitoring of the process of down-regulation, follicular growth, endometrial response and hormonal evaluation. This is also important to ensure modification of stimulation dose drugs to obtain optimum outcome to endure timely administration of hCG and avoid complications.

Criteria for Adequate Pituitary Suppression

Sonological

- Endometrial thickness <6.0 mm
- Follicles of size <10 mm
- No cysts of size >15 mm

Endocrinological

- $E_2 < 50$ pg/ml
- $H < 2.0$ IU/L
- $P_4 < 1.2$ pg/ml

Controlled Ovarian Hyperstimulation

An initial starting dose of gonadotropin is confirmed after a day 2/day 3 ultrasound examination and started accordingly. In our centre we call back the patient for a repeat ultrasound examination on day 6, day 8 and day 10 of stimulation and the dose adjustment is done based on the following criteria shown in the tabular columns (see Tables 2.5, 2.6, and 2.7). The dose adjustment is done by increasing or decreasing the gonadotropins by 37.5–150 IU/day depending on the clinical situation and response.

Table 2.5 Day 6 of stimulation

Increase the dose	Decrease the dose
Follicle number ≤4	Follicle number >8 of size 10 mm
Follicle size ≤5 mm	Lead follicle size >12 mm
E2 ≤125 pg/ml	E2 >500 pg/ml

Table 2.6 Day 8 of stimulation

Increase the dose	Decrease the dose
Follicle number <5 of size <10 mm	Follicle number >8 of size 14 mm
Follicle growth <2 mm/2 days	Follicle growth >6 mm/2 days
E2 <250 pg/ml	E2 >1000 pg/ml
E2 rise <100 %/2 days	E2 rise >200 %/2 days

Table 2.7 Day 10 of stimulation

Increase the dose	Decrease the dose
Follicle growth <2 mm/2 days	Follicle growth >6 mm/2 days
E2 <250 pg/ml	E2 >1000 pg/ml
E2 rise <100 %/2 days	E2 rise >200 %/2 days
Lead follicle size <16 mm	Lead follicle size >20 mm

Follicular Phase Progesterone Elevation [23]

Follicular phase elevation of progesterone is an important problem that can be difficult to tackle during batch IVF. Some of the strategies feasible to overcome this are to make stimulation milder and use minimum rFSH, or prepare for a "Freeze All" embryos (Deferred ET) option and repeat cryo-cycles, which will help in improving cycle outcome.

Criteria for Triggering Final Oocyte Maturation [24]

The following are the criteria for final trigger at our centre.
   When three or more follicles have reached a size of >18 mm of size.
   >50 % of the total growing follicles are of size >14 mm.

Triggering for Final Oocyte Maturation

When E_2 levels are <1000 pg/ml and total number of dominant follicles are <6, at our centre we trigger with 500 µg of rhCG. When E_2 levels are between 1000 and 3000 pg/ml and the total number of dominant follicles is between 6 and 15, the usual standard dose of 250 µg of rhCG is used for triggering final oocyte maturation. If E_2 levels are >3000 pg/ml and dominant follicle numbers are >15, usually a GnRHa (Decapeptyl 0.2 mg) is used for trigger followed by freeze all in an antagonist protocol and if it is a long agonist protocol, 5000 IU of HP-hCG is used for trigger and followed by a freeze-all embryo strategy.

Coasting of a Cycle

Deliberate withdrawal of gonadotropins during stimulation to reduce OHSS is known as coasting of a cycle. Coasting for 1–3 days can be done without compromising cycle outcome. Coasting is started when E_2 levels are >4500 pg/ml and or E_2 production is >150 pg/ml per each follicle of size 16–18 mm. Ideally once coasted, E_2 is measured on a daily basis to avoid skipping of an unexpected and unpredictable E_2 drop. Final trigger is administered when E_2 levels fall to <3500 pg/ml. But when an E_2 rise is above 6500 pg/ml and if >30 mature follicles are present and if coasting lasts for >4 days, the cycle has to be abandoned [25].

Donor–Recipient and Cryo Cycle Synchronisation in Batch IVF

Donor–recipient cycles are best done in a batch IVF programme or, in other words, it is always a batching and synchronisation of both cycles. Preparation of endometrium is the same for cryo-cycles as well as for the donor–recipient synchronised cycles.

Donors can be of two types:

1. Voluntary Oocyte Donor
2. Stimulated patients undergoing IVF amenable to oocyte sharing

Recipients can be classified according to the status of their uterus and ovaries.

Recipient Profile—Ovary
Without Ovarian Activity—Primary ovarian failure (POF); Menopausal woman
With Compromised Ovarian Activity—Perimenopausal woman; Young woman with poor ovarian reserve
With Normal Ovarian Activity—Undergoing heterologous ART for genetic diseases; Repeated poor cycle outcome, etc.

Recipient Profile—Uterus
Hypo-oestrogenic uterus—in POF; Menopausal woman
Normo-oestrogenic uterus without co-morbidities
Normo-oestrogenic uterus with co-morbidities (Adenomyosis, Fibroids)

In recipients without ovarian activity, we can directly start hormone replacement therapy without down-regulation. But when ovaries are active, we have to prevent the LH surge and hormone replacement should be started after down-regulation, especially in a Batch IVF programme. Scheduling is almost similar to synchronisation of patients for controlled ovarian stimulation. The sample calendar (see Table 2.8) can be used here for depiction of synchronisation of donor–recipient cycles in batch IVF [26].

Sun	Mon	Tue	Wed	Thu	Fri	Sat
		1	2	3	4 GnRHa Depot	5
6	7	8 Start GnRHa	9	10	11 Stop OCP	12
13	14	15	16	17 Start HRT Start Gonadotropin	18	19
20	21	22 Start Antagonist	23	24	25	26
27 Trigger	28	29 Availability of embryologist OPU ICSI Start P4	30 Availability of embryologist Continue P4	31 Availability of embryologist Continue P4 Embryo Trasfer		

Table 2.8 Sample BATCH calendar for donor–recipient cycle with D2 transfers

Basic Fundamentals of Endometrial Preparation in Donor–Recipient Cycles

1. Minimum duration of oestrogen exposure to induce endometrial receptivity is 8 days [27].
2. Maximum duration of oestrogen exposure that will not hamper endometrial receptivity is 42 days [27].
3. Dose of oestrogen required to get optimum endometrial thickness may vary from 2 to 12 mg [27].
4. Minimum endometrial thickness to achieve pregnancy is 6.0 mm [28].
5. Optimum endometrial thickness to achieve pregnancy is 8.0–12.0 mm [28].
6. Perform a mock HRT cycle in recipients before IVF cycle to decide the dose and duration of oestrogen therapy to induce optimum endometrial thickness.
7. Number of days of progesterone exposure for cleavage stage ET is 2–3 days [29].
8. P_4 Dose required per day for induction of endometrial receptivity is 50–100 mg IM injection/60 mg 8 % Gel/600 mg vaginal pessary.
9. Luteal phase in recipients should contain oestrogen and progesterone in the same dose and has to be continued till a minimum of 42 days following ET [30].

Advantages of Batch IVF Programme

The major advantage of batching is that it also facilitates provision of services in peripheral centres and makes ART more affordable and accessible to more people.
   The lab gets enough time to get ready with its logistics and QC.

The lab does benefit when there is a week which is cycle-free. Tasks such as incubator cleaning, calibrating, pH assessments, and sperm survival tests need a few work-free days. Doing all these tasks during an ongoing cycle is not always easily feasible.

If the number of patients recruited is in accordance with the number of incubators and other support, and the centre has a good vitrification plan, then cumulative pregnancy rates are not compromised in batch IVF.

Disadvantages of Batch IVF Programme

The biggest disadvantage is inflexibility in cycle management due to fixed and rigid time frames within which the entire process of batching has to be completed. A proportion of patients may not respond as expected and identifying such patients and their referral to centres better suited to them may become necessary. A few cases may end up with cancellation too. Antagonist protocols in particular may be difficult to control and synchronise.

When something goes wrong, it affects all at once.

The centre may have to use visiting embryologists whose accountability and skills may not always be assured.

There are potentially more chances for operator induced mistakes due to workload, including mixing of the patient's samples.

Difficulty with fixed protocols and programming—individualization of treatment according to the patient's requirement may be difficult.

Pretreatment with pills used for synchronisation may have an effect on cycle outcome and also increase the amount of gonadotropin required.

At times batching may turn out over-expensive if the consumption of media and consumables are not optimal.

Centres doing batches are under huge pressure because of predesignated dates of OPUs and ET depending on the availability of embryologist.

Incubator overload is also a concern when the centres are not well prepared.

Compromised culture conditions may also result due to work overload.

Rescheduling of some patients could be inconvenient and expensive for both the centre and the patient.

Centres doing batch IVF usually do cleavage stage D2 or D3 transfers due to time constraints enforced by the visiting embryologist. Blastocyst transfer, when required in an innate cycle is difficult and may lead to compromises.

Planning procedures such as TESE for those couples who may require it is cumbersome and can become difficult.

Freezing is also not always possible or compromised due to the time constraints.

QC may not be always optimal if the visiting embryologist needs to depend upon other technicians to maintain the incubators and laboratory equipment.

Inventory Management

Managing effective inventory control of laboratory as well as pharmacy supplies to IVF services facilitates timely and effective treatment for the patients. Effective inventory control ensure that equipment, drugs, reagents and consumables for the diagnosis and treatment of infertility patients are delivered in the right quantities, in the right condition, to the right place, at the right time and for the right cost-effective price. It is vital to rendering quality of services as well as optimising the profitability of the service by the clinic/establishment. Careful management of inventory helps to prevent waste, which can occur if reagents and supplies are stored improperly, or if reagents become out-dated before they can be used. In IVF units, inventory control is applicable to the drugs for clinical use, equipment, culture media and reagents, disposables, etc.

Good practice in inventory control management includes monitoring the storage conditions (temperature, humidity and exposure to sunlight, etc); keeping an eye on stock levels, conducting a physical inventory and keeping an update of stock every week/biweekly or monthly according to how the busy the unit is; disposal of time-expired media/reagents/drugs appropriately and safely; Each item can have a stock card with the following vital information—Date column, media/disposable/reagent/drugs name, stock at hand, stock received, stock issued, special storage requirements, lot number, expiry date, etc.

Cryo-stored gametes and embryos also need an inventory management system and currently many software systems are available to manage this area. Unlike the units performing regular IVF, batch programme units need a dedicated inventory management system since all the essential items for performing an IVF cycle are required at a particular time period and any fault in stock can affect the cycle of many patients.

Strategies to Optimise Outcome in Batch IVF

Ensure detailed assessment of the couple. This might include prior cycle-monitoring.

Optimise individualization of protocols based on overall patient profile and risk factors (combination of age, hormonal and ultrasound parameters to determine ovarian reserve).

Accurate estimation of the workload that the centre can handle.

Prompt identification and referral of those patients who may need care in a more structured setting.

Prompt system for referral/transfer of patients who may deviate from their expected course of stimulation or requirements to centres that may be able to cater to them better.

Well-trained counsellors to help cater to patients who may need in-depth explanation of the reasons for cancellation of cycle/ET by the centre both prior to starting the batch and after starting the batch.

Effective mechanism for liaison with the embryologist. Ideally the visiting embryologist should be involved in all the specifics of setting up of the laboratory. It also helps to stick to the services of the same visiting embryologist to ensure that proper systems are put in place and standardised, based on specific working needs.

Good vitrification programme often helps.

Well-planned billing system to minimise losses to the patient in the event of cycle cancellation.

Appropriate counselling systems in place to avoid patients losing confidence in the treatment strategy.

Minimising deviation by working up patients and being able to identify the minor differences based on down-regulation scans. With careful selection such deviations are minimum.

Individualise where necessary and standardise where necessary.

Regular auditing of work.

Maintain proper paperwork, labels and documentation.

Avoiding overcrowding of work-space.

Ensure proper documentation; photographic records of embryos. Assistant staff to help ensure that the process of documentation is complete and up-to-date.

Summary

Batch IVF outcome depends on the setting, specialists involved and their availability, planning and mechanisms in place to facilitate its smooth functioning, infrastructure and manpower. Clinicians and the embryologists and the staff should be passionately concerned and well trained and work as a team to prevent things going really wrong. Batch IVF can potentially be an economically viable option for start-ups provided everything is standardised with the minimum possible variables and the maximum possible benefit to the patients and the centre.

Troubleshooting in Batch IVF

Many times programmes doing exclusively batching of IVF come across problems associated with clinical or laboratory components. This is more evident in centres where the local expertise in infertility management is considerably low or where proper IVF training of the staff is meagre. If the unit employs visiting experts, problems may be identified very early and can avoid any mishaps. In fact, troubleshooting is an integral part of any batch IVF programme, especially at the beginning of the programme.

Hormonal Manipulation

Proper planning at least 2 months before the batch.
Awareness and understanding of stimulation protocols and rationale of each protocol.
In-depth understanding of the endocrinology of fertility.

Poor Follicular Growth

Check for proper injection technique.
Ensure availability of a specifically trained nurse for injections.
Check for proper storage of medicines.
Ensure UPS connections to refrigerators.
Review any inherent patient problems (age, poor responders).

Poor Oocyte Yield

Check for missed hCG.
Check for proper timing of hCG.
Ensure adequate dose of hCG.
Check for any break in cold chain.
Review any inherent patient problem.

Infection of Semen Sample

Consider freezing after semen culture.
Consider prior antibiotic therapy.

Problems with Aspiration Pump

Check for cracked tube.
Always keep all plug points connected to UPS.
Arrange for ready availability of additional pumps.
Be ready with mechanical suction if necessary. A 10 ml syringe connected to a needle should be kept handy.
Maintain cordial relationships with neighbouring IVF units who may be able to assist in case of any emergency.

IVF Culture Media

Measure pH with each new batch of media and regularly to verify physical parameters of the incubator, especially the gas calibration.

Check for optimal equilibration of oil and media.

If there is access to a blood gas analyser, this can be used to measure pH, or can use portable online pH analyzers, which may be expensive.

Check if the pH of buffers in handling media for use outside the incubator is appropriate.

Make sure that all culture dishes are prepared on a non-heated surface. Especially, microdroplet dishes should be prepared as fast as possible with oil overlay to avoid any drastic shift in osmolarity of media.

Infection of Culture Dish

Ideally prepare for one patient at a time. It has been noted in some batch IVF centres that the source of bacterial contamination in culture dishes as the air flow from low quality and non-replaced HEPA filters in laminar flow hoods where the culture dishes are prepared.

Ensure that pipettes are not reused. Aliquot media in small IVF grade test tubes and ensure that each one is used completely and exclusively for one patient.

Check semen culture sensitivity and consider pretreatment of infections.

Consistent Biochemical Pregnancies in Batch IVF

The air/gas environment in the laboratory needs proper quality checks. Most commonly the CO_2 gas supplying the incubators could be responsible for this. Procure medical grade gases from reliable sources and connect the gas lines with inline filters having activated charcoal. These need to be replaced on a frequent basis (3–4 months).

References

1. Kutty BA, et al. Batch in vitro fertilization: practical considerations. In: Rao KA, editor. Principles and practice of assisted reproductive technology, vol. 1. New Delhi: Jaypee Brothers Medical Publishers (P) Ltd; 2014. p. 827–33.
2. Das MC, et al. Batch IVF program. A practical guide for setting up an IVF lab, assessment of embryo culture systems and running the unit, vol. 1. New Delhi: Jaypee Brothers Medical Publishers (P) Ltd; 2014. p. 181–92.

3. Gianaroli L, et al. ESHRE guidelines for good practice in IVF laboratories. Hum Reprod. 2000;15(10):2241–6.
4. William L et al. Changing old trends in IVF laboratory cleaning and disinfection. 2011. www. gynemed.de.
5. Practice Committee of American Society for Reproductive Medicine; Practice Committee of Society for Assisted Reproductive Technology. Revised guidelines for human embryology and andrology laboratories. Fertil Steril. 2008;90(5):S45–59.
6. Higdon LH, et al. Incubator management in Assisted Reproductive Technology Laboratory. Fertil Steril. 2008;83(3):703–10.
7. Valasco JC, et al. To pill or not to pill: that is the question. RBM Online. 2015;30:39–42.
8. Duijkers IJ, et al. Ovarian function with the contraceptive vaginal ring or an oral contraceptive: a randomized study. Hum Reprod. 2004;19:2668–73.
9. Jenkins JM, et al. The development of functional ovarian cysts during pituitary down-regulation. Hum Reprod. 1993;8(10):1623–7.
10. Oyesanya OA, et al. Pituitary down-regulation prior to in-vitro fertilization and embryo transfer: a comparison between a single dose of Zoladex depot and multiple daily doses of Suprefact. Hum Reprod. 1995;10(5):1042–4.
11. Barmat LI, et al. A randomized prospective trial comparing gonadotropin-releasing hormone (GnRH) antagonist/recombinant follicle-stimulating hormone (rFSH) versus GnRH-agonist/ rFSH in women pretreated with oral contraceptives before in vitro fertilization. Fertil Steril. 2005;83:321–30.
12. Al-Inany HG, et al. GnRH antagonists are safer than agonists: an update of a Cochrane review. Hum Reprod Update. 2011;17:435.
13. Anderson RE, et al. Effects of norethindrone on gonadotropin and ovarian steroid secretion when used for cycle programming during in vitro fertilization. Fertil Steril. 1990;54:96–101.
14. Bermejo A, et al. The impact of using the combined oral contraceptive pill for cycle scheduling on gene expression related to endometrial receptivity. Hum Reprod. 2014;29:1271–8.
15. Griesinger G, et al. Oral contraceptive pill pretreatment in ovarian stimulation with GnRH antagonists for IVF: a systematic review and meta-analysis. Fertil Steril. 2008;90:1055–63.
16. Griesinger G, et al. Oral contraceptive pretreatment significantly reduces ongoing pregnancy likelihood in gonadotropin-releasing hormone antagonist cycles: an updated meta-analysis. Fertil Steril. 2010;94:2382–4.
17. Hauzman EE, et al. Cycle scheduling for in vitro fertilization with oral contraceptive pills versus oral estradiol valerate: a randomized, controlled trial. Reprod Biol Endocrinol. 2013;28:96–9.
18. Olivennes F, et al. Randomized, controlled, open-label, non-inferiority study of the CONSORT algorithm for individualized dosing of follitropin alfa. Reprod BioMed Online. 2015;30(3):248–57.
19. Yovich J, et al. Targeted gonadotrophin stimulation using the PIVEt algorithm markedly reduces the risk of OHSS. Reprod BioMed Online. 2012;24(3):281–92.
20. La Marca A, et al. Individualization of controlled ovarian stimulation in IVF using ovarian reserve markers: from theory to practice. Hum Reprod Update. 2014;20(1):124–40.
21. Wong PC, et al. Current opinion on use of luteinizing hormone supplementation in assisted reproduction therapy: an Asian perspective. Reprod BioMed Online. 2011;23:81–90.
22. Hill MJ, et al. Does exogenous LH in ovarian stimulation improves assisted reproductive technology success? An appraisal of literature. Reprod BioMed Online. 2012;24(3):261–71.
23. Venetis CA, et al. Progesterone elevation and probability of pregnancy after IVF: a systematic review and meta-analysis of over 60000 cycles. Hum Reprod Update. 2013;19(5):433–57.
24. Vanderckerhove F, et al. Delaying the oocyte maturation trigger by one day leads to a higher metaphase II oocyte yield in IVF/ICSI: a randomised controlled trial. Reprod Biol Endocrinol. 2014;12:31.
25. Ulug U, et al. The significance of coasting duration during ovarian stimulation for conception in ART cycles. Hum Reprod. 2002;17(2):310–3.
26. Galliano D, et al. ART and uterine pathology: how relevant is the maternal side for implantation? Hum Reprod Update. 2015;21(1):13–38.

27. Borini A, et al. Effect of duration of estradiol replacement on the outcome of oocyte donation. J Assist Reprod Genet. 2001;18:185–90.
28. Kovacs P, et al. The effect of endometrial thickness and IVF/ICSI. Hum Reprod. 2003;18(11):2337–41.
29. Haouzi D, et al. Endometrial receptivity profile in patients with premature progesterone elevation on the day of hCG administration. BioMed Res Int. 2014;2014:10. doi:10.1155/2014/951937. Article ID 951937.
30. Orvieto R, et al. Luteal phase support for patients undergoing frozen-thawed embryo transfer cycles—the required progesterone dose. Clin Exp Obstet Gynecol. 2007;34(1):25–6.
31. Kolibianakis EM, et al. Fixed versus flexible gonadotropin-releasing hormone antagonist administration in in vitro-fertilization: a randomized control trial. Fertil Steril. 2011;95(2):558–62.

Chapter 3
Risk and Regulation: The Role of Regulation in Managing an IVF Unit

John Peek

Introduction

This book is aimed at doctors running and managing IVF units. For some of you, your IVF unit will be located in a hospital which has its own its own management system, but many of you will be in private practice, running and possibly owning your own company. When it comes to quality management, there seem to be a bewildering number of things to consider. Probably foremost in your mind are the endpoints of a quality management system (QMS), such as designing the clinical and laboratory processes, setting clinical policies, writing Standard Operating Procedures (SoPs), setting up a method to control documents so only the most recent version is used, training staff, checking that staff are competent, joining a quality assurance scheme for semen analysis or embryology, internal auditing and possibly gaining certification. All these are important and necessary components of a QMS—and many are covered in detail in the chapter by Dr Jim Catt. On top of these, there may be laws and regulations with which you and your ART unit have to comply, or guidelines to follow.

A QMS and external rules both exist to reduce risk to your patients, yourself, and your organisation and its owners. You may be thinking that if you obey your local laws, regulations or guidelines then you have sufficiently addressed the problem of risk, and that you do not need a QMS. However, laws, regulations and guidelines only cover a subset of the risks that exist. Moreover, laws, regulations and guidelines are often silent or vague about how to address the risks they are designed to reduce.

This chapter does not summarise the laws and regulations about ART that exist in many countries, nor does it summarise the many guidelines that have been written

J. Peek, PhD (✉)
Fertility Associates, Level 3, 7 Ellerslie Racecourse Drive, Remuera,
Auckland 1051, New Zealand
e-mail: jpeek@fertilityassociates.co.nz

© Springer Science+Business Media New York 2016
S.D. Fleming, A.C. Varghese (eds.), *Organization and Management of IVF Units*, DOI 10.1007/978-3-319-29373-8_3

by scientific societies such as ESHRE [1] and ASRM [2] or local interest groups such as medical councils, colleges of obstetrics and gynaecology, or government health departments. There is enormous diversity between countries in what laws allow, and what regulations and guidelines address [3].

The focus of this chapter is about using regulations and guidelines from a variety of sources to help build a robust and useful QMS based on the real risks faced by an IVF unit. Regulations and guidelines can be more than just rules to obey; they are also a valuable source of ideas and solutions. This chapter draws on regulations and guidelines in place in the UK, Australia, and New Zealand and discusses the strengths and weakness of regulations as a resource for building a QMS.

What Are Regulations?

Briefly, regulations are rules which are mandatory because they can be enforced by law.

For instance in the UK, the practice of Assisted Reproductive Technology (ART) is directly governed by the Human Fertilisation and Embryology Act (2008). That Act of parliament established the Human Fertilisation and Embryology Authority (HFEA), which in turn publishes a Code of Practice [4]. The HFEA also inspects IVF units. The HFEA can close down IVF units that do not comply with the Code of Practice.

Often the link between law and regulation is less direct. In Australia, some state legislation and the federal *Prohibition of Human Cloning for Reproduction and Regulation of Human Embryo Research Amendment Act 2006* recognise an organisation called the Reproductive Technology Accreditation Committee (RTAC) as the body which accredits ART units in Australia. RTAC is a subcommittee of the Fertility Society of Australia (FSA); it issues a Code of Practice [5] and oversees the external auditing and certification of ART units. Through this chain of responsibility, RTAC sets some of the mandatory rules for IVF units in Australia, and issues a licence.

In the broad sense, *regulation creates limits, constrains rights, creates a duty or allocates a responsibility* [6]. As well as legal regulation, there can be self regulation through trade associations such as the regulation of doctors through a Medical Council. Apparent self-regulation is often linked to law; for instance in New Zealand and many other countries doctors are required to be registered and the Medical Council is recognised as the only body for administering this.

This chapter also considers guidelines. By definition, a guideline is not mandatory, and hence not binding or enforceable. In some countries, such as in Malaysia, local guidelines on ART are widely followed and determine what is allowed in the absence of laws or regulations. In other countries, some guidelines were generally ignored, such as guidelines in Thailand against paid donors and sex selection of embryos for social reasons. Although they are not mandatory, guidelines can also be an important resource for identifying risks and finding methods to reduce risk when building your QMS.

The Range of Regulations Relevant to an IVF Unit

If your country has laws specific to ART then there are probably specific regulations as well. However, specific regulations about ART might not be directly linked to legislation about IVF; an example is the National Health and Medical Research Council's *Ethical guidelines on the use of assisted reproductive technology in clinical practice and research* [7] in Australia.

Some types of ART regulation, such as the New Zealand Fertility Standard NZS8181 [8] are comprehensive and cover almost all aspects of running an IVF unit, including the patient's pathway from referral to consultation to treatment to discharge, running a day stay surgery, premises, and staff. Regulations in other countries may omit many of these topics, or only touch upon them obliquely.

In addition there are a wide range of regulations that are not specific to managing an IVF unit but which still apply. For instance, there is a requirement that doctors are registered, which in turn has an expectation of competence, which leads to requirements about continuing medical education. There are fire regulations about building safety, regulations about electrical safety, the occupational health of staff, and so on.

There are also regulations which have their origin outside health, such as the contractual obligation between a customer paying for a service and the organisation providing that service, such as the Consumer Guarantees Act in New Zealand. This legislation describes the rights a consumer automatically has when he or she buys goods or services, whether the goods is a new televisions set or the service is an IVF treatment. In a similar way the Human Rights Act in New Zealand applies equally to selling a television or providing donor egg treatment, so that an IVF unit cannot discriminate on the person's age, gender, martial status or sexual orientation (as well as on several other attributes covered by this legislation). The practical consequence for an IVF unit in New Zealand is that it cannot place an upper age on access to treatment, and cannot limit access to any type of treatment on the basis of a person's gender, marital status or sexual orientation.

Table 3.1 lists non-ART regulations that may be relevant for an IVF unit; these have been taken from a list of legislation and standards referred to in the New Zealand Fertility Standard. It is suggested that you make a list for your IVF clinic based on the laws, standards and regulations in your country. Next to each, write the associated risks that could arise in your ART unit, and how you are going to address those risks.

Table 3.1 Examples of non-ART regulations which may apply to an IVF unit, taken from New Zealand legislation, standards and regulations

Aspect	Areas of regulation
Medical safety	Infection control
	Management of healthcare waste
	Cleaning, disinfecting and sterilising reusable medical and surgical instruments and equipment and maintenance of associated environments in healthcare facilities
	Textiles for healthcare facilities and institutions—theatre linen and pre-packs
	Laundry practice
	Day-stay surgery and procedures
	Electrical installation
	Electrical installations—in-service testing
	Guide to the safe use of electricity in patient care
	Medicines regulations
	Technical management programmes for medical devices
Patients interests	Human Rights Act
	Registering children born from donor gametes, donor embryos or surrogacy
	Guide for removal, retention, return and disposal of body parts
	Health information and privacy
	Health records
	Protection of personal property
	Consumer Guarantees Act
	Fair Trading Act
	Advertising Standards Act
	Design for access and mobility—buildings and associated facilities
	Fire safety and evacuation of buildings regulations
Staff interests	Employment relations
	Occupational health and safety management
	Recommended practices for occupational eye protection
	Injury Prevention and Rehabilitation Compensation Act
Organisation	Risk management
	Business continuity management
	Resource Management Act

Different Approaches to IVF Regulation

The HFEA's Code of Practice in the UK and RTAC's Code of Practice in Australia exemplify two very different approaches to writing regulations to describe how IVF should be practised. Most other regulations and guidelines fall somewhere between these two extremes.

The HFEA and RTAC Codes of Practice cover a similar range of topics, such as the expertise staff need, counselling patients, giving patients information, ensuring patients can and do give informed consent, reducing the chance of multiple birth, looking after the interests of donors and children when donor treatment is used, safe handling of sperm, oocytes and embryos, storage of sperm, oocytes and embryos, patient and sample identification, traceability of materials that are used in treatment, and putting a QMS in place. The HFEA Code of Practice is highly detailed and proscriptive, meaning it tells you what to do and how to do it. It is a 230 page document of about 90,000 words. In contrast, the RTAC Code of Practice is very succinct. It states what has to be achieved in the form of criteria, and the measures you, or an auditor, will use to show that each criterion has been met. It is only 26 pages long, and has fewer than 5000 words.

Table 3.2 illustrates the RTAC's approach using Critical Criterion 5, covering identification of patients and samples. This Critical Criterion has 78 words, compared to the 3600 words in the HFEA's section on the same subject.

The RTAC Code of Practice has had an interesting history, which illustrates an evolving approach to quality management, starting with rules and moving to principles. In many ways this mirrors the evolution of quality thinking in the twentieth century, from quality control—checking that the service meets standards to defining what the customer wants and letting the organisation decide how to achieve it.

The RTAC Code started in 1986 as a compendium of practical rules issued by the FSA, growing to about 120 pages by 2005. The FSA then sought advice from the Joint Accreditation System of Australian-New Zealand, which is the government-appointed accreditation body which oversees all types of accreditation and certification in those two countries. As a result of the review, the RTAC Code of Practice was pared down into a number of simple critical and good practice criteria, each with measures that the IVF unit or an external auditor could readily audit. It was decided that IVF units should decide for themselves how to address each criteria. Only two areas were proscribed in some detail—the responsibilities, qualifications and training for the key personnel of medical director, scientific director, nurse manager and the senior counsellor; and the requirements for providing donor treatment. These two aspects were included as attachments in the Code. The FSA has recently published an international version of its Code of Practice for countries

Table 3.2 RTAC critical criterion 5, identification and traceability

Critical criteria	Measure
5. Identification and Traceability The organisation must ensure that gametes, embryos and patients are correctly identified and matched at all times.	Provide evidence of implementation and review of: • Policies/procedures to identify when, how and by whom the identification, matching, and verification are recorded for gametes, embryos and patients at all stages of the treatment process.
	• The process that constitutes the traceability of gametes and embryos at all stages of the treatment cycle.
	• Regular (at least annual) audit of the patient, gamete and embryo identification process.

outside Australia and New Zealand that accommodates local approaches to areas such as donor treatment. The RTAC Code of Practice was adopted by the Ministry of Health in Singapore in 2013. The RTAC Code of Practice can be supplemented by Technical Bulletins which give practical advice but which are not mandatory. In 2012 RTAC issued a Technical Bulletin on patient and sample identification [9].

The UK and Australia-New Zealand also have very different approaches to external audit of IVF units against their Codes of Practice. In the UK, inspection teams are organised by the HFEA, and some inspections are unannounced. There is a full audit every 4 years with a midway interim audit. Inspectors are engaged by the HFEA and can be accompanied by external advisors who include doctors, nurses, embryologists and counsellors.

Under the current RTAC Scheme, external audits occur every year, with the auditors looking at each of the 13 critical criteria that are related to patient safety, and a subset of the good practice criteria that cover running an IVF unit. All aspects of the good practice criteria are covered over a 3 year audit cycle. The IVF unit chooses which auditing company to use, has a say in the choice of auditor and the technical expert (embryologist, nurse or counsellor) who advises the auditor, and pays for the audit. Audits are planned well in advance. The audit has a dual focus on checking that an IVF unit meets the Code and on continuous improvement within the IVF unit. Many IVF units in Australia and New Zealand also hold ISO 9001:2015 certification, and combine their RTAC and ISO audits.

There are strengths and weaknesses associated with the UK and Australian approaches to ART regulation. A detailed Code captures and is explicit about more risks, and offers more solutions to mitigating the risks. On the other hand, it can limit people's thinking about risks and potential solutions—leading to people having the attitude that if it is not in the Code then it is not important. This may lead to a false sense of security because the IVF unit assumes that a detailed Code of Practice must have considered everything that is important. A detailed Code can also lead to inspectors auditing against the details of the Code and not the underlying risks, with all parts of the Code being given equal weight.

Limitations to Regulations for Containing Risk

There are important limitations to the extent that you can rely on regulations to contain risk in your IVF unit.

The first is that the major purpose of regulations of any sort is to reduce the chance of the big negative risks to the client of the service. These risks can cover physical safety, such avoiding Ovarian Hyper-Stimulation Syndrome or limiting multiple pregnancy, legal and psychological safety such as ensuring the correct gametes or embryos are used, and moral or cultural safety to ensure ART is used within the norms of society.

Of course there may be different opinions to what is considered safe—for instance twin pregnancy from IVF is considered more acceptable in the USA than in Australia or New Zealand even though the physical risks to mother and children are the same. The norms of society are particularly fickle—identifiable sperm donors are mandatory in Sweden but originally banned in neighbouring Norway. Norms can change with time—for instance sperm donation in Norway is now identifiable.

Often the risk is not explicitly stated when a law is created. For instance, New Zealand law forbids sex selection of embryos apart from preventing inheritable disease, but the law does not say what potential harm is being prevented. It is possible that legislation in India will require donors to be anonymous, presumably to prevent coercion of family members into agreeing to be donors. However, treating the symptom and not the cause may not prevent coercion in other circumstances.

While avoiding the big negative risks may stop your IVF unit from going out of business abruptly or from sustaining huge costs, most IVF units do not fail because they suffer a single catastrophic risk. IVF units that fail to prosper usually do so because of multiple and chronic shortcomings—lower than average pregnancy rates, poor customer service, inefficiencies that cost money or staff problems that sap energy and morale. In short, they do not give people what they want—patients, staff or other stakeholders. Regulations seldom address these problems sufficiently. Although many regulations such as the HFEA and RTAC Codes of Practice cover the key components of a QMS, the threshold for compliance in these areas is generally modest. Even in the UK, which is highly regulated under a detailed Code of Practice, pregnancy rates vary significantly between clinics.

A second limitation is that even detailed regulations can overlook risks, or be phrased in a way that may lead you to overlook a risk in your IVF unit. For instance, the HFEA Code of Practice has a very extensive section on patient and sample identification that includes a list of clinical and laboratory steps in which witnessing needs to take place to prevent mismatches. For instance assigning a donor code to a semen sample should involve checking by a second person—which is what the HFEA means by "witnessing".

This check is done in our own clinic. We also have a second person check when we remove the sperm donor's name from his hand-written non-identifying information and replace it with his donor code in preparation for typing the non-identifying information so that patients can use it to choose a donor. However until recently, we did not have a check to make sure a transcription error did not arise between the handwritten and typed information. So although we would have fulfilled the HFEA's Code, our process of typing up donor non-identifying information created an opportunity for an error, and hence the opportunity for a patient receiving the wrong donor sperm. If this had happened, the outcome would have been as serious as mislabelling the sperm itself. It is unrealistic to expect regulations to anticipate, and therefore cover, the many different ways clinics will structure their processes for doing things.

A further limitation is that the solutions put in place by regulations may not work as well as people intended. For instance, having two people check critical steps such as the movement of gametes or embryos between tubes or dishes is a standard solution against sample mismatch in many regulations and guidelines. The reliability of double checking has not been published for IVF. A paper on involuntary automaticity by Toft and Mascie Taylor [10] illustrates the practical shortfalls of double checking by health professionals. The authors cite a large study of almost 130,000 medication administrations, which found error rates of 2.98 per 1000 when one nurse checked the medication and 2.12 per 1000 when two nurses checked. While statistically lower, this difference hardly matters in practice. In preparing the RTAC's Technical Bulletin on Patient and Sample Identification, a working group of the RTAC committee created an anonymous web-based survey for embryologists to volunteer actual or near-miss identification errors they knew about in ART. There were 48 responses. In 58 % the error had arisen despite two person checking being in place. The most common reason suggested for these errors was the embryologist rushing, presumably due to external pressure from other staff.

Apart from some examples on the HFEA website, there is no systematic literature or repository of information on real problems that have occurred in IVF units, let alone an analysis to determine the root cause behind those problem. In the absence of such data, we have to conclude that most of the solutions put forward in regulations are not evidence based. Few will have been tested or piloted before being written into regulations or guidelines. While it is fortunate that major problems appear to be infrequent in IVF units, this also means that most IVF doctors and managers have no or little experience of investigating serious problems and determining why they have occurred using tools such as root cause analysis.

A fourth limitation to the effectiveness of regulations in reducing risk is that many problems arise because of the ways events unfold so that the clinic's normal processes are circumvented. Regulations seldom address how to react to unusual events or unusual circumstances. Common examples in IVF units are last minute changes to the order of patients having their egg collection or embryo transfer, the patient changing her mind about which donor to use after she has completed a consent form, or frozen material coming from an outside clinic labelled in an unfamiliar way. Two factors can come into play in these circumstances—staff being rushed or distracted, and staff following their usual process when the usual process is no longer appropriate.

What Regulations Do Not Address

Regulations do not ask the fundamental questions that your organisation needs to answer to be successful—what is the purpose of this organisation, who are its key stakeholders (eg. patients, staff, owners), and what would success look like from the perspective of each type of stakeholder? Regulators are generally not interested in your success, but exist to protect your customers and society from your potential failures. Good regulations require an IVF unit to have a QMS, and possibly to set quality objectives so that the organisation meets users' needs, mirroring the language of the ISO 9000 standards. Even so, it is likely to be "buried" towards the end of the document; in the HFEA Code of Practice it is section 23 of 31; in the RTAC

Code of Practice the elements of a QMS are among the good practice criteria, not the critical criteria.

Regulations are rather like the Road Code, itself a regulation that governs the way you drive. The Road Code sets down rules to minimise harm by preventing accidents—drive on the right (or left!) side of the road, stop at red traffic lights and stop signs, do not go faster than the speed limit. The Road Code does not answer the fundamental question about travel—"where shall we go?"

Following regulations will not make your clinic succeed and flourish, although it will make accidental failure or disruption less likely. At the most basic level of analysis, success arises from addressing two types of risk. The first is taking positive risks—identifying what to do that might lead to success. Positive risk taking needs to be planned and proactive, and is the responsibility of governance. An example of taking a positive risk might be to set up a new clinic. None of the regulations on ART that I have come across address good governance. The second is mitigating negative risks; stopping bad things from happening that would undermine you achieving success. Bad things can span from catastrophic events, such as wrong use of sperm or embryos or a patient dying from side effects of treatment, to chronic inefficiencies or poor customer service. Quality management systems address negative risks.

The next section outlines a simple risk-focussed approach to quality management in an IVF unit, which has at its heart a risk register. The following section looks at using regulations and guidelines to populate your risk register, both with the risks you face managing an IVF unit and ways of addressing those risks.

A Simple Risk-Focussed Approach to Quality Management in an IVF Unit

This section briefly outlines a risk-focussed approach to quality management in an IVF programme in five simple steps. It provides an easy way for all staff to see how the QMS works, and why each part of the QMS is useful to them. I have used examples from my own organisation, Fertility Associates (FA), to illustrate the concepts.

Setting Mission Statement, Goals, and Key Performance Indicators (KPI)

The first and most important first step is to define why the organisation exists (often captured by a mission statement), who its stakeholders are, and what it wants to achieve for its stakeholders (goals). Goals should be updated every year as previous goals are achieved and to meet the changing needs and expectations of stakeholders. FA's mission is customer focussed; *Together we will give you the best chance of a*

Table 3.3 Example of a Key Performance Indicator (KPI) dashboard for staff of an IVF unit

Area	Measures	Target	Clinic A	Clinic B	Clinic C	Clinic D	Period
Financial	Revenue, compared to budget	≥100 %	105 %	92 %	90 %	95 %	Mar
	Costs, compared to budget	≥100 %	96 %	86 %	90 %	100 %	Mar
	Fertility appointments, compared to last year	≥100 %	82 %	96 %	94 %	110 %	Mar
	IVF bookings, compared to last year	≥100 %	93 %	120 %	75 %	85 %	Mar
Product	IVF (implantation rate, women =<37 years)	≥45 %	41 %	52 %	46 %	35 %	Jan to Mar
	FET (implantation rate, women =<37 years)	≥40 %	38 %	40 %	48 %	34 %	Jan to Mar
	Donor IUI (pregnancy rate, women =<37 years)	≥20 %	17 %	25 %	35 %	18 %	Jan to Mar
	Partner IUI (pregnancy rate, women =<37 years)	≥20 %	14 %	9 %	15 %	18 %	Jan to Mar
Safety	IVF SET (women =<37 years)	≥85 %	87 %	88 %	88 %	86 %	Jan to Mar
	OHSS hospitalisations	<0.5 %	0.5 %	1.2 %	0.0 %	0.0 %	Jan to Mar
	Incidents	0	0	0	0	0	Jan to Mar
Service	Average satisfaction score (out of 10)	≥9	9.2	8.6	9.0	8.0	Jan to Mar
	Complaints/month	0	1.3	0.0	1.0	0.3	Jan to Mar
	Key			As expected			
				Keep under surveillance			
				Potential problem—needs investigation			
				Problem—needs fixing			

Abbreviations: *FET* Frozen embryo transfer, *IUI* intrauterine insemination, *SET* single embryo transfer, *OHSS* ovarian hyper-stimulation syndrome

healthy child through excellent care and technology. FA sets annual goals in five broad areas—pregnancy rates, patient safety, customer satisfaction, employee satisfaction and business performance. The goals are quantitative so they can be measured. The measures are called key performance indicators (KPI). Staff members collate statistics so actual performance can be checked against target every month. The main KPI are shown graphically and shared with staff. Table 3.3 shows a monthly "dashboard" for the main KPI that is shared with all staff. Because the data

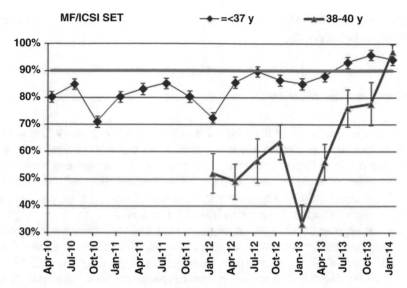

Fig. 3.1 Example of a Key performance Indictor (KPI) for staff of an IVF unit, in this example Single Embryo Transfer (SET), plotted over time for two patient groups, women age 37 and younger, and women aged 38–40, with the target of 90 % shown in *green*

in this dashboard comes from just 1 to 3 months, random variation needs to be considered when deciding whether a value is as expected or lower than expected. Figure 3.1 shows one particular KPI, the use of single embryo transfer as a measure for patient safety, over time to show staff progress towards a goal. Of course, there will be more detailed KPI in each area—for instance for the embryologists fertilisation rates, proportion of zygotes progressing to blastocysts, embryo utilisation in fresh transfer plus freezing, and many more—which will be shared within the embryology, nursing or medical team.

Incident Reporting

Incident reporting captures problems as they occur. It is helpful to call the process something other than "incident reporting" to broaden its scope. At FA it is called "Quality Response" and also includes reporting near misses, opportunities for improvement and good ideas. We have found that staff volunteer "Quality Responses" if they see that doing so helps solves problems for themselves and the organisation and comes without blame.

Incident reporting has three main purposes. It finds a solution to the immediate problem—such giving an explanation or a refund to an unhappy customer; fixing a malfunctioning piece of equipment; adding a missing step to a clinical process. If the problem is important or repeated, incident analysis should try to find the underlying or root cause of the problem to stop it happening again. Finally, incident reporting collects real-life problems that the organisation faces so these can be added to the risk register.

Creating a Risk Register

A risk register is a list of all the things that can go wrong in your IVF unit. While incident reporting captures risks as they occur, a risk register anticipates problems so you can put fixes in place before the problem occur. Risk registers are common in many areas of business and in project management, but sadly neglected in ART. They come with an objective way prioritising risks, which can help you decide where to spend your energy and attention on quality.

The risk register should contain all the things that you think could go wrong which could jeopardise the success of your IVF unit, all the things that have already gone wrong, and all the things you have heard about going wrong in other IVF units. The risk register should start out as comprehensive as possible. Items will include IVF-related risks—such as use of wrong sperm, oocytes or embryos, equipment failure or loss of patient information, and business risks—such interruption through natural disasters, bad publicity or shortage of staff.

It is most useful to express these risks as concretely as possible, for instance "transferring the wrong embryos" rather than "sample mismatch", "internal bleeding after egg collection" instead of "medical complications". The more specific your description of the risk, the more likely it is that your mitigant will address the specific risk. You can also use the risk register to decide what level of detail to include in your Standard Operating Procedures, and what can be left out.

There is a standard ways of assigning the likelihood of risks, the consequences of risks, and hence the severity of each risk. Table 3.4 shows FA's adaption for an IVF unit of the consequence and likelihood ratings published in the Australian-New Zealand Standard, Guidelines for Managing Risk in Health Care [11]. The consequence using costs, and of likelihood with respect to IVF cycles should be adjusted to the size of your IVF unit.

You will find that assigning likelihood will draw attention to some risks that are minor if they occur one by one, but which have a significant consequence if they occur often. Examples in our unit include breaches of privacy such as sending mail to the wrong person. Single lapses, such as a nurse not telephoning a patient when the patient expects them to seldom has much impact on the patient's confidence in the clinic, but several minor lapses in the same treatment cycle can lead to serious complaints.

Table 3.4 Example of a risk assessment matrix for an IVF unit

(a) Consequence scale

Consequence	Consequence factor	Examples for cost (e.g. replacement treatment)	Examples for running the unit	Examples for plant and equipment	Examples for patient care
Minimal	1		No one upset	Nothing damaged	Potential problem, but averted
Minor	2	<$1000	Unhappy staff member	Equipment failure	Unhappy patient, but satisfied by explanation; OHSS treated by bed rest in hospital
Moderate	3	$1000 to $50,000	Episode of unhappiness in team; ongoing shortages in team	Equipment failure during use	Unhappy patient not satisfied by clinic's response; OHSS needing intervention; outcome of treatment compromised; loss of sperm or embryos from one person
Major	4	$50,000 to $1,000,000	Disruption greatly affecting running of clinic; bad publicity	Key equipment unable to be substituted	Wrong use of sperm or embryos; permanent disability
Catastrophic	5	>$1,000,000	Survival of company	Clinic disabled by fire or earthquake; loss of whole sperm or embryo bank	Many patients' health seriously affected; death

(b) Likelihood scale

Likelihood	Likelihood factor	With respect to IVF cycles	With respect to other activities		
Happens all the time	5	1:10	More than every 2 weeks		
Likely	4	1:10	Every 2 weeks		
Moderate	3	1:100	Every 1–2 months		

(continued)

Table 3.4 (continued)

(b) Likelihood scale

Likelihood	Likelihood factor	With respect to IVF cycles	With respect to other activities		
Unlikely	2	1:1000	Every year or so		
Rare	1	1:10,000 or less	Every 5–10 years		

(c) Risk rating

Likelihood factor		Consequence factor				
		Minimal	Minor	Moderate	Major	Catastrophic
		1	2	3	4	5
Happens all the time	5	High	High	Extreme	Extreme	Extreme
Likely	4	Medium	High	High	Extreme	Extreme
Moderate	3	Low	Medium	High	Extreme	Extreme
Unlikely	2	Low	Low	Medium	High	Extreme
Rare	1	Low	Low	Medium	High	High

Notes on consequence:
- Choose the highest consequence if the issue can be evaluated against more than one area
- If more than five people are affected by the same incident, increase by one step
- If a near-miss is identified by some part of the quality system, decrease by one step

Risk Mitigation

Each risk should have one or more ways of reducing either its chance of occurring or its impact, if it did occur. This is called risk mitigation, and the things you do to reduce individual risks are called mitigants. You will already be familiar with many of the common risk mitigants. Some are specific to an IVF unit—such as single embryo transfer in women to virtually prevent the chance of multiple pregnancy, stopping stimulation or triggering with a GnRH-agonist to reduce the chance of Ovarian Hyper-Stimulation Syndrome. Others are generic to quality management— such as training staff so that they are competent, having a document control system so that only the newest version of a Standard Operating Procedure is used, or calibrating equipment so the you can rely on the temperature measurements of the incubators.

By listing risk mitigants in your risk table, you can see how well you are addressing each risk. It is common to be so focussed on doing all the things required of a QMS that you can forget why you are doing them and what risks they are designed to avert.

Internal Audit

Internal audit is about making sure that the risk mitigants you have put in place are still in place and working as you anticipated. Internal auditing is designed to find gaps before they cause a problem. The list of audits you do can be added to your risk register so that the register provides comprehensive overview of how you manage risk in your IVF unit. Table 3.5 shows a section of FA's risk register, listing risks, our estimate of their likelihood, their probably consequence, the risk rating, what we have in place to reduce the risk, and how we audit the mitigants we have put in place to reduce the risks.

Regulations as a Resource for Your Risk Register

Regulations and guidelines can be used in two ways to populate your risk register. First, they can help identify risks. For instance, many of the criteria in the RTAC Code of Practice and the sections of the HFEA Code of Practice correspond to particular risks, such as—staff not having the appropriate training, sample mismatch, multiple pregnancy, patients experiencing a medical emergency after egg collection, patients having side effects from drugs.

Second, some regulations such as the HFEA Code of Practice provide ways of addressing particular risks. For example, to address the risk of sample mismatch, the HFEA Code includes independent checks by two people (witnessing), training the witnesses, defining a critical work areas, making sure the critical work area is empty before using it for the next patient, etc.

If there are regulations in your country, you will have to include the regulation's solutions among your mitigants. If you do not have regulations, or your regulations are not comprehensive, then look for potential solutions from other regulations or guidelines.

Summary

Regulations can help you build your QMS, but regulations themselves cannot be relied upon to provide a broad and robust framework for addressing quality for your clinic to prosper—they have gaps, they probably do not cover all the things you do or the way you do them, their solutions are seldom evidence based or tested. Regulations are unlikely to encompass the positive risks you need to take for continuous improvement; they focus on keeping you out of trouble, not on being successful.

Table 3.5 Example of part of a risk register for an IVF unit

Area of risk	Risk	Consequence	Likelihood	Risk rating	Risk reduction strategies	Audits
Untoward outcomes after medical procedures	Serious haemorrhage after ectopic	3	1	M	Pregnancy monitoring by serial hCG until <5 iu/l; risk and symptoms of ectopic pregnancy described in patient information	hCG forms show hCG tracked until <5 iu/l in failed pregnancies
	Serious haemorrhage after egg collection	3	2	M	Monitoring blood pressure, pulse, oxygen saturation until stable; physical appearance; doctor to discharge	Record audit of sedation and discharge records (part of Record audit of IVF cycles)
	Vasovagal reaction at egg collection, embryo transfer, IUI	2	1	L	Doctor and nurse training; emergency drugs; emergency call bell; second person in clinic when procedures done	Training records of simulated emergencies; contents of emergency trolleys; response to call bell; number of nurses rostered when inseminations done
	OHSS leading to prolonged hospitalisation	3	2	M	Dose of FSH and stimulation algorithm; when to freeze all embryo and not to trigger guidelines; risk and symptoms of OHSS described in patient information; weight gain measured daily after egg collection; guidelines on how manage OHSS for doctors	IVF tracking sheets to check appropriate FSH dose and stimulation; freeze-all and trigger limits followed; weight measured at egg collection
	OHSS leading to serious morbidity	4	1	H		
	OHSS leading to death	5	1	H		
	Infection after egg collection, embryo transfer or IUI	2	2	L	Screening tests; guidelines when to give prophylactic antibiotics; sterile and aseptic techniques; symptoms of ectopic pregnancy described in patient information	Incidence of infection from ORs; watch egg collection, embryo transfer and IUI techniques; check patients with indications are given antibiotics

References

1. De Los Santos MJ, Apter S, Coticchio G, Debrock S, Lundin K, Plancha CE, Prados F, Rienzi L, Verheyen G, Woodward B, Vermeulen N. Revised guidelines for good practice in IVF laboratories (2015). Hum Reprod 2016;31(4):685–6.
2. Practice Committee for American Society Reproductive Medicine: Practice Committee of Society for Assisted Reproductive Technology. Revised guidelines for embryology and andrology laboratories. Fertil Steril. 2008;90(5 Suppl):S45–59.
3. Mansour R, Ishihara O, Adamson GD, Dyer S, de Mouzon J, Nygren KG, Sullivan E, Zegers-Hochschild F. International committee for monitoring assisted reproductive technology world report: Assisted Reproductive Technology 2006. Hum Reprod 2014;29(7):1536–51.
4. Code of Practice. London: The human fertilisation and embryology authority; 2015 Oct. Available from: http://www.hfea.gov.uk/code.html.
5. Code of Practice for Assisted Reproductive Technology Units. Melbourne: Fertility Society of Australia; 2015 Aug. Available from: http://www.fertilitysociety.com.au/wp-content/uploads/RTAC-COP-2015.pdf.
6. Regulation. http://en.wikipedia.org/wiki/Regulation.
7. Ethical guidelines on the use of assisted reproductive technology in clinical practice and research. Canberra: National Health and Medical Research Council; 2007. https://www.nhmrc.gov.au/_files_nhmrc/publications/attachments/e78.pdf.
8. NZS 8181:2007. Fertility Services Standard Handbook Wellington: Standards New Zealand; 2007.
9. RTAC Technical Bulletin 4 patient and sample identification. Melbourne: Fertility Society of Australia; 2012 Sep. Available from: http://www.fertilitysociety.com.au/wp-content/uploads/20120924-RTAC-Technical-Bulletin-4.pdf.
10. Toft B, Mascie-Taylor H. Involuntary automaticity: a work-system induced risk to safe health care. Health Serv Manag. 2005;18:211–16.
11. HB 228:2001. Guidelines for managing risk in Healthcare. Canberra: Australian Standards', Standards NZ; 2001.

Part II
Total Quality Management

Chapter 4
Risk and Disaster Management for the IVF Laboratory

Charles L. Bormann and Erin I. Lewis

Introduction

Since 1978 with the first documented live birth via in vitro fertilization (IVF), the assisted reproductive technology (ART) field has grown to become a commonplace practice. Clinics and laboratories dedicated to the cultivation and cryopreservation of embryos, oocytes, and spermatozoa are now found in most parts of the world, not just developed countries [1]. With this widespread presence of assisted reproduction comes the responsibility to protect fresh and cryopreserved human tissue and maintain continuity of patient care in the event of a natural disaster or other destructive events upending the normalcy of clinics and hospitals. Critical for handling these types of disruptions is an emergency plan to first and foremost (1) protect laboratory personnel and patients, (2) preserve cryopreserved gametes and embryos, and (3) safeguard patient information, financial and operational documents, and laboratory equipment [2]. An effective emergency plan sets out, in writing, the actions to be taken by an IVF program during an emergency or natural disaster.

Creating an Emergency Plan

Regulatory Agencies

The first step in formulating an emergency plan requires IVF programs to contact local, and country-specific authorities to ensure protocols include mandated requirements in the event of a natural disaster [2]. Furthermore, plans should include

C.L. Bormann, PhD, HCLD (✉) • E.I. Lewis, MD
Department of Obstetrics, Gynecology and Reproductive Biology, Brigham and Women's
Hospital, Harvard Medical School, Boston, MA 02115, USA
e-mail: cbormann@partners.org; eilewis@partners.org

© Springer Science+Business Media New York 2016
S.D. Fleming, A.C. Varghese (eds.), *Organization and Management of IVF
Units*, DOI 10.1007/978-3-319-29373-8_4

recommendations given by licensure bodies that oversee laboratories and hospitals. In America, these organizations include the Centers for Disease Control (CDC), the Joint Commission, the Clinical Laboratory Improvement Amendments (CLIA), and the College of American Pathologists (CAP). In the UK these supervisory bodies include The Human Fertilisation and Embryology Authority (HFEA) and Medicines and Healthcare Regulatory Agency (MHRA). In countries where the IVF laboratory is novel and rare, and no regulatory bodies yet exist to govern their emergency preparedness, information can be obtained from more established locales. Specifically, for the past 30 years the Joint Commission has required American healthcare providers to have strong emergency management protocols and a record of practicing these protocols through drills, exercises, and scenario-based training [3]. The set standards and guidelines from the Joint Commission are publically accessible at http://www.jointcommission.org, and list documents that represent some of the best of America's knowledge, suggestions, and requirements for exceptional preparation and response to emergency situations.

In order to develop an emergency plan appropriate for its needs, an IVF program should take into account the possible scenarios that may lead to or cause disruption to its operations. Each IVF laboratory should tailor their specific emergency plans to their geographic location, and which types of natural disasters are most likely to occur. Prior to preparing an emergency plan, specific infrastructure and equipment need to be purchased to minimize damage. For example, California and Japan are predisposed to large earthquakes as they lie on fault lines, northeastern USA must address frequent blizzards, and southeastern USA such as Louisiana are prone to hurricanes. Some disasters can uniformly affect all IVF laboratories regardless of location, such as floods, fires and terrorist attacks. It might be prudent to prepare different variations of emergency plans to address each disaster. Below are several well documented emergency events that greatly affected ART facilities around the world. These examples serve as a reminder of how important it is to be well prepared for an emergency event.

Earthquakes: IVF laboratories in areas susceptible to earthquakes should include close inspection of the laboratory's infrastructure to ensure the building is up to code and able to withstand significant tremors as part of their emergency preparedness. After Japan experienced the 7.2-magnitude Great Hashin Earthquake in 1995, many IVF laboratories had invested in anti-tremor workbenches and devices to prevent falling laboratory equipment [4]. Although 65 out of 78 IVF clinics implemented some emergency power supply in the 9.0-magnitude Great Eastern Japan Earthquake of 2011, many were unprepared for the prolonged power outages incurred. Emergency power supply was short-term in many cases and unequipped to deal with unstable voltage supply and unexpected fuel shortage for generators [4]. Furthermore in 2011 when a 6.3-magnitude earthquake hit Christchurch, New Zealand, emergency power supply failed to perform as the severe shaking disturbed sump sludge within the diesel tanks and the generators failed several times [5]. In the literature documenting affects of earthquake on laboratories and hospital, insufficient backup power supply was the culprit to many failed emergency plans. In earthquake prone areas, IVF laboratories should ensure their emergency power supply is able to withstand protracted power outages as well as tremors, or prepare for failure of these backup systems.

Hurricanes: Much of what we know about the management of IVF laboratories in natural disasters stemming from turbulent weather emerged from the catastrophic Hurricane Katrina that struck New Orleans, Louisiana on August 29, 2005 [6]. Unlike earthquakes, hurricanes often come with several days warning from meteorologists. This can provide for planning and movement of cryopreserved specimens. For one clinic, The Fertility Institute of New Orleans, IVF laboratories were located on the ground floor of two hospitals [6]. Given risk of severe flooding if levees broke, liquid nitrogen tanks storing embryos were moved to the third floor of both hospitals [6]. Similar to post-earthquake experiences, electric power and telephone lines remained out of commission for prolonged periods (up to 12 weeks post-Katrina). After the city was closed to reentry for 5 days by civil and military authorities, backup generators soon ran out of diesel fuel and supplies were unable to be delivered [6]. No one at the time could foresee the degree of disruption severe flooding caused, which prevented embryologists from entering the laboratory without risking their lives. Unfortunately some developing day 2 and day 3 post-retrieval embryos were unable to be saved [7].

Terrorism: Prior to 9/11, American hospitals and laboratories lacked the infrastructure to respond to large-scale terrorism disasters. In 2002, the US government developed the Hospital Preparedness Program (HPP) to improve this response ability by developing disaster plans, collaborating with local agencies, preparing for a bioterrorism attack, and improving communication within the hospital and the community [8]. Terrorism is one calamity that usually occurs without notification in advance, and measures must be put in place to protect cryopreserved specimens as well as deal with ongoing fresh cycles. In the Boston Bombings in April 2013, a lockdown was placed on Boston residents while the terrorism suspects were at large. This precluded personnel from coming into the IVF laboratory to perform fertilization checks, embryo culture and embryo evaluation. Furthermore, since residents were restricted from leaving their home, oocytes were unable to be retrieved. In some ways IVF laboratories can prepare for these large-scale events by placing cryopreserved specimens in safe predetermined locations, but without a doubt some fresh IVF cycles cannot be rescued. Moreover, bioterrorism can potentially have a serious affect on the IVF laboratory with the inadvertent introduction of microorganisms or viruses during processing of oocytes, semen, and embryos [9].

Elements of an Emergency Plan

Safety and Protection of Program Personnel and Patients

The principal part of any emergency plan is protection of program personnel and patients. The American Society of Reproductive Medicine (ASRM) lists essential elements of an emergency plan as:

1. Procedures for reporting a fire or other emergencies
2. Procedures for emergency evacuation, including type of evacuation and exit route assignments
3. Procedures to be followed by employees who remain to operate critical laboratory operations before they evacuate
4. Procedures to account for all employees performing rescue or laboratory duties
5. Procedures to be followed by employees performing rescue or laboratory duties
6. The name or job title of every employee who may be contacted by employees who need more information about the plan or an explanation of their duties under the plan

It is the responsibility of the laboratory director to review the emergency action plan with each staff member. This review should cover the following topics:

1. Description of the various hospital emergency codes and the appropriate response for each scenario
2. Information on how to report an emergency

    (a) Hospital security phone numbers
    (b) Location and use of Fire and Panic Alarms

3. Description and map of the staff and patient evacuation plan

    (a) Employee meeting locations for various emergency scenarios

4. Description and map of the frozen reproductive tissue evacuation plan
5. A list of laboratory procedures that may be performed by essential employees
6. An updated copy of the laboratory phone tree and instructions for maintaining communication during a critical event

A copy of the emergency action plan should be given to each employee and a copy must be maintained in the laboratory at all times. In addition, a list of hospital codes, emergency contact phone numbers, locations of emergency alarms and clearly labeled evacuation plans must be posted in and around the laboratory. Lastly, in order to ingrain the emergency plan, both unannounced and announced drills should take place. The purposes of these drills are to educate staff on the facility's safety features and exits, and to test the ability of institutional personnel to implement the center's emergency plan. These drills will ensure that exit corridors and stairwells are clear and that all emergency exit doors open properly. For these reasons it is essential that staff must actually exit the area in order to properly educate them on these procedures. Paper or computerized testing of an individual's emergency safety knowledge is not sufficient [2]. It is important to note that many of the IVF laboratory and hospital accrediting agencies only require that there is evidence or documentation that employees participate in a fire drill on an annual basis. However, it is necessary to prepare your staff to respond to a variety of emergency drills, some of which may require you to identify an alternative safe location for staff to meet.

Staff Communication

Another important part of the emergency preparedness is maintaining communication throughout the emergency. Each laboratory should have a phone tree in place to communicate an emergency situation and to account for each member of the laboratory staff. Personnel should be able to report their status as soon as possible after reaching a place of safety and if they are able to report to work. It is important to know the best method for communicating with each member of your team. Create a list of the preferred method of communicating outside of working hours for each of your staff members. Be sure to know which email address each member of your staff utilizes when off work. Also, be sure to know which members of your staff accept text messages or allow communication via social media networks when outside of work. One or more persons should be designated as a key contact member, and they should be equipped with both a satellite phone and a computer in the event of a cellular phone service is not working.

Continuity of Patient Care

The safest course of action in the event of a disaster may be to discontinue treatment of that cycle. If the patient wishes to continue treatment and the ART facility is not able to safely do so, patients can be given the option of completing their IVF or intra-uterine insemination (IUI) cycle at another center. Patients may be either directed to a specific facility or instructed to find a clinic in the area to which they have relocated. It is the responsibility of each IVF clinic to have a written agreement with a nearby facility to provide continuity of care for patients during a crisis situation. It is important that these agreements are well-documented in the emergency plan and that all parties have a clear understanding of their roles if they find themselves in this type of situation. In most cases the use of another facility is only for a short period of time and patients ultimately resume care with their original providers. Therefore, it is critical that your IVF consents contain language which describes the transfer of care to another facility and that their cryopreserved reproductive tissues may be transported between the facilities during that period of time. If your facility uses a specific courier for transporting reproductive tissues, it is necessary that you also have patients sign the courier service's transport consent prior to providing them with treatment.

ART Procedures

It is the responsibility of the laboratory director for communicating which ART procedures should be performed during an emergency situation. In cases where there is sufficient time to prepare for an emergency event, such as a hurricane or a blizzard the laboratory director and medical director may decide to cancel procedures such as semen analyses, endocrine assays, ultrasounds, IUIs, embryo transfers, gamete and embryo imports and exports, and only accept patients undergoing oocyte retrievals and other time sensitive procedures that cannot be postponed. By reducing the number of procedures that need to be performed during this period of time, the laboratory director may reduce the number of essential staff required to complete these operations.

The amount of notice you receive before an emergency event takes place will affect the way you are able to manage patient cycles. Depending on the situation, there may be adequate time to cryopreserve all the specimens in the laboratory before needing to exit the facility. However in other situations there may not be sufficient time or an ability to gain access to the laboratory to cryopreserve patient specimens. If you are permitted access to the laboratory within a few days of the incident, it may be possible to salvage some of the embryos left in culture during this period of time. In these cases it is the responsibility of the medical and laboratory directors to determine how the specimens are going to be managed.

Cryopreserved Specimens

Cryopreservation of human tissue is an integral part of the modern-day IVF laboratory. In the past, cryopreservation was done solely via a slow-freeze method, but with the application of vitrification for cryopreservation an increasing number of laboratories are now using this technology. Recent meta-analyses have demonstrated improved implantation rates with frozen embryo transfers utilizing vitrification versus slow-freeze methods [10, 11]. Similar improvements have been shown when comparing vitrified oocytes with slow frozen oocytes [12]. While most people acknowledge that there is a benefit to vitrifying oocytes and embryos, there are still many programs that have not adopted this technology and continue to use slow-freeze methods for preserving these tissues. One major drawback for using slow-freeze technology during a crisis situation is that this equipment relies on electricity to perform the lengthy freezing process, which may take as long as 2 h to complete. This is in stark contrast to many of the vitrification methods which do not require any electricity and can be performed in less than 15 min. For programs that have not adopted vitrification as their primary method of freezing, strong consideration should be given to utilize this method of freezing in an emergency situation where there is limited time and/or electricity available to preserve patient specimens.

To minimize damage to cryopreserved tissue in the IVF laboratory, liquid nitrogen storage tanks should be well maintained. These tanks should be equipped with their own alarms, notifying laboratory personnel if there is a change in temperature or a problem with the system. A set of duplicate records identifying ownership of the tissue must be kept at a separate site. In the event of an emergency, a specific plan for frozen tissue evacuation should be in place. With enough advance warning tissue storage tanks can be filled with liquid nitrogen and moved to another location.

This location might change depending on the type of disaster. For instance in Hurricane Katrina, cryopreserved embryos were transferred to a higher floor given risk of flooding affecting the ground level [6]. When cryopreserved tissues are moved to a location that they do not ordinarily occupy, an attempt should be made to notify the appropriate personnel that the tissue has been moved. If time permits, the new location should be secured and the tanks marked appropriately so that they can be easily identified by nonmedical personnel (police and other institutional and/ or municipal authorities). Following an emergency situation, reasonable efforts should be made to notify patients regarding the location and status of the cryopreserved tissue in as timely a manner as possible. If the tissue has been compromised or destroyed, this information should be communicated to the patient and documented in the medical record. In addition, efforts to contact patients and the results of this communication should be documented in each individual patient's medical record [2].

Off-Site Tissue Storage

Many IVF programs are ill-equipped to safeguard their frozen tissue inventory and/or safely evacuate these specimens in a crisis situation. Failure to maintain proper security, appropriate alarm monitoring, and adequate levels of liquid nitrogen can quickly result in the loss of numerous patient specimens. To help minimize this liability, many programs rely on commercial storage facilities to maintain specimens long-term. For many of these companies, storing reproductive tissues is their primary service and their facilities are specifically designed to protect frozen specimens from many of the natural disaster events described in this chapter. The use of an outside facility to store patient specimens will not completely eliminate your need for developing an evacuation plan for your frozen inventory, as most programs typically have specimens from patients who are currently undergoing treatment or have recently completed a cycle stored on site. However, reducing the number of frozen specimens stored on site will significantly decrease the time it takes to evacuate specimens in an emergency situation.

Laboratory Infrastructure

Laboratory Design

Each geographical location presents its own unique set of challenges for an IVF laboratory. With proper planning many of the risks associated with these locations can be greatly reduced. If you are fortunate enough to be a part of the planning process for a new IVF laboratory or clinic, there are several precautionary measures you can take to minimize the chances of having your IVF laboratory affected by a natural disaster. For instance, if you are located in an area susceptible to flooding, the IVF laboratory should be constructed outside of a floodplain. If your facility cannot be developed outside of a floodplain then it is important to construct a laboratory above the first floor level of an existing building. Additionally, all medical gases, backup power generators, and embryo and gamete storage tanks should be housed above the basement or ground floor level of facilities located in these susceptible regions.

For centers that are located in an area susceptible to wildfires, Safe Rooms can be developed that are able to endure temperatures of 1200 °C for up to 3 h. ReproTech, a long-term storage facility for reproductive tissues constructed such a facility in Nevada. In addition to their Safe Room they also included a defensible space buffer and hydrants along the perimeter of the facility to help safeguard against this potential disaster (http://www.reprotech.com). Similarly, Category 5 hurricane Safe Rooms or EF-5 tornado Safe Rooms can be developed to protect the laboratory and tissue storage areas from these disasters. Guidelines for constructing Safe Rooms that meet the Federal Emergency Management Agency (FEMA) regulatory standards can be found at: http://www.fema.gov/safe-rooms.

Not all emergency situations are a result of a natural disaster or event. In fact, many emergency situations arise from structural issues within the facility, such as an electrical fire or a water line break. To help safeguard against these disasters, it is important that your engineering services conduct routine inspections of the facility and follow an active preventative maintenance schedule. In addition, it is important that the engineering team is effectively educated on the nature and sensitivity of the IVF laboratory. This point cannot be understated. It is critical that the laboratory director and the facility engineers have a direct line of communication. The laboratory director should always be kept informed on the following events: construction in an adjacent room or floor, heating, ventilation and air-conditioning (HVAC) changes or testing, power supply testing, any issues with water or plumbing, and any interior or exterior construction that may affect the laboratory environment. It is the responsibility of the IVF laboratory director to educate the facility engineers on how all of these factors can affect embryo development.

Below is a list of other laboratory design and organizational considerations that may help reduce the amount of loss or damage during an emergency event:

1. Minimize or eliminate the number of windows or glass in an IVF laboratory
2. Do not store items on open shelves, especially above workspaces
3. Ensure that all items attached to a wall are securely fastened and are not at risk of falling during a crisis event
4. Keep all power cords and electrical devices off of the floor
5. Do not store any equipment or supplies on the floor
6. Store laboratory supplies in plastic airtight bins to guard against water and smoke damage
7. Fasten all storage tanks to a wall so that they cannot be inadvertently overturned during an emergency situation

8. Incubators should be kept on a fixed counter space to help maintain stabilization

    (a) For those incubators stored on movable carts, additional precautions should be made to secure the incubators to a wall and reduce jostling and to prevent the incubator from being overturned during an emergency

9. Maintain a laboratory free of clutter and keep all entrances and exits accessible during an emergency event
10. Maintain up-to-date electronic medical records and laboratory databases on an external server to ensure patient information is safeguarded and readily accessible in case of an emergency

Laboratory Equipment

It is important to carefully consider your region and emergency risk factors when selecting equipment for your laboratory. Laboratories located in areas prone to seismic activity may require a specific anti-vibration surface for safely performing micromanipulation procedures. Similarly, laboratories in these areas may benefit from using heavy large water-jacketed incubators as these incubators are less affected by vibrations compared to small lightweight benchtop incubators. Alternatively, areas susceptible to flooding may opt to have small benchtop incubators that can be readily relocated if there are signs of water damage. Among the large variety of benchtop incubators available, there are some that can be connected to tri-mixed gas tanks while others require separate CO_2 and N_2 gas cylinders to balance their atmosphere. There may be a benefit to having benchtop incubators that can be connected to a single gas cylinder if they need to be relocated at short notice.

The location of the practice may also influence the source of nitrogen use for incubators and anti-vibration platforms. Liquid nitrogen vapor is a great source for nitrogen if there are no concerns with receiving and maintaining an adequate gas supply. However if you are in a region where this supply is inconsistent, you may want to consider using a nitrogen generator or choose to order a large supply of tri-mixed gas tanks that can last long periods of time without the need for reordering. The size and location of your practice may also influence the type of tanks used for long-term storage of reproductive tissues. Auto-fill liquid nitrogen tanks are able to maintain appropriate levels of liquid nitrogen on their own while smaller dewars require continuous maintenance by staff members. Large auto-fill tanks have the capacity to hold thousands of patient specimens, but can be difficult to relocate in an emergency situation. Small dewars have much smaller storage capacity, but can be easily moved in an emergency situation. Both types of storage tanks have advantages and disadvantages that must be carefully considered when selecting them for your practice.

Testing Laboratory Equipment

Once you have selected the equipment appropriate for your region, it is important to test its performance in a "mock" emergency situation. All equipment used in an IVF laboratory should be connected to a backup power generator. Each new piece of equipment should be carefully monitored when switching between the main power supply and the backup generator power supply as even a 1 s delay between power sources can greatly affect the function of your equipment. For instance, there is some temperature sensitive equipment, such as certain makes and models of incubators and stage warmers that will automatically turn on when the power source switches over to the backup power supply. However, some of these pieces of equipment will quickly elevate their temperature well above the targeted set-point before they gradually lower the temperature and normalize to the appropriate settings. Without carefully monitoring the temperature of these pieces of equipment, it would be easy to overlook this occurrence. To overcome temperature shifts caused by switching between power sources, these pieces of equipment may be connected to an uninterrupted power supply (UPS) battery backup system to guard against voltage spikes or sustained overvoltage. It is important to note that like all batteries, UPS devices must be monitored and replaced as needed.

It is also important to test your equipment to see how long it can be sustained in a crisis situation. For instance, each laboratory should know how long their backup generator and/or UPS battery supply are able to maintain equipment before they lose function. This information may influence how you respond to an emergency situation. Laboratory staff should also know how long each incubator can be maintained without changing gas supplies. Similarly, it is important to know how long each reproductive tissue storage tank (liquid or vapor) can be safely maintained without refilling it with liquid nitrogen.

Equipment Records

It is important to keep a detailed record of all equipment and supplies in your laboratory. These records should include the make and model, purchase and service dates, as well as any special notes regarding its function in the laboratory. These records are critically important if you're in a situation where any of these items need to be relocated, stored, or replaced. In addition to a detailed log of your equipment, a photo inventory of all your supplies and equipment is extremely valuable when working with an insurance adjuster and/or vendor to replace items that were destroyed in an emergency situation. The laboratory director should also maintain an updated floor plan of the laboratory space. This plan should include details about the electrical outlets, data ports, gas lines, lighting, plumbing, and HVAC system. These records should be updated every time there are changes made to the existing floor plan. Having these records readily accessible will greatly expedite the process of rebuilding your laboratory following an emergency event.

Post Emergency Considerations

Rebuilding an IVF laboratory following a disastrous event can be an extremely challenging situation as there is pressure to rebuild the facility and have it operational in a very short amount of time. To add to this complexity, the process of rebuilding involves numerous personnel, such as hospital administrators, medical directors, general contractors, equipment vendors, insurance adjusters, and regulatory inspectors. Below are steps that may help expedite the rebuilding process:

1. Have copies of your facility's floor plan, equipment list, supply list, and vendor contact information readily accessible
2. Record and photograph all items that were damaged or relocated

    (a) Do not discard any items without photographing the damage

3. Secure a climate controlled storage facility to maintain your equipment and records

    (a) Identify an appropriate storage location for all protected health information (PHI)

4. Identify independent IVF equipment vendors to assess the damage and have them provide you with a quotation and lead time for replacing equipment
5. Work directly with the insurance adjuster and point out all damage to your equipment

    (a) Consider having an IVF vendor participate in this inspection as well

6. Educate the insurance adjuster on the sensitivity of performing ART procedures and the importance of maintaining a sterile environment for human embryos to safely develop

    (a) Provide the insurance adjuster with contact information for experts in the field of IVF Laboratory Quality Management and Safe Environmental Practices

7. Establish a direct line of communication with the general contractor and physically oversee every phase of construction
8. Require vendors to include the dates your equipment will be delivered as part of your purchase agreement

    (a) Require vendors to provide you with alternative equipment if the anticipated time of delivery cannot be met

9. Allow sufficient time for all equipment to be validated and quality tested before resuming clinical activities

No response to an extreme circumstance is complete until the participants have moved to the recovery phase, including reestablishing the medical and health infrastructure, both physically and in human resources, disrupted by the disaster. This does not necessarily require fully returning to the pre-emergency status quo (e.g., in the case of major damage to a facility) but simply achieving a level of staffing and supplies that justifies returning to an ordinary level of care for most, if not all, patients and redirecting those not being served locally to a suitable alternative facility [13].

Summary

Extreme conditions may arise with or without warning, due to weather, geology, utility failure, industrial explosion, transportation crash, or deliberate human action. The response of the entire health workforce may make the difference in the rate at which recovery occurs. Being ready to adapt and provide essential care under extreme conditions is a professional responsibility. It is a responsibility that can be better met if health professionals have considered the issues in advance, participated in planning and practice, and remained committed to delivering the best care possible in the circumstances [13].

References

1. Wang J, Sauer MV. In vitro fertilization (IVF): a review of 3 decades of clinical innovation and technological advancement. Ther Clin Risk Manag. 2006;2(4):355–64.
2. Practice Committees of the American Society for Reproductive Medicine and the Society for Assisted Reproductive Technology. Recommendations for development of an emergency plan for in vitro fertilization programs: a committee opinion. Fertil Steril. 2012;98(1):e3–5.
3. Emergency Preparedness and the Joint Commission. Addressing Joint Commission Requirements. www.jointcomission.org.
4. Ishihara O, Yoshimura Y. Damages at Japanese assisted reproductive technology clinics by the Great Eastern Japan Earthquake of 2011. Fertil Steril. 2011;95(8):2568–70.
5. Ardagh MW, Richardson SK, Robinson V, Than M, Gee P, Henderson S. The initial health-system response to the earthquake in Christchurch, New Zealand, in February, 2011. Lancet. 2012;379:2109–14.
6. Dickey RP, White C. The ART program during a natural or human-made disaster. In: Sharif K, Coomarasamy A, editors. Assisted reproduction techniques: challenges and management options. 1st ed. West Sussex: Blackwell Publishing; 2012.
7. Dickey RP, Lu PY, Sartor BM, Dunaway HE, Pyrzak R, Klumpp AM. Steps taken to protect and rescue cryopreserved embryos during Hurricane Katrina. Fertil Steril. 2006;86(3):732–4.
8. Hartwell C. The effects of 9/11 & Katrina on hospital preparedness. Continuity insights. 2012. http://www.continuityinsights.com/articles/2012/08/effects-9-11-katrina-hospital-preparedness.
9. Bielanski A. Biosafety in embryos and semen cryopreservation, storage, management and transport. Reproductive sciences in animal conservation. New York: Spring Science+Business Media; 2014.
10. Loutradi KE, Kolibianakis EM, Venetis CA, Papanikolaou EG, Pados G, Bontis I, et al. Cryopreservation of human embryos by vitrification or slow freezing: a systematic review and meta-analysis. Fertil Steril. 2008;90:186–93.

11. AbdelHafez FF, Desai N, Abou-Setta AM, Falcone T, Goldfarb J. Slow freezing, vitrification and ultra-rapid freezing of human embryos: a systematic review and meta-analysis. Reprod Biomed Online. 2010;20:209–22.
12. Smith GD, Serafini PC, Fioravanti J, Yadid I, Coslovsky M, Hassun P, Alegretti JR, Motta EL. Prospective randomized comparison of human oocyte cryopreservation with slow-rate freezing or vitrification. Fertil Steril. 2010;94(6):2088–95.
13. Gebbie KM, White KM. Adapting standards of care under extreme conditions: guidance for professionals during disasters, pandemics, and other extreme emergencies. Washington, DC: American Nurses Association; 2008. p. 1–24.

Chapter 5
Staff Management: Leading by Example

Steven D. Fleming

Introduction

Just before I started my first position in senior management, someone told me, "it's much harder to tell someone to do something than it is to do something yourself". Therein lies the essential challenge posed in staff management—how can we effectively communicate with others to encourage them to become accomplished in their chosen profession? The task is complicated by various factors, including differences in character and personality amongst individual staff members, differences in the demands and expectations of staff in different disciplines and at different levels of career progression, and differences between public, private and corporate business cultures. Very rarely does a clinical, scientific, nursing or administrative manager enter a position within senior management pre-armed with the knowledge and training necessary to excel in the role, though short courses in management do exist, such as those provided by the Australian Institute of Management (http://www.aim.com.au). If one is fortunate enough to have learned the art of man-management from a mentor or supervisor then those lessons can prove invaluable. Notwithstanding prior training for the role, there is no single correct style of staff management and leading by example is as good a starting point as any.

The responsibilities of staff management are complex and numerous, so it can be useful to break down the tasks involved into the separate stages of employment, from recruiting the best available staff for different positions through to maintaining a professional relationship with staff once they have moved on in their career elsewhere. Regardless, the principles of decency, clarity, transparency, fairness and

S.D. Fleming, BSc (Hons), MSc, PhD (✉)
Discipline of Anatomy and Histology, School of Medical Sciences, University of Sydney, Sydney, NSW 2006, Australia
e-mail: blueyfleming@gmail.com

© Springer Science+Business Media New York 2016
S.D. Fleming, A.C. Varghese (eds.), *Organization and Management of IVF Units*, DOI 10.1007/978-3-319-29373-8_5

honesty should prevail in all dealings with staff at all stages of their careers. Providing staff are treated with respect, appropriate supervision and training, and are provided with clear objectives and the means to achieve them, there remains every opportunity for them to excel in their role and remain positive and productive, leading to retention of good staff and enhancement of the institution's reputation. In this respect, it is worthwhile bearing in mind that it can be much harder and can prove more expensive to replace a fully trained, experienced and valued staff member than it is to retain their services.

Staff Recruitment

It is often stated that, "an organisation is only as good as its staff", so the recruitment of the most able and appropriate staff for each position is vital to ultimate success. The recruitment process includes workforce planning, advertising, interviewing and vetting of applicants, as well as the administrative requirements of employment.

Workforce Planning

Prior to advertising positions of employment, it is worthwhile carefully thinking through precisely how the organisation will function best, what the chain of command will be, what level of experience and qualifications are required for each position, and how many staff are required to cover the workload, workflow and provision of cover for staff who are on-leave or not well enough to work. The drawing up of a staff chart is a useful aid in workforce planning and is usually a requirement of quality management (Fig. 5.1). The layout of the staff chart will vary according to the range of clinical services provided and the complexity of the organisation but should accommodate all staff members, from Directors down to Trainees. Once determined, the process of advertising the various positions to be filled can commence.

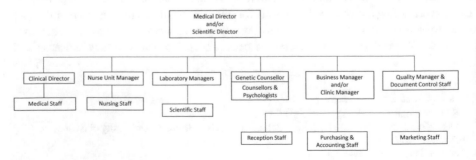

Fig. 5.1 IVF Centre staff chart

Advertising Staff Positions

Composing an accurate, factual and informative advert for a position is important if one wishes to limit the applicants to those who would be most desirable. In order to attract suitable applicants and discourage unsuitable applicants, it is wise to state position selection criteria including all limitations and restrictions associated with the position, with respect to salary, qualifications, experience and eligibility to work within a given state or country (Table 5.1). If advertising space permits, it can be worthwhile including a job description or statement of duties so that any individuals considering applying for the position know exactly what will be expected of them in advance (Table 5.2). In the advert, it is advisable to request that applicants specify their suitability for the position with respect to the selection criteria in their application. To avoid discrimination and meet equal opportunity requirements, it is advised to avoid stereotyping and the use of any wording that may be construed to discourage minorities and other groups from applying.

The various avenues for advertising include local and national newspapers, journals, professional meetings and conferences, national and international professional society email alerts, special interest group blogs such as EmbryoMail (www.embryomail.net) and IVFnet (www.ivf.net), and online via national and international job vacancy advertisers such as "Seek" (www.seek.com.au). Some of these sources for advertising are free of charge. Naturally, the position to be advertised will determine the most suitable avenues. For example, if advertising for an embryologist to work in Australia, one might choose to advertise via the scientific arm of the Fertility Society of Australia (FSA), Scientists in Reproductive Technology (www.sirt.org.au), "EmbryoMail", "IVFnet" and, if the timing was right, during the FSA annual conference. Alternatively, if advertising for a receptionist within Australia, it would probably be more effective to advertise in the local newspaper and via "Seek".

Table 5.1 Example of a generic advert for a clinical embryologist

An exciting opportunity has arisen to join a team of proven professionals, providing fertility services within a major teaching hospital of the University. Applicants should be registered with their professional body, hold an undergraduate degree in science and have at least 2 years experience in clinical embryology. An ability to communicate effectively and empathise with couples seeking fertility treatment is a prerequisite. Duties will include all aspects of clinical andrology, embryology and endocrinology plus active participation in the quality management system and clinical research. An ability and willingness to work flexible hours is essential as working early mornings and evenings is occasionally necessary, and the successful candidate will be required to work weekends every 3 weeks, taking time off in-lieu. Salary is in the range, $65,000–$85,000, according to qualifications and experience, consistent with our fair work enterprise agreement for clinical scientists. Applications will only be considered from citizens and permanent or temporary residents holding a permit to work in this country. *Selection criteria*: Degree in Science; Minimum of 2 years working experience as a clinical embryologist; Professional registration (if applicable in your country); Excellent communication and customer service skills; Flexible work ethic.

Informal enquiries are welcome and should be directed to the Scientific Director. A letter of application, addressing the selection criteria, and a full CV should be submitted to the Human Resources Manager by the closing date, which is May 1, 2016.

Table 5.2 Example of a generic statement of duties for a clinical embryologist

To assist with and perform all aspects of clinical andrology including semen analysis, anti-sperm antibody testing, sperm DNA analysis, surgical sperm recovery, semen cryopreservation and sperm preparation for IUI, IVF and ICSI.
To assist with and perform all aspects of clinical embryology including oocyte retrieval, preparation and insemination by IVF and ICSI, fertilisation and cleavage assessment, assisted hatching, embryo transfer, biopsy and vitrification.
To perform all aspects of clinical endocrinology including receipt, preparation and hormone assay of blood samples for AMH, E_2, FSH, hCG, LH and P_4.
To assist with and undertake all aspects of clinical data entry, audit and review for internal quality assurance and submission to external accreditation bodies.
To communicate in a timely and effective manner with administrative, scientific, nursing and medical staff and management as part of the ART team.
To comply with the legislative framework governing ART, occupational health and safety requirements, smoke-free environment policy, equal employment opportunity policy, and the institution's standard operating policies and practices.
To participate in monitoring and maintenance of laboratory equipment and audits, in conjunction with various quality control and development programmes.
To be fully conversant with emerging concepts and developments within ART, engage and participate in clinical research, marketing and public relations for the benefit of patient treatment and to promote the institution as a centre of excellence.

Interviewing and Vetting of Applicants

Once all applications have been received and a short-list of the most suitable applicants has been drawn up, the process of interviewing and vetting of applicants can proceed. As a matter of courtesy, those not selected for interview should be notified to that effect. Depending upon the limitations of time, distance and expenses, interviews may be held face-to-face or via Skype or teleconference. Face-to-face interviews may be held either at the place of work or at a conference venue and, if desired, allow an opportunity for members of staff not on the interview panel to informally meet and assess the personality of each applicant. Ideally, an interview panel would include the line manager for the position advertised plus someone from Human Resources (HR). Naturally, the various directors of the IVF centre, whether medical, scientific or nursing, would normally make up the main core of an interview panel but an ideal number of interviewers is probably three, which is less cumbersome yet allows for a majority decision where disagreement may exist. Once the interview panel has been formulated, interview dates and times can be organised. If the interviews are to be held face-to-face then the applicants should be asked to bring along at least three forms of legally acceptable identification, such as a passport, driving licence and national public health card.

For a fair and transparent interview process, the questions to be asked of each applicant should be the same, so it is advisable to thoroughly think through the most important qualities required for the position advertised in order to formulate the key questions (Table 5.3). Also, it is important to identify the main strengths and weaknesses of each applicant as well as their availability for employment. Questions can

Table 5.3 Example of open questions to ask candidates at interview

1. What aspects of this position in particular encouraged you to apply for it?
2. In what ways do you think you are particularly suited to this position?
3. Which components of your previous studies do you believe have best prepared you for this position?
4. Can you describe the various techniques that you have experience in?
5. How have you learned good communication skills and in which ways do you think good communication is important for this position?
6. How have you learned good teamwork and in which ways do you think good teamwork is important for this position?
7. What is the extent of your experience with patient contact?
8. What would you say are your main strengths and weaknesses?
9. What would you say has been your greatest achievement to date?
10. What would you like to have achieved over the next 5 years?

be specific or open-ended but the latter tend to be more effective in elucidating the most information from the applicant. However, applicants should not be asked about any disability or other health issues prior to an offer of employment, about current or intended pregnancies, and any matters relating to age, race, religion, sexual orientation or gender reassignment. Furthermore, it is important to encourage each applicant to ask any questions they may have towards the termination of the interview. In order for the interviews to remain as objective as possible, each member of the interview panel should make notes and/or scores against each question asked of each applicant. At the conclusion of the interview, if held face-to face, each applicant should be asked for proof of identity, usually to be checked by someone from HR.

Once all the interviews have been held, the interview panel can debate their scores and opinions in order to reach a conclusion concerning their preferred candidate for the position, including their second preference, should their preferred candidate decline to accept the position offered. Should other members of staff have had the opportunity to meet the applicants for the position, the interview panel may be well advised to seek their opinions before reaching a final decision. Offer of the position to the successful applicant may be in person immediately following the interviews but is usually made in writing within a specified timeframe of which the applicants should be made aware. It is important that any offer of employment is made subject to satisfactory references and other clearances being received, so it will be necessary to ask the successful applicant to provide the contact details of at least one professional referee and one personal referee, and written permission to conduct background checks (e.g. www.gov.uk/disclosure-barring-service). As with interviews of applicants, it is advisable to formulate key questions to be asked of their referees and it may be more enlightening to ask predominantly open-ended questions. References may be sought in writing via letter or email, though referees may be less guarded and more forthcoming during a telephone conversation. It is also important at this stage to check the applicant's nationality and eligibility to work within a given state or country, criminal record plus working with children and vulnerable adults clearance (e.g.

Enhanced Certificate in the UK; Positive Notice in Australia), the veracity of any relevant qualifications held by the applicant and the applicant's registration with national professional bodies (e.g. Health & Care Professions Council in the UK), their general health and their immunisation status with respect to Tetanus, Tuberculosis, and Hepatitis A and B. Employment of someone ineligible to work in a given state or country may constitute a criminal offence, subject to fines or imprisonment. Should all conditions of employment be satisfied, a written formal offer and contract of employment may be made. Again, as a matter of courtesy, all unsuccessful interviewees should be notified to that effect.

Employment Contracts

In order to maintain transparency, employees should be provided with an employment contract to be signed and accepted prior to commencing their employment. An employment contract should state whether the employment is part-time, full-time, temporary or permanent, and whether it is a fixed-term, rolling or renewable contract. It should state both the title and duties of the position and, since IVF is a rapidly evolving profession, it may be wise to state that the employer reserves the right to modify the job description as necessary. The contract should include key details relevant to the position, such as the agreed date of commencement of duties, the place of work, the length of any probationary period during which the employer reserves the right to terminate the employment, the normal hours of work including any overtime or weekend work, entitlement to holidays, sick leave and other forms of leave such as study leave, maternity, paternity and parental leave, remuneration including overtime, expenses, superannuation, pension and any other benefits, and the period of notice that must be given by either party prior to termination of employment, during and after the probationary period.

The employer may wish to include further contractual rights and responsibilities of the employer and employee within a contract of employment such as those concerning staff, patient and business confidentiality and data protection including post-termination competitive restraints, the usage, ownership and distribution of any equipment or intellectual property, the usage and monitoring of email, social media and the Internet in general, grievance and disciplinary procedures, and any agreements concerning external consulting or professional duties including any deductions from pay associated with such activities. By spelling out in full detail a contract of employment, to which the employer and employee agree to be bound, there should be greater likelihood for a positive working relationship between employer and employee.

Staff Induction, Training and Performance Appraisal

Appropriate and thorough induction, training, development and appraisal of staff should be considered of utmost importance, especially within an IVF working environment. It is important to appreciate that the quality of the system depends upon the provision of appropriate access to training and development, and continual feed-back from staff undergoing these processes, so any constructive criticism should be encouraged and welcomed. Indeed, this is an effective means in which the services provided to clients and patients may be continually reviewed and improved.

Staff Induction and Orientation

The induction of all new staff into the workforce is a vital first step to ensuring they fully understand the institution's objectives, culture, ethics, organisation, operation, and the interaction between different staff members and specialities. An orientation manual and/or staff handbook, detailing these aspects, is a useful source of informa-tion that can be provided to all new staff on or before their first day of work, with the proviso that they sign-off on having read and understood its contents. Naturally, most aspects will be common to all new staff whereas others will be specific to dif-ferent sections, whether administrative, nursing, scientific or clinical. Nevertheless, "staff shadowing" is an effective means of ensuring that new staff better understand the roles, responsibilities and lines of communication between staff from different sections. For example, a new embryologist might spend a given period of time in the shadow of a receptionist, followed by a consultant gynaecologist, followed by a nurse. Likewise, new admin, nursing and clinical staff might spend a given period of time shadowing an embryologist plus other staff outside of their own section.

For the purposes of contact, remuneration, superannuation and taxation, all new staff should be required to provide various information upon enrolment, including their full name, date of birth, home address, telephone number, personal email address, emergency contact (usually next of kin), marital status, national insurance or tax file number, bank account, pension scheme and previous employment details. This information should be recorded in the staff member's file and treated as confi-dential. A good starting point for orientation of new staff is to gain an appreciation of the lines of management via the staff chart (Fig. 5.1) and it should be the respon-sibility of their line manager to introduce them personally to all the other staff members. In particular, they should spend time with the Clinic Manager or Quality Manager, who is better placed to introduce new staff to the general organisation, security and operation of the institution, including the usage of institutional tele-phones, email and databases, and the various codes and passwords necessary for access. It is also important that all new staff are familiarised with general health and safety, first aid and emergency procedures and facilities, and know who the desig-nated Health & Safety Officer is. Prior to provision of access to patient data, it should be compulsory for all new staff members to sign a confidentiality agreement and to fully understand the gravity and legal implications of any breach in patient confidentiality, as mandated by national regulatory bodies such as the Human Fertilisation & Embryology Authority and the National Health & Medical Research Council. Similarly, it is important to document other aspects of staff induction and orientation by means of a signed and dated checklist that can be maintained and updated in the staff member's file (Table 5.4).

Table 5.4 Example of a generic induction checklist for new staff

Staff orientation	Staff sign/date	Manager sign/date
Confidentiality, privacy and dignity		
Institutional layout and staff structure		
Institutional culture, mission and policy		
Access keys, codes, security and alarms		
Fire, emergency and first aid training		
Occupational health and safety training		
Quality management system policies		
Punctuality, staff rosters and absences		
Working hours, tea and lunch breaks		
Internal and external communication		
Email, database and intranet training		
Regulation and ethics of treatment		
Patient communication and consent		
Complaints and non-conformances		
Corrective action and improvement		
Annual, parental, sick and study leave		
Expenses, timesheets and remuneration		

Staff Training and Competency

Regardless of previous experience, all new staff should be trained according to the processes, procedures, methods and equipment used to perform their duties within their particular section of the organisation. It should never be assumed that they are competent until they have demonstrated their understanding and ability to follow prescribed protocols. Therefore, adequate time needs to be allowed for the assimilation of regulatory codes of practice, policies and procedures, and one-to-one training. Ideally, new staff should observe all other staff within their section so that they can assess for themselves which techniques are optimal. A good way of familiarising new staff with various procedures is to have them conduct an audit, where they check that what they observe is consistent with the documented standard operating protocol for a given procedure. Indeed, the dogma of "observe one then do one (under observation)" is a good starting point in order to assess the procedural competence of experienced staff. However, inexperienced trainees will require greater supervision and their learning curve will be longer. As with staff induction and orientation, it is important to document, file and update staff training and assessment of competency. In this respect, checklists specific for competency amongst administrative (Table 5.5), nursing (Table 5.6), scientific (Table 5.7) and medical (Table 5.8) staff are useful and should be signed and dated by both the new staff member and the people responsible for their training and assessment.

Logbooks for recording ongoing competency in the full range of standard scientific procedures are available from national professional bodies such as the Association of Clinical Embryologists and SIRT. However, many institutions

Table 5.5 Example of a generic competency checklist for administration staff

Administration staff competency	Staff sign/date	Manager sign/date
Patient reception and appointments		
Patient information brochures and flyers		
Patient demographics data entry		
Photographing patients for ID records		
Preparation of patient notes and records		
Email and telephone calls and messages		
Receipt and sending of faxes and mail		
Typing, photocopying and scanning		
Office equipment servicing and supplies		
Treatment costs, invoices and payment		
Payment data entry and records		
Petty cash and banking records		
Public and private health claims		
Account data entry and records		
Overdue payment communication		
Staff communication and meetings		
Meeting agendas and minutes		

Table 5.6 Example of a generic competency checklist for nursing staff

Nursing staff competency	Staff sign/date	Manager sign/date
Patient communication and interviews		
Patient body mass index measurements		
Phlebotomy for assays and screening		
Patient treatment cycle planning		
Instruction in hormone administration		
Dispensing of pharmaceutical hormones		
Cycle scanning and follicle assessment		
Interpretation of hormone assay results		
Infectious screening results and records		
Recording patient consent to treatment		
Assisting with intrauterine insemination		
Assisting with surgical sperm retrieval		
Assisting with oocyte retrieval		
Assisting with embryo transfer		
Clinical data entry and reports		
Patient information and support		
Drug stock takes and clinical audits		

Table 5.7 Example of a generic competency checklist for scientific staff

Scientific staff competency	Staff sign/date	Manager sign/date
Data entry, retrieval and interpretation		
Patient lab records and paperwork		
Infectious screening and consent checks		
Patient communication and ID checks		
Lab cleanliness and aseptic technique		
Equipment records and maintenance		
Preparation of culture consumables		
Semen analysis, freezing and thawing		
Assisting with surgical sperm retrieval		
Sperm preparation for IUI, IVF and ICSI		
Oocyte retrieval, denudation and maturity		
IVF, ICSI and fertilisation assessment		
Embryo culture, grading and biopsy		
Assisted hatching and embryo transfer		
Oocyte and embryo cryopreservation		
Oocyte and embryo thawing/warming		
Import/export of gametes and embryos		
Clinical data audits, analysis and reports		

Table 5.8 Example of a generic competency checklist for medical staff

Medical staff competency	Staff sign/date	Manager sign/date
Patient consultation and consents		
Patient treatment cycle planning		
Clinical management of COH		
Cycle scanning and follicle assessment		
Interpretation of hormone assay results		
Clinical management of OHSS		
Patient communication and ID checks		
Administration of local anaesthesia		
Administration of sedation		
Intrauterine insemination		
Surgical sperm retrieval		
Ultrasound guided oocyte retrieval		
Ultrasound guided embryo transfer		
Management of early pregnancy		
Patient treatment review and support		
Patient information sessions		
Clinical data audits, analysis and reports		

prefer to develop and utilise their own form of documented ongoing competency. Internal quality control and external quality assessment are an integral component of quality management, and demonstration of staff competency within and outside of an organisation has become mandatory for accreditation within some countries. To meet this requirement, various recognised external quality control programmes have been initiated, particularly within the medical sciences. For example, there is the External Quality Assurance Schemes for Reproductive Medicine in Australia (www.eqasrm.com.au) and the National External Quality Assessment Service in the UK (www.ukneqas.org.uk). Acceptable differences in results achieved by various staff members both within and between institutions are based upon either biological variation, generally considered to be approximately 10 %, or statistical variation, the limit of acceptability usually being two standard deviations either side of the mean.

Performance Appraisal

A formal performance appraisal of all staff should be carried out at least once per annum. It presents an opportunity for two-way feedback, from management to staff and from staff to management. If it is to prove of some value and use to the recipient, it is important for feedback to be constructive and truthful, though delivered with respect and sensitivity. Achievements should be recognised and suggestions for improvement should be made where necessary. In particular, staff should be encouraged to air any concerns they may have and outline their aspirations for the year ahead. Therefore, adequate time needs to be made available between the initial appraisal and any response to the feedback received by both parties, it being a somewhat limited exercise if no response is forthcoming within a reasonable period of time. The performance appraisal should be documented using an open questionnaire and stored within the staff member's file for review prior to the next appraisal (Table 5.9).

Staff Working Hours and Absences

Bearing in mind that all staff will have various demands upon their lives, whether it be in relation to other members of their family, friends or outside interests, it is important to act in a fair and balanced manner when organising who should do what, when and for how long. Hence, a sensible, reasonable, balanced approach is necessary if such decisions are to be perceived by staff as properly weighted and fair to all.

Table 5.9 Example of a generic performance appraisal form

Staff qualities	Employee's comments	Manager's comments
Punctuality		
Time management		
Teamwork		
Technical skills		
Attention to detail		
Customer care		
SOP conformance		
OHS conformance		
Achievements		
Improvements		
Concerns		
Positive aspects		
Signed and dated by employee:		
Signed and dated by manager:		
Response to appraisal		
Signed and dated by employee:		

SOP: standard operating procedure, *OHS* occupational health and safety

Staff Rosters

Staff rosters determine who is responsible for what, when and for how long. Smaller organisations with fewer staff and less workload have the advantage that rosters can be more spontaneous but, conversely, may be more restricted by shortage of cover in the event of unexpected staff absences due to sickness as well as in planning annual leave. Larger organisations with larger numbers of staff have greater flexibility in terms of filling in for staff absences at short notice and providing cover for staff that are on leave. In either event, it is important to appreciate that once treatment has been offered, planned and paid for by a patient then it effectively becomes a binding contract, so adequate staffing and resources must be made available. Therefore, any organisation attempting to operate with a skeleton staff without any emergency external support runs a considerable risk of failing to meet their contractual obligations. Hence, the availability of two members of staff for each clinical speciality, whether medical, nursing or scientific, should be considered an absolute minimum.

When planning staff rosters, the physical and temporal demands of each activity to be undertaken need to be taken into consideration since it is impossible for one person to be in two separate places at the same time and the time required for some procedures are less predictable than others, e.g. a surgical sperm recovery can take anything from 20 min to 2 h, depending upon its difficulty, whereas a semen analysis rarely takes longer than about 20 min. Furthermore, some activities require more than a single member of staff, so allowance needs to be made within the roster for such instances, e.g. physical double-witnessing during biopsy for pre-implantation

Table 5.10 Example of a 42-day rolling roster for three scientific staff

Period	Scientist A	Scientist B	Scientist C
March 1–5	Embryology	Andrology	Embryology
	7.00–16.00	7.30–16.30	8.00–17.00
March 6–7	Weekend off	Weekend cover	Weekend work
March 8–12	Andrology	Embryology	Embryology
	7.30–16.30	8.00–17.00	7.00–16.00
March 13–14	Weekend cover	Weekend work	Weekend off
March 15–19	Embryology	Embryology	Andrology
	8.00–17.00	7.00–16.00	7.30–16.30
March 20–21	Weekend work	Weekend off	Weekend cover
March 22–26	Embryology	Andrology	Embryology
	7.00–16.00	7.30–16.30	8.00–17.00
March 27–28	Weekend off	Weekend cover	Weekend work
March 29 to April 2	Andrology	Embryology	Embryology
	7.30–16.30	8.00–17.00	7.00–16.00
April 3–4	Weekend cover	Weekend work	Weekend off
April 5–9	Embryology	Embryology	Andrology
	8.00–17.00	7.00–16.00	7.30–16.30
April 10–11	Weekend work	Weekend off	Weekend cover

genetic screening (PGS) of oocytes and embryos. Rosters may be designed such that all staff begin and finish work at the same time but flexi-time rosters provide staff coverage over a greater period of time as well as allowing staff more variation and flexibility over their working day. For example, with three staff members working an 8-h day, a rolling flexi-time roster enables an institution to provide a longer clinical service, with two staff members available to work together for longer than an 8-h period. By rotating staff weekly through such a roster (Table 5.10), the necessity to start work early or work late and the opportunity to start work late or leave early are equally shared, as is any weekend work.

Staff Workload

The hours of work that can be expected from staff are regulated in many countries, e.g. Working Time Regulations in the UK (1998). However, some institutions get around such regulations by including a waiver in staff contracts, requesting that staff accept that their average working time may exceed, for example, 48 h in any consecutive 7-day period. Furthermore, some institutions adopt the practice of batching their patient throughput, such that 1 month's activity may be condensed into just 2 weeks, effectively doubling the workload. Also, the proportion of more demanding, complex work undertaken by some institutions is greater than that of others, e.g. some institutions treat more patients requesting PGS and surrogacy. Allowances also need to be made for individuals who are undergoing training, as training demands the availability of staff and is always more time consuming. Hence, it is possible for staff to be placed in a position where they are expected to work very long days, well in excess of 8 h, consecutively. However, the risk of errors occurring increase with increasing uninterrupted hours of work and tiredness, which can increase progressively when working consecutive long days. Therefore, assuming an institution wishes to minimise the risk of litigation should an avoidable error occur, it is advisable to impose formal limits upon the number of hours each staff member is permitted to work without any break and the number of hours permitted to work each day and over any consecutive number of days or weeks. In this respect, adequate time needs to be allowed for appropriate lunch and "tea" breaks.

Sickness Leave

Inevitably, we all suffer from some form of illness or sickness eventually, so allowances have to be made for the possibility that staff will be absent from work for one or more days from time to time. Unfortunately, there are those that consider it acceptable, either personally or culturally, to feign sickness in order to take time off work in addition to annual leave. Such an attitude should be strenuously opposed in order to protect other staff from being unfairly burdened with the additional workload of their colleagues and to maintain a harmonious working environment. Therefore, it is good policy to insist upon telephone notification of management by any member of staff too sick to come to work as soon as their condition is realised, and certainly no later than their normal starting time, on the understanding that failure to do so may result in loss of entitlement to sick pay. Staff should appreciate that it may be expected of them to provide details relating to the nature of their illness, their expected duration of sick leave and a medical certificate from their General Practitioner, covering their period of absence. On returning to work following a period of sick leave, it is good practice for management to hold an interview with the staff member, recording the believed cause of illness and working dates absent in their file.

Holidays and Annual Leave

Bank holidays, public holidays and annual leave are generally considered a normal staff entitlement. The duration of annual leave granted varies according to country, state, position, and whether the institution is in the public or private sector. However, to protect the institution from sudden or chronic shortage of staff, it should be clearly stated in the staff member's contract that holidays and annual leave can only be taken provided sufficient notice has been provided to management and at times that do not significantly inconvenience other staff members. There are staff leave management computer programs, such as "Breathe", that provide a documented framework within which staff may apply for leave and for management to more easily overview staffing logistics during the period of leave applied for prior to granting or refusing the application. To further protect the institution, it is good policy to include in all employment contracts that holidays may not be taken during any period of employment termination notice unless "gardening leave" is required by the institution. To avoid accumulation of excessive entitlement to annual leave, it is wise to have a policy whereby holidays cannot be carried over from one calendar year to the next.

Conflict, Grievances and Misconduct

Sadly, conflict, grievance and misconduct are all part of human nature, so there will be instances where steps must be taken by management in order to resolve disputes and deal appropriately with misconduct. A grievance could be any concern or complaint raised by a member of staff related to various issues including their conditions of employment, health and safety, equal opportunity, harassment, and any organisational or operational changes. It is usually preferable for disputes and grievances to be fairly resolved by those directly involved and at the level of staff management at which they arise. However, senior management should take responsibility for dealing with all matters related to staff misconduct. Fortunately, guidance is available for dealing with issues of this nature, such as the ACAS code of practice on disciplinary and grievance procedures (http://www.acas.org.uk).

Conflict and Grievance Resolution

It is vital to promptly restore workplace harmony whenever a conflict or grievance comes to light. Usually, staff concerned will speak for themselves but occasionally they will choose someone, such as a trusted colleague or their line manager, to represent them. Should an informal discussion amongst the parties concerned fail to resolve the issue, staff should submit their grievance to their line manager in writing. On receipt of written notice, the line manager should attempt to isolate and resolve the dispute as soon as possible by arranging a formal meeting, preferably within one week. In this respect, it should be made clear and agreed that it is in the best interests of both staff and management that the matter must not be discussed more widely in the meantime. Should the outcome of this preliminary meeting fail to satisfy all concerned, the matter may be referred on to the line manager's director. If the conflict or dispute concerns a line manager, staff should submit their grievance directly to the line manager's director. Prior to reaching any decision, it is important to fully establish the facts by reassuring staff that, as far as possible, all discussions will remain confidential and allowing them ample opportunity to set out their grievances. Staff should also be encouraged to suggest their own recommendations for resolving the dispute. The director should inform staff of their decision in writing as soon as possible, preferably within one week. Staff should be given an opportunity to appeal against this decision if wished, on the understanding that an appeal hearing would be held at the very highest level within the institution, after which there will be no further recourse.

Misconduct and Disciplinary Procedures

All staff should be expected to maintain appropriate standards of attendance, conduct and performance. In the event of allegations of misconduct, it is important to ensure a fair, prompt and confidential process in fully investigating them, the primary objective being to encourage and help staff improve their behaviour. Trivial issues can be dealt with informally but more serious matters should be dealt with in writing. Therefore, it is necessary to provide sufficient time in which an employee may consider and respond to any issue raised. If necessary, preferably within one week, a disciplinary meeting should be held with the staff member concerned to address their attendance, conduct or performance under review. Afterwards, the employee should be provided with any decision arising from the meeting in writing, including whether any further action is necessary or justified. As with grievance meetings, the employee has the right of representation and appeal, on the understanding that there will be no further recourse following the decision of an appeal hearing. Except in cases of gross misconduct, employees should not be dismissed following an initial breach of discipline or unacceptably poor performance of their duties. In some circumstances, however, the institution may consider it appropriate to suspend an employee with pay until a disciplinary meeting has been held or a final decision reached following an appeal.

To ensure veracity, staff disciplinary procedures should be supported with sufficient details regarding the alleged misconduct or poor performance, including any written evidence or statements. Ideally, those making decisions of a disciplinary nature should be different to those investigating the issue and should have the authority to dismiss an employee if deemed necessary. Any actions or sanctions should be made in writing and kept in the staff member's file, whether informal or formal. Informal records may be subsequently disregarded, subject to satisfactory staff behaviour and performance. However, if the matter is of a more serious nature or if no improvement has occurred following informal discussions, a written warning should be issued to the staff member by their manager. A written warning should include details regarding the alleged misconduct or failing in performance, any recommendations for remedial counselling or further training recommended, and a timeframe for improvement, including due notice that any subsequent written warning may eventuate in reallocation of duties, demotion, suspension without pay or dismissal.

Gross Misconduct

Gross misconduct covers a range of serious misdemeanours that usually result in summary dismissal of staff without any due notice or pay in lieu of notice. Such activities include bullying, harassment, victimisation, discrimination, assault, theft, fraud, breach of confidentiality, falsification of records, alcohol or drug induced intoxication, wilful or negligent loss, damage or injury, and other serious breaches of policy regarding decency, discipline, health and safety that would be likely to bring the institution into disrepute.

Employment Termination and Post-employment Relationships

Termination of employment is the natural culmination of an employment contract and comes about for a variety of reasons including staff reaching the end of a fixed term contract that is not renewed, resignation of staff opting to further their career elsewhere, redundancy and retirement. Whatever the reason, it is important to handle the process in an appropriate and thorough manner in order to minimise disruption to the ongoing functioning of the institution and maintain a good relationship with past staff.

Termination of Employment

To protect the institution from sudden loss of staff without adequate provision for their replacement, employment contracts should state the period of notice required upon resignation. Adequate notice can be typically anything from 1 week to 3 months, depending upon the level and experience of the employee, and should be considered legally binding by both staff and management. In order to be legally binding, notice should be written, signed and dated. It is good practice to hold an exit interview at some stage during the period of notice in order to ascertain whether the employee is leaving on good terms, to ensure the employee passes on any knowledge and expertise necessary for the smooth transition of their responsibilities, and to make sure that all property and possessions belonging to the institution are handed back, including all means of security access such as keys and staff ID. Institutional security, email and database managers should be advised of the last day of work of the departing staff member so that they may be inactivated accordingly. Those managing staff salaries, wages, superannuation and taxation should also be informed so that departing employees are paid the balance of any expenses, holiday pay, sick pay and salary, and are issued with a final summary of those various accounts along with any relevant certificates of employment and taxation. A termination checklist is helpful in this respect (Table 5.11). Equally important, is a formal personal farewell from management, recognising and appreciating the departing staff member's contribution to the institution.

Table 5.11 Example of a generic employment termination checklist

Procedure to complete	Staff sign/date	Manager sign/date
Return of staff ID badge		
Return of staff access cards and keys		
Return of staff locker keys		
Return of staff car keys		
Return of staff uniforms		
Return of staff mobile phone		
Return of staff laptop computer		
Notification of institute security		
Notification of IT manager		
Notification of webmaster		
Notification of payroll manager		

Post-employment Relationships Between Staff and Management

A positive ongoing relationship between staff no longer employed and management is beneficial to both parties. To protect the institution it is advisable to state various restrictions and post-employment non-competition clauses within an employment contract to which the staff member is obliged to sign their acceptance prior to employment. These might include the disclosure of any confidential information concerning the institution, its employees and its clients, and any attempt to work in direct local competition with the institution or recruit other staff members within a given period following termination of employment.

At some stage during a period of notice or at any time following termination of employment, previous staff members may request management to act as referees on their behalf. In most instances this is a perfectly reasonable request and management should feel obliged to cooperate and support past employees' applications for future employment elsewhere. However, if any manager feels that they are unable to provide an honest assessment of a previous staff member, they should decline their request.

Summary

Employment and management of staff is a complicated skill, requiring a wide range of abilities and experience in understanding what inspires and motivates different individuals. This is the reason why no single style of management can be considered the best. Nevertheless, leading by example and being accessible, accountable, authentic, compassionate, empathetic, engaging, fair, grateful, honest, respectful and enjoyable to work with are certainly keys to success. The responsibility of staff management is considerable but the rewards can be great with good, professional relationships built upon mutual trust and respect yielding optimal performance and better outcomes for all parties concerned.

Chapter 6
Patient Management: A Nursing Perspective

Denise Donati

Evolution of the Fertility Nurse's Role in IVF Clinics

Despite a nurse being at the forefront in the development of Assisted Reproductive Technology (ART), there was little order in the way that the ART nurse's role evolved; in fact, like many areas of nursing, it advanced through trial and error [1–4].

The nurses' role during the early days was largely confined to the usual practices in the ambulatory care setting of outpatient clinics. As identified by de Lacey [5], these roles included traditional nursing functions of chaperone, clinic management and supervision of patient investigation and data. The outpatient clinic fostered a situation in which couples came to consult with their physician and only had brief dealings with the nurse. The nurses' role in patient care was nominal and secondary. Since these days pressure has been exerted from within the discipline to improve the professional status of the ART nurse [6].

The sudden explosive increase in patients seeking fertility treatments in the early to mid-80s led to extraordinary demands on the medical profession. As a result there was an increased demand for nursing intervention. Doctors were able to provide for the medical needs of their patients but were simply unable to provide for their physical and psychological needs. Out of necessity rather than planning, a team approach to human fertility evolved in many clinics [7]. James [8] proposes that nurses working in ART need to be multiskilled, incorporating a multitude of multidisciplinary functions to their practice.

Other authors [9, 10] have discussed the role of the ART nurse to include that of 'physician extenders', phlebotomists and ultrasound technicians. They refer to nurses scrubbing in theatre, coordinating team meetings, participating in decision-

D. Donati, RN, CM, BAppSc, (Nsg), MN (✉)
Fertility Solutions, Sunshine Coast Clinic, Suite 22 Nucleus Medical Suites,
Bldg B, 23 Elsa Wilson Drive, Buderim, QLD 4556, Australia
e-mail: denise@fssc.com.au

© Springer Science+Business Media New York 2016   103
S.D. Fleming, A.C. Varghese (eds.), *Organization and Management of IVF Units*, DOI 10.1007/978-3-319-29373-8_6

making, conducting research, performing intrauterine inseminations and running artificial insemination programmes. In addition to all this, the ART nurse is also encouraged to engage in professional activities such as publishing, presenting at scientific assemblies, continuing education activities and to have involvement in professional associations, be a patient educator and provide emotional support for patients.

It is recognised, however, that not all ART clinics operate similarly and therefore not all nursing practice requirements are the same [11]. To some extent role requirements depend upon the type of treatment being provided; for instance in some clinics the nurse's role is that of organising appointments and 'chaperoning' doctors, whilst in others the role of the nurse is much more diversified where they monitor ovarian follicle growth with ultrasound scanning methods, perform intrauterine insemination assist in oocyte retrievals and in some cases, perform embryo transfers.

In order to provide effective and comprehensive care to patients undergoing fertility treatment, nurses, clinicians and other health care providers must embrace the opportunity to collaborate with each other. No one discipline can claim total authority over the other; instead each should strive for the ideal where all work together for the benefit of the patient. Each profession requires different areas of professional competence and expertise which, when combined together, will provide care that is based on best practice which leads to excellence in the fertilty care delivered.

Managing Patient Expectations

Managing patient expectations is perhaps the most important skill (and often the most difficult) you can acquire as an infertility health care practitioner. Of course, it is important to be confident and competent with your clinical skills but communication skills are equally important. Remember, patients come into contact with not just their doctor and the nurses but the scientific and administration teams as well. Each member of the team has a responsibility to be able to present information to the patient in such a way that it assists them manage their expectations throughout their journey.

When expectations are realistically managed then the patient journey too becomes easier to manage. This is particularly true for new patients and one of the key roles that the nurse plays is providing information to patients so that expectations can be realistically set, right at the very beginning of treatment. Irrespective of the amount of knowledge that the patient has when presenting to the clinic it is extremely important, that you are always thinking of assisting them to manage their expectations realistically when providing them with information about their specific situation. In order to do this the health professional needs to ensure that they provide information that is evidence based, relevant to the situation at hand and is timely so as to allow assimilation of the information along with possible implications prior to decision making. Maintaining these principles will ensure that the patient and their expectations are managed competently and professionally.

It is extremely important that we adequately prepare our patients for the fact that many ART treatments will fail. The reality is that human reproduction remains very inefficient.

Essentially we set our patients' expectations by the language that we use. The language used whilst meant to provide the patient with a positive outlook can in fact leave them with the feeling that the cycle is bound to work and as a result their expectations are set at an unrealistic level. It is therefore important to use language that conveys a cautious level of optimism.

For cycles that result in failure of implantation, the most honest answer that we can and should provide our patients is that we do not know why the embryo did not implant. There is no rationale to manufacture reasons to placate the patient. It is important to only provide information that is factual and supported by evidence. If you do not know the reason, tell the patient this.

It is important to inform patients going through IVF that it may be that several cycles/embryo transfers will be required before a pregnancy occurs (if in fact one does). Although a number of people do experience a pregnancy after the first cycle, the fact is that the majority need to go through several transfers before achieving success.

The only real solution to this problem is to prepare patients before the cycle starts. The patient has a right to know exactly what the limitations of today's technology are. Then, when the cycle is not successful, the patients' expectations are realistic because they have been adequately prepared even though they will be emotionally upset and disappointed.

Communication

In order to facilitate continuity of care effective and efficient communication between all parties is paramount. The patients themselves are also an active participant in their care and must be included in the consideration of the communication pathways. The rapid development of information technology is opening up new opportunities to facilitate communication, which also carry their own disadvantages and risks. It will be an ongoing challenge to maintain and develop good communication.

When communicating with others it is important to consider the following:

- *At all times, patient confidentiality must be considered.* This includes being aware of who else is present when conversations are occurring, and whether it is possible to be overheard by an unseen observer.
- *Electronic/hard copy* patient files when not in use should not be left open where the contents can be seen.
- *Written communication* has the advantage that a copy can be kept for future reference long after a conversation has taken place. It is therefore important to document all conversations with the patient or about the patient.

All formal discussions with a patient or about a patients' care should occur with the patients' history open for reference and any communication/alterations to management being made within 24 h of the communication taking place.

In an attempt to minimise communication error some clinics operate using a Primary Nursing Care concept. One nurse, (often working with other nurses), provides complete care for a small group of patients attending the clinic for treatment. The primary nurse is then responsible for coordinating all aspects of the patients' care and treatment in discussion with the patients' doctor. This approach assists in the patient receiving accurate and consistent information along with best practice care.

E-mail has taken on increased significance as a mode of communication that is readily available to patients and healthcare practitioners. With the continued increase in usage of computers and mobile devices e-mail can be a valid, simple, convenient and inexpensive form of communication. At the same time, issues of privacy, confidentiality and security must be addressed to ensure the effectiveness of e-mail. It is also important to ensure that a copy of any e-mail communication with the patient is kept usually using the bcc (blind carbon copy) function.

Society has enthusiastically embraced social media communication such as blogging, personal websites, and online social networking. It is often easy for patients to find those who are providing medical care for them on various social media sites. Inappropriate online behaviour can potentially damage personal integrity, nurse/doctor–patient and nurse/doctor–colleague relationships, and future employment opportunities.

Nurses, doctors and health care providers have an ethical and legal responsibility to maintain their patients' confidentiality. A must-read for all who use any form of social media is "Social Media and the Medical Profession" [12]. A summary of what is suggested when using social media is as follows:

When using social networking sites, think before putting up a post or sharing information about unprofessional activities or accepting a patient as a friend or fan—ask yourself "Is it appropriate and within my professional boundary?"

New communication technologies must never replace the fundamental interpersonal communication methods that should be used as the very basis of the relationships we build with patients.

Medico-legal Aspects

It is important that patients are fully aware of the fact that any form of medical treatment carries with it inherent risks and ART treatments are no exception. It is therefore important for practitioners to communicate to their patients that ART treatments are often unsuccessful and things can go wrong. Some of the areas for consideration include but are not limited to:

(a) Adverse events
(b) Open disclosure
(c) Patient privacy
(d) Informed consent
(e) Welfare of the child

By no means an exhaustive overview of the medico-legal facets facing practitioners working in ART, however those working in this field should, at the very least, be familiar with and aware of the following:

Adverse events can be classified as either a serious adverse event or a serious notifiable adverse event.

A serious adverse event is any event associated with ART treatment which either causes or potentially causes harm, loss or damage to patients or their reproductive tissues, and/or results in hospitalisation following, and as a result of, the treatment, e.g. OHSS, pelvic abscess.

A serious notifiable adverse event on the other hand, is an abnormal unintended outcome associated with ART treatment which might result in the transmission of a communicable disease or might result in death or a life-threatening, disabling, or incapacitating condition arising from a gamete or embryo identification error.

Open disclosure is the discussion of an incident that results in harm to a patient while receiving health care. The elements of open disclosure are an expression of regret, a factual explanation of what happened, the potential consequences and the steps being taken to manage the event and prevent recurrence.

Patient privacy is a universal concept that, in many countries, is enshrined in legislation, e.g. Australian Privacy Act 1988. Privacy issues include the requirements of information collection, use, disclosure, storage, maintenance, access and correction.

Clinics and practitioners can request personal, sensitive, health and genetic information from their patients. Obviously this information is confidential and has to be protected from disclosure.

Informed Consent. It is the clinician's obligation to obtain informed consent from the patient; it is often the nurse who is asked for clarification around treatment procedures and the consenting process. It is commonplace that the nurse operates as patient advocate and as such it is important that the nurse be familiar with the consenting process so that there is no doubt that the patient has been provided with adequate information to enable them to provide informed consent to their treatment/procedure.

It is important that patients have given written consent to their treating specialist or clinic before any disclosing information is released to their GP or any other recognised third party. In general, when obtaining informed consent, practitioners should consider the following key points:

Consent must be obtained from a competent adult patient before they are examined or treated.

It should be noted that patients may be competent to make some health care decisions but may not be competent to make others.

Patients can change their mind and withdraw consent at any time.

Best practice is that the person treating the patient should actually be the one to seek the patient's consent.

Patients are required to receive sufficient information before they can decide whether to give consent; this would include information about the benefits and risks of the proposed treatment.

Consent must not be given under any form of duress.

Consent can be written, oral or non-verbal. The consent form indicates that the patient has recorded their decision and also that discussions have taken place.

No one can give consent on behalf of an incompetent adult.

All patients are given samples of relevant consents to review prior to treatment commencing. There must be enough time for the couple to be able to clarify any issues and ask questions before treatment commences.

Counselling should be offered regarding the implications of the treatment.

Gametes and embryos cannot be used or stored unless the provider has given competent consent to that use or storage.

Consent forms must be dated and signed by both partners in the presence of a witness as stipulated in the clinic's policies.

Patients must be offered a copy of their signed consent forms.

The consent form must be signed by the patient and clinician immediately after stating that an explanation has been given, and that the form has been read and understood.

When patients are consenting to the storage of their gametes or embryos they must indicate the fate of them in the event that one or both are unable to vary or revoke consent because of death or another occurrence.

At the time of initiating storage of gametes and embryos, patients must also be made aware of any time limitations associated with storage and what the clinic's position statement is relating to this issue.

Reaffirmation of written consent to treatment from both parties (if applicable) should be considered under a number of circumstances including each new Frozen Embryo Transfer treatment cycle, change of clinician or treatment i.e. from IVF to ICSI and any documentation change.

Consent to use donor material is very regionally orientated varying from complete bans, through non disclosure to mandatory disclosure and is really beyond the scope of this chapter except to say that fertility nurses will be involved in whatever the process is.

Welfare of the Child. ART clinics must provide a non-discriminatory access to treatment in line with what is occurring within the community. Refusing treatment on the grounds of race, sex, marital status, sexual orientation, gender or disability is usually against legislation. However, clinical decisions must respect, primarily, the interests and welfare of the person/s who may be born, as well as the long-term health and psychosocial welfare of all participants, including gamete donors. As such, fertility clinics are also required to consider the welfare of any child who may be born as a result of the treatment and of any child who may be affected by the birth. Clinics can reserve the right to refuse fertility treatment where there is deemed to be an unacceptable risk of harm to the physical, psychological and/or social well-being of a child (or any other participants involved in the treatment).

Amongst other possible causes, a risk of harm may arise from issues related to medical conditions, psychological stability, cognitive impairment that significantly impairs decision making and parenting capacity, and/or a significant child protection history.

Minimising Risk

It is a practitioner's responsibility to inform patients that no medical treatment is entirely free from risk and infertility treatment is no exception to this rule. Whilst it is important to provide information about the risks of treatment, it is also important to appreciate that most women go through IVF and other assisted conception treatments without serious problems. It is imperative that clinics have policies and procedures around minimising risk and ensure that all practitioners are familiar with and adhere to these policies.

Essentially the risks of treatment can be work-up and screening, medications, abnormal offspring, surgical and pregnancy risks.

It is part of a nurse's duty to be aware of such risks and be able to discuss these with the patient as required. Should a nurse identify that the patient is unclear on any aspect of treatment, it is their responsibility as patient advocate to ensure there is an opportunity for them to discuss any concerns or seek clarification with their clinician.

Pretreatment and screening risks are largely centred around the discovery of underlying pathology such as disease status or an unexpectedly poor semen analysis. These risks are best mitigated by prior patient education and nurses play a central role in this education.

The main medical risk due to medication is ovarian hyperstimulation syndrome (OHSS). This is best mitigated with patient monitoring with a defined management plan for those patients most at risk. These mitigations are best overseen by fertility nurses as they have day to day contact with the patients.

The risk of having an abnormal baby is probably no greater than in the general population but this needs continual monitoring, usually by nurses due to them following up on established pregnancies.

There is always a risk of complications post oocyte pick-up and indeed post embryo transfer and again the fertility nurses are usually the first line in reporting any untoward outcomes.

The biggest risk of pregnancy that is specific to ART is the establishment of twin or higher order pregnancies and ectopic pregnancies.

Many couples are unaware of the serious nature of the risks of a multiple pregnancy and the frequency with which these complications can occur. Risks to the mother include a higher rate of miscarriage, preeclampsia, gestational diabetes, birth intervention and maternal mortality. Risks to the child include premature birth (with all its sequelae), increase in neonatal intensive care, respiratory distress and cerebral palsy (4–6 times the risk than in singleton births).

Each of these risks are exponentially increased when higher order multiple pregnancies occur. It should also be remembered that while the success rates in older women may be improved by multiple embryo transfer (or insemination with a higher number of follicles), the consequences of a multiple pregnancy in an older mother are much more serious.

The main risk mitigation for multiple pregnancies is to educate patients about not transferring more than one embryo at a time. In Australia, the risks of multiple pregnancy is regarded as so dangerous that the RTAC code of practice [13] specifies that multiple pregnancies have to be kept at less than 10 %.

Medication Management

Historically, nurses have supplied patients with medications in IVF clinics once they have received a written (or verbal) order from a medical officer. The nurse would then provide the patient with the required medication and also instructions on how to use the medication including dose, method and mode of administration, commencement dates and storage method.

As of July 2015 medication dispensing changed in Australia to a more recognised system used by the Pharmaceutical Benefits Scheme (PBS) where patients are now provided with a streamlined authority or private script for their fertiltiy medications with medications being provided from a pharmacy. Due to the risks involved in drug administration patients have a right to:

* be informed of the name, purpose, action and potential side effects of drugs
* refuse a medication regardless of the consequences
* receive labelled medications safetly
* be adequately informed of the experimental nature of any drug and sign a written consent to use
* not receive unnecessary medications

It is important that the clinician provides the nurse with instructions on the type of medications to be used, the mode of administration, frequency and dosages. Medication orders are legal documents and must be completed accurately and unambiguously in order to ensure that patients receive safe and optimal drug therapy.

Registered and endorsed enrolled nurses are legally responsible for the correct administration of drugs. This includes ensuring that the seven "rights" of administration have been established:

1. Right patient
2. Right drug
3. Right dose
4. Right route
5. Right time (as per Table 6.1)
6. Right documentation including the use of acceptable abbreviations (as per Table 6.2)
7. Right to know the effects and side effects of the medication

The nurse is also responsible for ensuring that they have thorough knowledge of the medication to ensure the correct administration of the drug. This includes

Table 6.1 Accepted abbreviations in medication administration frequency

Abbreviation	Meaning
Mane	Morning
Midi	Midday
Nocte	Night
BD	Twice a day
TDS	Three times a day
QID	Four times a day
STAT	Give immediately
PRN	As required
ac	Before meals
pc	After meals
q.h or 1/24	Every hour
q2h or 2/24	Every 2 h
q4h or 4/24	Every 4 h

Table 6.2 Accepted abbreviations in medication routes of administration

Abbreviation	Meaning
BUC	Inside cheek
O	Oral
S/L	Sublingual
ID	Intradermal
IMI	Intramuscular
SC	Subcutaneous
IVI	Intravenous injection
IVT	Intravenous therapy
Neb	Nebuliser
PR	Per rectum
TOP	Topical
PV	Per vagina

knowledge of the how the drug works and its interactions with other medications. It is imperative before the administration of any medication that the nurse checks with the patient if they have any known drug allergies. Finally, the nurse should also be aware of the need to monitor the effect of the drugs that are administered to a patient, in particular if any adverse reactions occur. In this instance this should be documented in the patients' notes and their treating clinician notified immediately.

Psychological Sequelae of ART Treatments

Counselling is an essential component of the services provided by any ART clinic/organisation. All counsellors/psychologists are expected to be a member of their professional body.

Fertility counselling generally includes crisis counselling, decision-making counselling and implications counselling. It may also include supportive and therapeutic counselling.

Counselling is helpful when experiencing stress, depression or anxiety due to infertility, treatment and treatment outcomes, relationship and support issues, or just to assist in coping from time to time. Patients experiencing failure of fertility treatment, adverse responses to treatment, miscarriage, stillbirth or other losses may greatly benefit from counselling. Some patients benefit from or need ongoing supportive counselling. Infertility and treatment at times involves grief and loss, and grief counselling may be appropriate. Discussion of available options and counselling regarding future treatment or cessation of treatment assists in decision-making for clients. Referral to appropriate other support organisations is expected.

The main job of a fertility nurse in counselling is to recognise any potential need for counselling, have initial conversations with the patient and then refer them (if necessary) to professional counsellors.

Counselling is a mandatory component of treatment when any donor gametes or embryos are being used or when planning surrogacy. It is often mandatory depending on jurisdiction and is a specialised area of counselling beyond the scope of this chapter.

Conclusions

Fertility nursing is a relatively new field which offers a diverse and challenging environment in which a nurse can work. This is why we have become a sub-speciality, formally recognised by the Fertility Society of Australia as the Fertility Nurses Australasia. The work of a fertility nurse is varied involving many disciplines, skills and peculiar situations with the scope of practice continuing to expand to accommodate rapid developments in reproductive technologies, along with societal pressures and expectations. Nurses should be encouraged and supported to extend their roles and rather than be considered as 'mini doctors' they should be assisted in becoming 'maxi nurses'.

References

1. Barber D. Continuity of care in IVF: the nurse's role. Nurs Times. 1994;90(45):29–30.
2. Barber D. Nurses performing embryo transfers: successful outcome of in-vitro fertilisation. Hum Reprod. 1996;11(1):105–8.
3. Barber D. Use of competencies in training fertility nurse in clinical practice. Hum Fertil. 1997;2:5–9.
4. Barber D. Research into the role of fertility nurses for the development of guidelines for clinical practice. Hum Reprod. 1997;12(11 Suppl):195–7.

5. De Lacey S. The nurse's role in assisted reproduction: visions for the future. Fertility Nurses of Australasia Newsletter (1998). August 1999;9(2):6–10.
6. Birch H. The extended role of the nurse—opportunity of threat? 14th International conference for nurses and support personnel in reproductive medicine. Arizona: Phoenix; 2001.
7. Bernstein J. Development of the nursing role in reproductive endocrinology and infertility. In: Garner C, editor. Principles of infertility nursing. Boca Raton, FL: CRC Press; 1992. p. 169–78.
8. James C. The nursing role in assisted reproductive technologies. NAACOG's Clin Issues. 1992;3(2):328–34.
9. Ashcroft S. Developing the Clinical Nurse Specialists' role in fertility: do patients benefit? Hum Fertil. 2000;3:265–7.
10. Barber D. The extended role of the nurse: practical realities. Hum Fertil. 2002;5:13–6.
11. Denton J. The nurse's role in treating fertility problems. Nurs Times. 1998;941(2):60–1.
12. Social Media and the Medical Profession. A guide to online professionalism for medical practitioners and medical students. A joint initiative of the Australian Medical Association Council of Doctors-in-Training, the New Zealand Medical Association Doctors-in-Training Council, the New Zealand Medical Students' Association and the Australian Medical Students' Association. Pub. Australian Medical Association 2010.
13. Reproductive Technology Code of Practice. 2014. http://www.fertilitysociety.com.au/wp-content/uploads/RTAC-COP-Final-20141.pdf.

Chapter 7
Low-Risk Laboratory Management

Simon Cooke

Introduction

There are a lot of texts on management techniques, so in this chapter the main difference that I have focussed on is discussing and explaining the low-risk approaches to running human IVF laboratories. Some items may be similar to what you are doing now, and some may be challenging to your beliefs; however that is exactly the reason for this chapter. This then becomes a chapter to help Laboratory Managers determine the best low-risk practice to employ in their system, and not a document that simply tells people one method of running labs.

Any suggestion of good versus bad management can be more appropriately looked at from the concepts of:

- Low versus elevated risk
- Efficient versus non-efficient systems
- Proof of items happening versus assumptions
- Known problems versus methods around them
- Ensuring equipment is operating within correct parameters versus not checking, and
- Using Laboratory Performance Measures (LPM) and Benchmarking to increase control over a laboratory and reduce the risk

For many of the areas in this chapter, I have taken the perspective from a large laboratory system, employing a large number of staff across multiple laboratories. As an example, in 2015, I have a laboratory system with six embryology laboratories (of varying sizes) performing over 5000 fresh and 2500 frozen cycles per year, nine accredited diagnostic andrology laboratories performing over 8000 andrology

S. Cooke, BSc Agr, PhD (Med) (✉)
IVF Australia, Level 3, 176 Pacific Highway, Greenwich, NSW 2065, Australia
e-mail: simon.cooke@ivf.com.au

© Springer Science+Business Media New York 2016
S.D. Fleming, A.C. Varghese (eds.), *Organization and Management of IVF Units*, DOI 10.1007/978-3-319-29373-8_7

tests per year, and a reproductive hormone laboratory performing over 250,000 tests per year. The staffing to run this, 7 days a week all year, across many physical laboratory sites, is approximately 60 laboratory staff, filling 40 full-time positions (comprised from full-time staff, part-time staff, and staff currently on maternity leave).

This may sound like a large IVF system, so the main aim of this chapter is efficient, reproducible, consistent, low-risk laboratory management, with ease and use of accepted systems, without having to reinvent the wheel. The risk items will concentrate mostly on IVF laboratories, however the system can be used to cover any type of medical laboratory.

In general, if the low-risk laboratory management items work efficiently for a large laboratory, it will work for a smaller laboratory...however, the reverse is not always true.

Starting to Reduce Risk Using Quality Systems

Medical pathology and clinical IVF laboratories have a specialised set of customer service, laboratory outputs, operating techniques, and technical competence requirements that set them apart from other Industries.

A good way to reduce laboratory risk is to find an applicable internationally recognised standard, and hopefully exceed the requirements in that standard.

Most IVF laboratories have some form of national accreditation documentation to follow; however, these usually follow the form of a Code of Practice (i.e. RTAC Code of Practice [1] in Australia, or HFEA Code of Practice [2] in the UK) or mandated general rules (i.e. European Union Tissue Cell Directive [3]); however, these are not international standards. They cover a little bit from multiple areas of the clinics, but do not cover a lot of areas well. National accreditations require some form of training and laboratory quality control (QC), however there is no documentation or table to interpret exactly what QC schedule of calibration or checking should happen.

This is where actual International standards become more important. They take the QC and quality management systems required by the national accreditation programmes, and ensure it is formalised. However, what type of international standards are the best for different laboratories to follow?

Generic QC programmes, such as the ISO9001 [4] series, are good to ensure all areas of the clinic are operating to an international standard level (far superior to a national accreditation level), but the ISO9001 series of documents is not specific to IVF or pathology. In fact, ISO9001 is applicable to all types of different companies (i.e. cleaning contractors, transport companies, consumables goods suppliers), as well as to medical clinics and laboratories. Unfortunately, this standard has no documentation to suggest the frequency, or the type of QC calibrations. Despite this, as a quality system to follow it is a fantastic system to ensure all parts of the system are moving in the correct direction, and it has risk minimisation processes inside this standard.

A standard such as ISO15189 [5] is a superb standard to follow for medical pathology laboratories, as it is a technical competence standard that is aimed at controlling risk by minimising laboratory error, and assesses the qualifications, training and experience of staff; correct equipment that is properly calibrated and maintained; adequate quality assurance procedures; appropriate sampling practices, and so on. Some countries (i.e. Australia) have a system that requires their certification for pathology laboratory accreditation is based on the relevant international standard (e.g. ISO15189). So the methodology, results and the individual are assessed in this technical competence standard.

Whilst it has clear benefits for pathology laboratories, its usefulness may not be as strong for IVF laboratories. In these laboratories, the process of human embryo culture is not often based on completely proven methodology. Whilst culture media bottles and freeze-thaw kits will have instructions-for-use, most of the embryo manipulation and consumables certainly do not, and they are best described as *in-house methodology*.

For IVF laboratories, following one or both international standards as well as the required national accreditation codes, is a great way to ensure the laboratory is running to a standard that is reproducible, and ensures that the *minimum* standard of laboratory care (i.e. Generally, the national accreditation codes for IVF laboratories, are the minimum standard of accreditation) is being exceeded.

Regardless of what system is followed, the national accreditation codes and the international standards will start controlling laboratory risk at its most basic level, and try to eliminate system errors via:

- Identifying outdated documents, policies, procedures, consents or forms
- Ensuring a clear consistent source of information
- Requirements for sample identity, and even techniques on how to reduce sample errors
- Ensuring staff are proven to be trained to a documented level, and can be recertified at that level yearly
- Ensuring there is continual education, sufficient and appropriate managerial oversight and backup of staff, and
- Equipment works, is suitable for the task, and is fit for purpose before use that day

These are start points though, and a laboratory MUST be doing more than this to control risk.

It is better to run a laboratory safely using some form of international standard wherever possible, which is in addition to any mandated national codes. If there is an international system available and a certification body to accredit you, then always use it. That way you are covering multiple forms of risk and error.

You will be operating well above any minimum laboratory requirements, and that is a positive thing to do when managing human IVF laboratories.

If the risk minimisation was efficient in these international codes or local laboratory standards, then medical laboratories would never make mistakes. However, as laboratories are human based systems, and humans are predisposed to make errors, this chapter will look at some methods to ensure these errors occur less frequently or, if possible, are almost eliminated.

I would be the first to acknowledge that running a low-risk laboratory management model is not cheap, is not easy, and is a luxury that may not be easy to achieve for all people in all countries. Whilst I have been given great company management support and flexibility to mould a system, these luxuries do come at a cost. This is a financial cost of staff, cost of resources and equipment, operating cost of consumables, and a cost in accreditation compliance and QC. It is accepted that running low-risk systems requires a huge personal and mental investment in time and effort.

Whilst risk minimisation does have a financial cost, that cost in the total scheme of the system is minimal, so should never be used as a reason not to perform a low-risk version of any process, and should not be used as a reason to avoid extra accreditation.

If you were the patient, you would expect that the clinic is operating with the lowest risk method possible, has obtained the highest quality standard possible, and you would expect that a laboratory can achieve the hardest accreditation that is available. You certainly would not accept that a clinic or a laboratory is happy to just do the minimum it can, to get basic accreditation.

Staffing an IVF Laboratory

One of the best ways to run laboratories with multiple outputs such as IVF laboratories with multiple specialist techniques (i.e. IVF, ICSI, PGD, TESA, etc.), diagnostic andrology laboratories (i.e. Full semen analysis, DNA analysis, etc.), or endocrine pathology laboratories (covering multiple scope or testing areas), is to ensure you have good staff in key positions.

In most systems, there is a single Scientific Director, or Laboratory Director who takes overall responsibility for the process in operation. Certain standards or regulatory bodies use different terminology for these same roles so, in this chapter, I will call them the Scientific Director. In this chapter, the phrase "laboratory management" can essentially be viewed as the Scientific Director's role. Interestingly, the Scientific Director's role, responsibilities and requirements are often set by legislation or standards or codes [1–3, 5, 6]; however, the number of laboratory scientists varies widely inside each laboratory, and inside each type of laboratory. Some countries have national registration of clinical laboratory scientists (i.e. Singapore, UK, NZ); however, the majority do not, and some countries such as Singapore have minimum staff numbers needed to be on-duty at any one time, which can alter the staffing ratios that we will cover later.

Whilst Directors are key staff in the running, organisation, development, direction, and quality management of laboratories, they cannot be everywhere at any given time, nor can they do everything. It is also clear from personal experience, that as laboratories approach 2000 fresh cycles, or multiple laboratories come under the Director's responsibility, then the time spent actually doing bench work in laboratories diminishes rapidly. So, the Scientific Director must be supported by good staff, who actually process the laboratory work. Spreading these good staff around to the important areas is crucial to controlling risk in laboratories. Skilled Laboratory Supervisors or Senior Scientists are terribly important to maintaining a quality process in an IVF laboratory.

Laboratory Supervisor

Each laboratory in the system needs to have staff that are trained, encouraged and empowered to make the correct choices. Having efficient, knowledgeable Laboratory Supervisors is crucial to this, and is a fantastic risk minimisation process. They give consistency of information to the Scientific Director and to the medical professionals using that laboratory, consistency of direction and training to their staff, and can deal with small items that appear during daily work in a smooth, efficient, knowledgeable and patient focussed way.

With IVF laboratories, I see it as a requirement that every human embryo culture laboratory needs a Laboratory Supervisor (or depending on size and staff numbers, an empowered Senior Scientist) to manage this process daily with some clear authority. The choice of personality in a Laboratory Supervisor is also very important. Having a Supervisor who simply says "yes" to everything the Scientific Director says, is a system designed for disaster. One of the key roles and risk minimisation strategies of senior laboratory staff is that they give "feedback" and can assess technical decisions and suggest alternative methods.

The Laboratory Supervisor then becomes a sounding board for ideas, technical knowledge on whether items are feasible at the bench, a lead training resource when new or altered techniques are devised and implemented, and holds a key role to ensure that the laboratory does not progress aimlessly down a pathway without some form of continual review. Senior staff that simply say "yes" are almost as dangerous as a Director that doesn't listen. Having multiple Laboratory Supervisors is an even stronger management system, as some will have strengths in different areas, and may give more robust feedback than their peers. Now it is true that some feedback can be very challenging, sometimes not expected, or very poorly delivered and quite confronting; however, that is the beauty of the system. Constructive feedback is a positive and essential risk-minimisation process, and is essential in ensuring low-risk laboratory management.

The Laboratory Supervisor also has a huge role in empowering their staff to discuss and to watch out for risks during daily laboratory tasks, and to bring these potential risks to the attention of laboratory management. The development of this internal laboratory discussion process is discussed later in this chapter under human factors training.

When any technical processes (i.e. standard operating procedures, work instructions or policies) are written, the Laboratory Supervisors are invaluable. Documents may be written by a wide range of people, however it is the technical review of the document that becomes important. The Laboratory Supervisor with help from their staff must be able to review the content, discuss the process, and be able to give their technical and safety feedback. This creates ownership of the process, knowledge of the process and in most cases, the desire to follow the process and to teach and implement it efficiently; because they helped write it.

Some laboratories also use the Laboratory Supervisor as the main sign-off mechanism for staff laboratory training, and some facilities may share this training officer role with other senior laboratory staff. They also take responsibility for ensuring the laboratory QC tasks that we will cover later are completed correctly and on time.

Laboratory Staff Numbers Required

Managing laboratories and working out the staffing required for different size and different type laboratories can be quite difficult.

With IVF laboratories, it is not as easy as breaking down the number of yearly cycles and dividing by the number of staff, and using that formula to work out the staff sizes for your laboratory. A suggested number is one full-time embryologist for every 125 fresh cycles performed [7], but this is heavily influenced by:

- The culture techniques and processes in operation at the time the book was written.
- The skill level of the staff.
- The number of days that the staff are able to work in a week, and the length of their day.
- The complexity of task (i.e. is it basic IVF and ICSI, or is the laboratory performing lots of high complexity tasks such as PGD or IMSI, that are very labour intensive?).
- Whether the egg collection facility is close to the laboratory, or does it take a large amount of staff time to move between work locations?
- Whether the laboratory has mandated that there be a requirement for identity double witnessing of all gamete movement stages, or does the accreditation provider insist on a certain staff ratio in the laboratory?
- Whether the laboratory uses electronic methods to perform this identity witnessing to allow a lower staffing number?
- How many cycles does the laboratory perform? A chosen number of staff can process a small amount of work or a much larger amount of work. This forms "Economies-of-Scale" where a larger number of cycles can get processed without an increase in staff numbers or overall cost or risk.
- What other tasks take staff time in the laboratory (i.e. Embryo thaws; do they also run diagnostic andrology clinics too, etc.?)

Consider the staffing ratios of six actual laboratories below. These are broken down into Full Time Equivalent (FTE) staff.

- For the calculation of 1.0 FTE, it is taken as being 5 days cover from the staff member (i.e. where there is 38 h work in a week). So, if one staff member works 3 days a week (that is $3/5 \times 1.0$ FTE=0.6 FTE worked by that staff member), and if one staff member works 4 days a week (that is $4/5 \times 1.0$ FTE=0.8 FTE). That means that to achieve 7 days full laboratory cover when you allow staff to take breaks and weekends off, actually requires=1.4 FTE staff. And that is only if you have one staff member working at any given time.

In Table 7.1, there is a basic number of FTE staff needed for varying size laboratories. All these laboratories have a requirement for double witnessing of every vessel change at every time (regardless of the day of the week). There must clearly be a minimum level of staffing for embryology laboratories, so some laboratories such as Laboratory D, must have the minimum number of staff, even if their cycle

Table 7.1 Fresh cycles performed per Full Time Equivalent (FTE) Laboratory Staff member

Embryo lab	Identity witnessing	Fresh cycles	FTE in lab	Fresh cycles per FTE
A	Manual	1650	9.6	172
B	Manual	1640	9.2	178
C	Manual	770	5.1	151
D	Manual	150	1.7	88
E	Manual	470	4.0	118
F	RFID	320	1.8	178
Total		5000	31.4	159

Table 7.2 Fresh and frozen cycles performed per Full Time Equivalent (FTE) Laboratory Staff member

Embryo lab	Identity witnessing	Fresh cycles	Frozen cycles	Total fresh + frozen cycles	FTE in lab	All cycles per FTE
A	Manual	1650	880	2530	9.6	264
B	Manual	1640	750	2390	9.2	260
C	Manual	770	490	1260	5.1	247
D	Manual	150	110	260	1.7	153
E	Manual	470	250	720	4.0	180
F	RFID	320	20	340	1.8	189
Total		5000	2500	7500	31.4	239

Note the standardisation of work-flows for Laboratory D and E, when frozen cycles are included in the data

number is not great. This is because one person cannot be at work for many days in a row as that is a source of fatigue and errors.

When only the fresh numbers of cycles are included in these ratio calculations, it looks like Laboratory D and E are underworked compared to Laboratory A, B and F.

The cycle:staff ratio of 125:1 (i.e. one full-time embryologist for every 125 fresh cycles performed) suggested in Mortimer and Mortimer [7] appears to be quite low. The ratio seems accurate in the traditional smaller laboratory size using conventional manual-human witnessing processes.

Table 7.1 only covers the number of fresh cycles. There are more laboratory techniques that are involved in standard operations that take up staff time. Table 7.2 is an adjusted model that covers more of the tasks that happen in a laboratory, and covers more of the risk. This table is for the same laboratories as in Table 7.1, only now the workload associated with frozen embryo cycles is taken into account. As you can see, Laboratory D, E and F are now very similar in the work performed by this staff. This is because Laboratory F is a new laboratory that has not yet built up a lot of frozen embryos to then perform thaw cycles upon.

It is also interesting to note the difference in FTE staff that can be used when a laboratory uses an electronic RFID witnessing system (RI Witness™), instead of traditional human double witnessing; which allows the use of lower numbers of staff to be present processing more cycles, whilst still giving no reduction in patient safety for identity witnessing.

The three smaller laboratories (D, E and F) have similar FTE/cycles when fresh and frozen cycles are included (between 150 and 190 cycles per staff FTE).

The bigger laboratories (A, B and C) can achieve "economies-of-scale" by their size and staff availability, and achieve similar FTE/cycles when fresh and frozen cycles are included (between 245 and 265 cycles per staff FTE).

So, by working out:

(a) The size of your laboratory
(b) What laboratory tasks it is planning on performing, and whether you will be including frozen embryo cycles in the calculated workload of the laboratory as well as fresh cycles, and
(c) What is the chosen method of identity witnessing

you can compare staffing ratios that match the size of the desired laboratory. It becomes clear that a single arbitrary cycle:staff number will not suit multiple different laboratories, workloads or even different laboratory sizes, and staff ratios/cycle is affected by the techniques the laboratory is performing and the type of identity witnessing used in that laboratory.

How Often Should Staff be Working and for How Long?

If the aim of laboratory management is to have staff who are engaged in their task, not rushing, fully concentrating, and not likely to make fatigue based mistakes, then another low-risk laboratory management strategy to use to help guide staffing ratios, is to set clear rules.

In Australia, national employment standards that form the minimum work conditions allowed do not cover items such as staff breaks. Based on their specialty though, IVF scientists often have more complex Enterprise Agreements or other agreements that formalise these breaks that are crucial to risk minimisation. Enterprise Agreements [8] are held in a freely accessible format controlled by the Australian Federal Government. Irritatingly, all items that companies negotiate on behalf of their own staff, are then accessible to everyone else using the internet. However, some items are not suitably covered by Enterprise Agreements, so need to be covered by written policies in the workplace.

To overcome staff fatigue, some suggestions could be:

1. Rules on how many days in a row a staff member should be at work:

   • Set a maximum such as cannot work more than 7 consecutive days, and in a 2 week period need to take 4 days off.

2. Rules on what is the maximum time staff should be concentrating for in a day or without a break:

   • Breaks are required to avoid fatigue. Lunch breaks can have a minimum length of 30 min, and one suggestion is staff should not to work for longer than 5 h without a break. The maximum hours in any working day for concentration could be set at 10 h.

3. Rules on how many breaks staff should get to allow staff to have a mental "refresh", and to help ensure that lab concentration is maintained.

   - If staff work for under 7.5 h a day they get one extra break, and if staff work over 7.5 h they get two extra breaks.
   - Ensure that all work breaks are taken outside the laboratory, to allow a change of environment and change of sensory information.

4. Rules on what tasks staff are allowed to perform if any of points 1, 2 and 3 are exceeded:

   - If staff ever work >7 consecutive days, they are restricted to low risk activities and support roles.

Whilst the Employment Agreements and Work Health Safety criteria in Australia may appear to be very generous compared to work hours and practices in other countries, it is clear that anything that increases patient risk by ignoring items that are easily controlled (such as fatigue and breaks) is a system that will fail. These four suggestions above may change the number of staff needed in your facility, however the staff ratios suggested earlier in Tables 7.1 and 7.2 were obtained using these fatigue minimisation rules. There is no doubt that staff can process more work than suggested in Tables 7.1 and 7.2; however, as with everything, it comes with risk that has to be identified, and accepted or minimised.

Laboratory Equipment to Reduce Risk

When it comes to low-risk laboratory management, the laboratory needs to have a numerical grading system that can be used to allocate a score based on good and bad areas of certain laboratory equipment. Based on this score, the laboratory can choose equipment, with the knowledge that they have applied science and risk to their choice of equipment.

In relation to equipment chosen to do a task, it comes down to looking at several principles. Regardless of whether it is an IVF laboratory or a pathology laboratory (such as diagnostic andrology or chemical pathology), the processes are similar.

1. Is the equipment already in service in your system? If not in service, has it been tested and validated in your hands, or have your staff previously used this equipment?
2. Does it allow a work-flow that is not overly complex, containing additional handling stages that could lead to a sample being dropped or spilt?
3. In an IVF setting, does the equipment allow conditions that maintain temperature and pH stability, or do small process changes need to occur?
4. Does it overcome errors or uncertainties that have already been highlighted in current laboratory process working?
5. Is the design, setting and use of the equipment ergonomic to staff, and overcomes staff pain and discomfort when using it?
6. Is there a competent and speedy service and maintenance system available in your city or country?

These days, it would be hard to implement equipment changes or implementations that do not cover all of these process steps.

It is important to use a comparison scoring system that can allow you to either compare two different new pieces of equipment, or compare new equipment against existing equipment in your laboratory. If you are comparing new equipment against existing equipment, then only the new equipment can have a score change. Using a system that increases/reduces the scores when items have known laboratory risk is quite useful, as is increasing the scores allocated to embryo culture risk, as compared to staff comfort. It is pointless awarding similar "scores" to items that carry different risk to the products being manipulated.

As an example, consider the shaded example in Table 7.3. This was a multiple stage comparison of equipment grading of two standard laboratory items (K-systems bench versus Humidicrib), with alterations that happened over multiple years (A, B and C).

- A = K-systems workspace versus old version Humidicrib
- B = K-systems workspace versus new version Humidicrib (Emcell)
- C = K-systems workspace versus new version Humidicrib (Emcell) with service facility now unavailable

When comparing equipment, you have to set rules on how you will do the scoring. If testing against an existing piece of equipment, the new item can only have three options. It can only be:

- Better
- The same, or
- Worse than the existing equipment

So in this logic, only one score can increase for each item. For example, if an existing piece of equipment is poor at maintaining heat and the new equipment is tested to be better, then the new equipment will have the altered score and the existing equipment will be "the same". If you have existing equipment going down in score and the new equipment increasing in score for the same column heading, the differences will be unrealistically large.

In Table 7.3, the columns titled 'Lower-Risk Workflow' and 'Temp-pH Stability' cover embryo risk items, so actually carry double scoring points. Interestingly, whilst the Humidicrib systems are significantly better for temperature and pH stability for the embryos, the Humidicribs loose points because the embryo dish in use had to be passed through a quite small circular hole that has a membrane sleeve covering. This increases the risk of bumping the dish and moving the fluid and losing embryos, or actually dropping the dish. So whilst the embryos are better managed inside the chamber, there is a higher risk in moving items into and out of the chamber. This concept cannot be ignored.

When the chamber had a design alteration (see recording "A" to "B"), the chamber is now at different seating heights, has access to ergonomics, movable arm-holes, etc. This makes it more comfortable for staff to use, and they have less health issues (i.e. head, neck, shoulder pain), so the score changes and makes it a more preferable laboratory process to use.

Table 7.3 Risk scores for two standard equipment items, with alteration of that equipment over multiple years (A, B and C)

	Item being decided	1 = Yes, 2 = No Tested-validated	1 = Better; 3 = Same, 5 = Worse Lower risk workflow	1 = Better; 3 = Same, 5 = Worse Temp-pH stability	1 = Better; 3 = Same, 5 = Worse Overcomes known problems	1 = Better; 3 = Same, 5 = Worse Ergonomic	1 = Better; 3 = Same, 5 = Worse Service	Lowest is best Total
A	K systems workspace	1	3	3	2	2	2	13
	Closed Humidicrib-IVFCrib	1	5	1	1	3	2	13
B	K systems workspace	1	3	3	2	2	2	13
	Closed Humidicrib-Emcell	1	5	1	1	2	2	12
C	K systems workspace	1	3	3	2	2	3	14
	Closed Humidicrib-Emcell now	1	5	1	1	2	3	13

What is interesting to note though is that risk and acceptability of a product can change based on local conditions and experiences, and the laboratory has to be able to respond accordingly. Recording "C" in Table 7.3, shows the change in scores that happen as a country loses its factory backed service. Actually, both items in this comparison lost their manufacturer and factory-backed support so they both had an increase in score.

It must be remembered, that any score must be attributed by the laboratory using their own processes and testing of the equipment. A score from two separate labs in two separate countries cannot be compared. The location of the laboratory around the world will change the scores during these comparisons. An item that may rate very highly in equipment comparisons in Europe (because the manufacturer is in Europe) would rate very poorly in other regions. With laboratories based on the other side of the world, getting factory service and replacement for items that are made in Denmark and are in high use in Europe (i.e. K-Systems products), is almost impossible in Australia in 2015 when service, spare parts and distribution companies have stopped operating. Scientific Directors may wish to use different equipment, however if they are not available or able to have service, then that will ensure your choice of equipment may have to change.

Similarly, some laboratory equipment that is available one year may not be available next year, so new products and suppliers have to be located, tested, appraised, purchased and scored. The luxury of purchasing the same systems year after year, with the same degree of knowledge and factory backed service, is not available in some areas of the world.

This has a huge effect on new laboratories starting up, and the acceptance of this new equipment when improving existing laboratories with other manufacturer's products in use. This leads to different equipment now in operation inside the same laboratories, and some staff choosing "favourite" equipment to work on.

Other laboratory items can be assessed in this same manner before being chosen (but with different column headings for the scoring). Some starting suggestions could be:

Culture Incubators

- Is the temperature and pH stable?
- Does the incubator directly heat the dish surface?
- Which has the shortest time to regain desired temperature/pH after opening?
- Ability to run low oxygen gases?
- Holding capacity suitable?
- How much power is needed by your uninterruptable power supply (UPS) to run the incubators for a selected time if mains power is interrupted?
- What are the known pregnancy rates out of the incubators?
- Can alarms be triggered easily to test incubator monitoring response?
- Does the incubator have any user-operated diagnostic software to help in determining problems?
- Has the incubator been tested to be free of odours and volatile organic compounds (VOC's) etc?

Uninterruptable Power Supply

- Have you decided what length of time your UPS needs to operate?
- Have you ensured that the UPS+battery pack will last at least the entire night (i.e. 15–20 h), so staff never have to attend and perform culture tasks, if the lights are not working?
- Has this been tested, and proven in your hands?
- Can the battery pack be extended as your system grows?
- Is the battery pack so heavy that it needs relocation close to a weight bearing support pillar, if your laboratory is not on a ground floor?
- Does the system come with a speed charger to reduce charging time if UPS has been in use?
- Does the system have an alarm relay card so you receive alarms and activation signals if power is interrupted?
- Is there rapid service (i.e. 2 or 4 h technician response) that can be included in a service maintenance programme, etc?

Laboratory Equipment Monitoring Programmes and Software

- Will they cover multiple recording areas (i.e. fridge, freezers, liquid nitrogen vessels, incubators, stage warmers)?
- Is the software user-friendly?
- Will the software auto-graph items monthly or are graphs manually obtained?
- Is it easy to adjust the equipment alarm settings and levels?
- Can you easily change the people receiving the alarm and is it independent of a secondary monitoring system or company?
- Is there a global system for mobile networks or multipath equipment to allow signals to transmit to software if internet power is interrupted?
- Are the transmitters wireless or do they need Ethernet+power cables attached, and if so, is this a trip hazard in the laboratory, etc?

Identity Witnessing Systems (Human or Electronic)

- Does your system use two humans, or human+electronic witnessing?
- In a "2-human" system, do you check identity by reading aloud, silently, or together or independently?
- Does the system incorporate identity detection for frozen samples as well as fresh culture samples?
- Does the system allow samples belonging to more than one patient to be brought into a work area without an alarm automatically sounding?
- Does the system require the detection device to be picked up/brought over to the sample, or the sample to be specifically brought to the detection device, or does it automatically register the presence of a sample/tag?
- Does the system track where the sample is inside a defined workflow process?
- Can the software provide lists/views on uncompleted processes for busy labs to follow?
- Can the software be easily altered to follow changes to your work flow process?
- Can the software provide specific mismatch data for tasks, frequency numbers, and operator staff at the time of mismatch in an easily obtainable manner, etc?

Dealing with Laboratory Risk

Human Factors Risk

Since 1980, aeroplane pilots have been exposed to training procedures for use in high-risk environments where human error can have devastating effects. This was called "crew resource management" [9]. More recently the name of this training system has been accepted as the more general "human factors" training. The term "human factors" refers to the wide range of issues affecting how people perform tasks in their work environments. The study of human factors involves applying scientific knowledge about the human mind, to better understand human capabilities and limitations so that there is the best possible fit between people and the systems in which they operate. Human factors are the social and personal skills (i.e. communication and decision making) that complement technical skills, and can be used to reduce the likelihood of errors and at the same time build a more error resistant, and therefore more resilient, system [10].

The system was initially designed for air-crew training, to ensure all crew are empowered to help the overall running and safety of the plane and to eliminate autocracy. This process also can help medical and laboratory staff communicate and not accept error.

Helmreich and Merritt [11], stated that the causes of human error include:

- Fatigue
- Workload
- Limitations of human cognitive processes
- Poor interpersonal communications
- Flawed decision making processes
- Leadership problems, and
- Team work issues

As such, it is perfectly sensible to follow human factors communication processes and techniques in medical laboratories. Especially in human embryo culture laboratories where almost all techniques involving embryos, genetics and patient identities are performed by humans, and patients face huge emotional burdens in the event of an error. Staff must be empowered with freedom of comment and the ability to "stop processes" and to notice errors, and to intervene, to ensure safety and overcome poor techniques.

In medical laboratories, staff training historically centres around technical or scientific tasks, and not around risk averse training methodologies and interpersonal communication strategies. Whilst basic laboratory training obviously still needs to occur, laboratory management is gradually changing, as laboratories concentrate on minimising the potential for the huge patient risks that can be involved if mistakes are made.

For example, "human factors" systems can take as few as two simple steps, such as:

1. *Team briefings*: These will occur with the staff that are about to perform a laboratory task, and the briefing lasts no more than 30–90 s. Cover the processes that are

about to be performed, who is doing it, any problems anticipated. Anyone can talk or add details that are relevant. Always end with "are there any questions?" so you are testing and receiving feedback that they understand the task they are being briefed about. The aim is for everyone to have the same knowledge of what everyone is doing, and who can help if needed.

2. *Team debriefings*: These occur after the task has been completed. Aim is to discuss any unusual events and whether the outcomes are consistent with what was expected in the briefing. In IVF laboratories, this can also act as a QC measure to recognise if fertilisation, cleavage or blastulation is unusually low. Team members can discuss what went well or went poorly, what needs to be improved and the best way forward, and if any extra equipment could help. These do not have to take a long time, and can focus on discussion of technical and process events.

The presence of the briefings and debriefings for each task being performed, and done by the group actually performing that specific task, creates situational awareness where all in the laboratory understand what is happening and can anticipate what should happen next. It also means the Laboratory Manager/Supervisor is not the only person thinking and processing information. The whole team is now empowered and involved in the laboratory's direction, and any unusual events are immediately processed by all in the group. This situational awareness has been shown to encourage staff to speak up if something is not happening correctly. It is important when a laboratory task is being performed, that staff prioritise the task, and do not let disruptions or distractions force them to lose situational awareness.

In 2015, there are courses available modelled upon human factors training that have been aimed mostly at nursing systems and operating theatre teams to improve communication. Whilst these are not yet structured towards medical laboratory systems, the content format is simple and relevant in a laboratory setting.

Laboratory Design and Reducing Risk

Modern low-risk laboratory management also covers items such as laboratory design, construction, reduction of walking with culture dishes and ergonomics for staff.

Local standards, such as *AS/NZS 2982:2010, Laboratory design and construction* [12] give good guidance on some important laboratory design criteria. For example, they give relevant information on floor types, bench heights and ergonomics, safe distances between work stations and passage ways when staff are working or where corridors are located, laboratory lighting, basic ventilation, hazardous storage, and even details for biological/plant/radioactive and secondary school laboratories. However, there is nothing that is specifically designed on how to build a modern, efficient, safe, clean and functional human culture laboratory.

A suite of international standards such as *ISO 14644 Cleanrooms and associated controlled environments* [13], give fantastic technical and mechanical requirements on how to build laboratories to specific air cleanliness standards, and are a wonderful suite of standards to ensure the build, compliance, testing and validation of high-end clean air laboratories meet international criteria. These can be linked to other local documents [3], but by themselves, each document is helpful as a guide during the design of IVF laboratories.

Generally, IVF laboratories have physical needs on air-flow direction and speeds, and cooling drafts near some incubator models or warm benches or ICSI equipment, and certain practicalities such as patients entering rooms where embryo transfer will occur. These types of physical items are easily combined with international standards, and modern laboratory equipment and testing to ensure that the laboratory is both functional, practical and meets elective air quality levels that are far higher than standard laboratories.

However, IVF laboratory design also needs to overcome specific laboratory work logistics that are outside the scope of normal laboratory design standards, such as:

- Suitable distance between workstations and incubators (to reduce embryo dish cooling when being carried, and maximum distances for carriage to eliminate staff tripping-bumping or dish dropping).
- There is also the important inclusion of the actual planned work-flow that incorporates the physical size of the laboratory, how many cycles the laboratory will be expected to perform (as a maximum planned cycle throughput over time), how many staff are inside the laboratory, and sensible access to equipment.
- Access to items in storage, and liquid nitrogen rooms.
- Access to embryo transfer rooms and how to carry embryos from laboratory to transfer room.
- Security monitoring, and best practice for securing laboratories, and frozen embryo storage areas.
- Location of alarm panels and monitoring of incubators and location and type of UPS system (and size of battery pack to provide a defined length of power), etc.

Unfortunately, these logistical needs are normally only obtained by experience, and having had the ability to design and build many laboratories. If your unit does not have this depth of internal knowledge in laboratory design-build, then it is always well worth the money to travel to some colleague's facilities, and view their laboratory logistics, and ask what works well or poorly in each design you see.

By amalgamating multiple standards, local regulatory requirements and logistical knowledge of how equipment functions a good laboratory system can be designed and built to your specifications, however, thought is needed on how to minimise risk in laboratories that are already built. Existing laboratories experiencing cycle growth cannot always find extra space for workstations and staff, so items with elevated risk are incorporated and must be managed. This may require a change in workstation type-size, and a retraining exercise to ensure this changeover in workstations does not affect outcome.

Some examples of controlling risk in existing laboratories may be:

Minimising walking distances and staff movements in small areas: To overcome human error and bumping/dropping culture dishes, some laboratories have actively redesigned their laboratories to reduce dish movement distances that could lead to staff tripping/bumping/dropping of embryo dishes. Some examples of this are self-sufficient work pods containing culture incubators, heated workbenches and microinjection

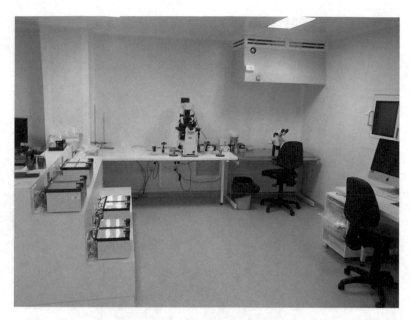

Fig. 7.1 Work-pod in an ISO14644 compliant clean room. Culture Incubators, ICSI microscope, Biopsy laser, Dissecting microscope, and K-Systems workbench are all located together for minimal dish and staff movement. Five work pods like this exist in a laboratory performing over 1800 fresh cycles (photo courtesy of IVFAustralia)

equipment (Figs. 7.1 and 7.2). These can be laid out in a right-angle so items are at a 90° turn, or at a 180° turn to eliminate the possibility of staff walking behind you (Fig. 7.3).

Placing culture incubators away from staff movement areas: In laboratories, there will always be staff and Doctor movement. One of the design challenges in different shaped buildings is to ensure that any laboratory access path between different rooms or locations happens away from where culture incubators are accessed. This can be from a dedicated movement channel on the opposite side of the culture incubators (Fig. 7.4), or can be merged with some of the criteria mentioned in Fig. 7.1, if the room dimensions are such that the self-contained work areas can have culture incubators right next to the workstation.

Choosing smaller workstations: Depending on the shape of some laboratory areas and the size of some laboratories, best use of space to minimise risk of having only one workspace, can occur by selecting different size workstations. There can be quite significant differences in the required space for two workstations, so selecting a narrower workstation may allow you to have two or even three workstations in the same space (Figs. 7.5 and 7.6), and increase your productivity whilst improving culture conditions or safety.

Liquid nitrogen tanks in the same room as staff: It is always preferable to place liquid nitrogen storage tanks for gametes/embryos in a separate room away from staff, however in some laboratories the lack of space means it is difficult for this to occur, and tanks are often located under work benches in the laboratory. If you are

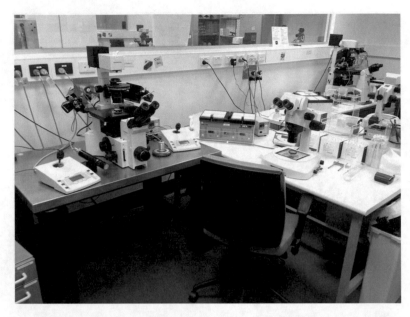

Fig. 7.2 Work-pod in a standard air laboratory. Bench-top incubator to use at work-pod, ICSI microscope and Dissecting microscope workbench, all located together for minimal dish and staff movement (photo courtesy of Melbourne IVF)

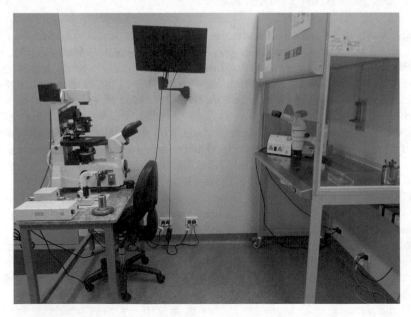

Fig. 7.3 Single person work area in a standard air laboratory, incorporating an ICSI microscope, a Dissecting microscope, and K-Systems workbench all located close together, to eliminate staff movement behind you (photo courtesy of IVFAustralia)

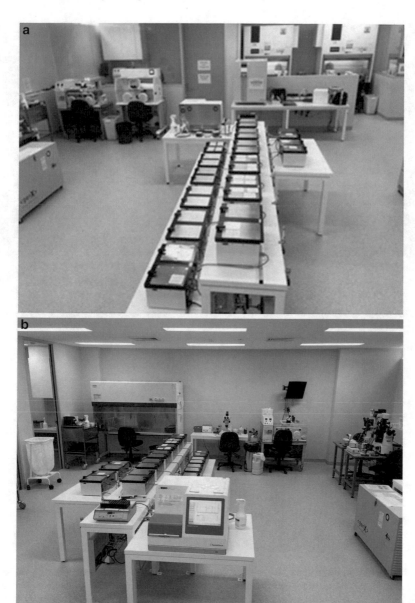

Fig. 7.4 (**a**, **b**) Incubators face towards an internal culture access system (incubators, worksta-tions, ICSI areas). Staff access for areas not involved with embryo culture (i.e. embryo transfer rooms, culture media preparation areas, media equilibration incubators, fridges, and sperm prepa-ration areas), happens on the other side of the incubator bench (photo courtesy of IVFAustralia)

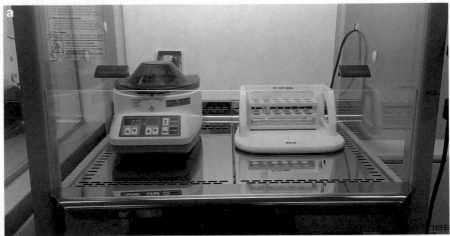

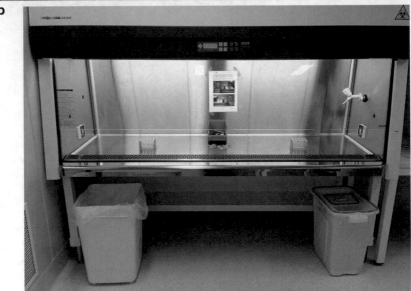

Fig. 7.5 (**a**, **b**) Relative width of two different sperm preparation workstations. Selecting narrower workstations, can allow more work areas in the same size laboratory. A 2 ft wide Class II cabinet (*top*) enclosed with centrifuge and tube rack, and a 6 ft wide Class II cabinet (*bottom*) without centrifuges. Whilst the 6 ft cabinet, is three times the size, it does not hold three times the workspace in a safe, well-separated manner (photos courtesy of The Fertility Centre and IVFAustralia)

trying to overcome historical room usage systems, and wish to separate storage tanks from staff, if the room is available there is no reason why a separate locked room can't be used that is external to the laboratory, or even in a separate part of the facility. Risk control can involve methods of moving selected frozen material to-from the storage room, and the new room can be fitted with appropriate hard-wired oxygen monitoring

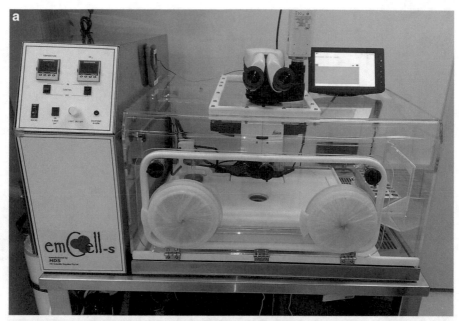

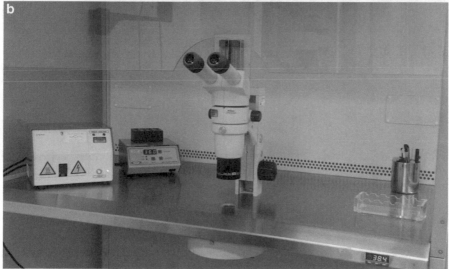

Fig. 7.6 (**a**, **b**) Relative width of two different workstations. Selecting narrower workstations, can allow more work areas in the same size laboratory. The enclosed crib workstation is narrower than the open K-system workbench (photos courtesy of The Fertility Centre and IVFAustralia)

and exit breathers for staff in the laboratory. As the storage tanks are now outside of the view of staff, effective external monitoring of the integrity of the tanks linked to external warning systems (Fig. 7.7) can be used to ensure staff always know (a) the integrity of the tanks before entering a room or whilst a room is in use, and (b) the maximum temperature of the internal environment of the tank.

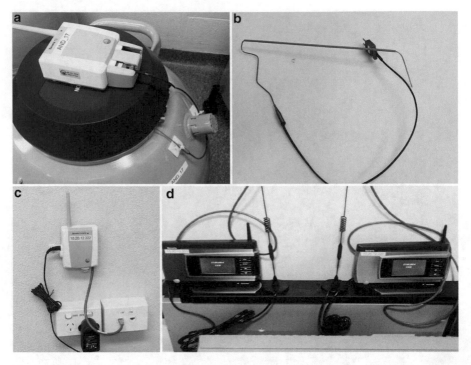

Fig. 7.7 (**a–d**) TESTO Saveris Liquid Nitrogen Tank Monitoring, for constant monitoring of tank contents and temperature (photo courtesy of IVFAustralia)

Sample Witnessing Risk

When practising low-risk laboratory management, a "zero tolerance" approach to dish identity needs to be adopted. This means having robust, enforced, strict rules ensuring all changes of dishes-tubes-vessels are always double witnessed by a second person (or electronics) BEFORE the items are moved. This also means understanding that there are no processes where failing to double witness is acceptable.

This must happen regardless of how busy the laboratory is, the time of the day, or the day of the week, every time, no excuses. If you cannot prove something is double-witnessed, then it hasn't occurred.

Now that takes time, effort and acceptance, however there is no point following all the other low-risk systems in this chapter, and allowing identity checking to be a high-risk area where mistakes can happen.

Ensuring the genetic integrity of patient's gametes and embryos is the constant risk that all human culture laboratories have to face. Whilst it is accepted that witnessing is important, it is disturbing that there is no universally accepted process or methodology to follow for accreditation in many countries around the world.

Some accreditation codes-of-practice state standard wording such as:

- "Centres must have in place robust and effective processes to ensure that no mismatches of gametes or identification errors occur" [3] or
- "Provide evidence of: "policies/procedures to identify when, how and by whom the identification, matching, and verification are recorded for gametes, embryos and patients at all stages of the treatment process" [1]

Both the HFEA and RTAC also provide excellent documents that state exactly what has to happen at each stage of culture to ensure identity is known [14, 15].

Despite the RTAC Technical Bulletin 4 [15] stating everything required for double witnessing, and being approved by the RTAC of Australia, this fantastic identification document (that was researched, written and negotiated by active members of Australian IVF laboratories, not by a government department), has been deemed as "non-enforceable". This means that as at 2015, Australia has no requirement for double-witnessing and as such, no active, accurate, reproducible or national method required by accreditation to reduce identity risk. This is a disturbing state of affairs.

Other countries such as Singapore, have followed in the HFEA's footsteps by enforcing identity stages, exactly what must happen, and have also enforced it by writing it into their Licensing Terms and Conditions [16].

And therein lies the problem. In many countries, there are:

- Differing methods of performing checks
- No requirements in some countries to perform them in a standardised manner
- No controls over how manual identity checks are actually performed, and
- No directives to stop clinics choosing which witnessing stages or events they want to follow

Some countries have allowed a system to develop where the licencing process only enforces minimal identity witnessing, and does not enforce a robust, widespread and consistent identity witnessing and proof methodology across all clinics.

The major items for a low-risk laboratory management process to review in regard to sample identity are:

1. Is double witnessing of all stages and vessel changes mandated before the sample is moved, and what is your second witnesser (manual or electronic or video-camera, etc.)?
2. What methodology do you use for human double-witnessing, and if two staff are used, how do they interact to ensure the sample is correct?
3. How are you reducing the possibility of involuntary-automaticity (i.e. when something is incorrect, but since the staff member is expecting the item to be correct, they do not actually recognise that the identity name or ID number is incorrect)?
4. How are you recording this double witnessing has happened? Without a permanent record, there is no proof it has happened.
5. Can you use other methods of broadcasting an image to a second human that may not be in the laboratory?
6. Do you allow any deviations in your witnessing system, or is the process the same on a weekday and weekend?
7. What do you do when the double-witnesser (human or machine) fails?

8. What is the error rate of a human based system, and are all "near-misses" accurately recorded currently?
9. What is the cost of various witnessing systems, and are witnessing systems scalable for bigger or smaller laboratories?

If we accept in this chapter that low-risk laboratory management ensures that all vessel changes at every stage are double witnessed, then a comparison table (Table 7.4) shows how some of the risk areas can be overcome using different methods or technology.

Liquid Nitrogen Frozen Sample Storage Risk

All established IVF laboratories or andrology laboratories have large stocks of frozen gametes and embryos, and most clinics store these samples onsite.

The cumulative replacement value of frozen material inside each storage tank is substantial, and this can be multiplied by the number of tanks in the system. It is fair to assume that apart from severe events (i.e. fire, earthquake, criminal activity, etc.) it is unlikely that multiple tanks will fail at any given time. It is controlling the remote risk of a tank failure that is important in low-risk laboratory management, and ensuring at any given time, you know what temperature the contents of the liquid nitrogen tank are at. Lots of laboratories will record their culture media refrigerator temperature, but not their liquid nitrogen storage tanks. One has minimal risk and one has huge risk.

Historical liquid nitrogen monitoring has comprised of daily or even twice weekly monitoring of storage tanks by means of measuring liquid nitrogen depth in a tank (and comparing to what it should be reading), or even viewing the external surface of a liquid nitrogen storage tank for any water or condensation. Whilst these checks can be suitable, they do not provide long term or even 24 h monitoring, and there is every chance that a tank can fail in between the times tanks are viewed, or most likely in the vast bulk of the day-night when staff are not present.

In 2015, with staff owning smart phones, tablets and laptops; electronic monitoring offers a far better method of managing the risk involved with liquid nitrogen storage. Electronic monitoring will give 24 h a day, 7 days a week monitoring.

Tanks that store samples using vapour freezing are often attached to large feeder fluid tanks, and they usually have inbuilt volume sensing and are hard wired to power points to provide the power to drive the sensor. If a main vacuum jacket fails, or the feeder tank is empty, the storage tank is still monitored.

However, most of the storage tanks sold worldwide are in the 35–50 litre size range, containing liquid nitrogen (not vapour), and most of these tanks do not have any depth or temperature monitoring systems. By their size and nature (i.e. mostly on roller base frames) they are designed to be moved, and there are many stored in a single location, so hard wired electricity and data sockets are not all that efficient.

Table 7.4 Major risk items to consider from a laboratory management pathway (split by the method of double witnessing)

Method of witnessing?	Scientist + second responsible person	Scientist + electronic image broadcast method	Scientist + electronic witnessing
What days of the week?	All days should be viewed the same. Weekends are no different to weekdays, and witnessing must occur in the same manner.		
How is witnessing performed?	• Second person does not always have to be a trained laboratory staff member • Make use for administration, nursing or specifically trained laboratory technician staff	• Internet camera • Use of telephones with FaceTime, voice and/or image capture for attachment to practice software • Second person can be providing the service to multiple small laboratories	• RFID systems • Bar Coding systems
What stages are witnessed	Labs should resist trying to determine what are "high risk" processes and then only trying to double witness those. Take the holistic approach, and enforce mandatory double witnessing, on all vessel changes, at all times, including loading into freeze straws/vessels.		
What is the witnessing methodology of the second person or electronics?	Which method covers the risk appropriately: • Both people reading ID silently? • One reading ID aloud, one listening/watching? • Two people reading ID, but at different times, after process has occurred? • Two people reading ID aloud and together? • Who signs laboratory worksheet or do both sign? • If images are broadcast, whose job is it to ensure all the electronics/images/videos/SMS are entered into the patient's records?		• Is the workspace active? • Will it immediately identify any tagged/barcoded vessel entered into the workspace? • Does the staff member have to lift a receiver or take a vessel to a reader to activate the system? • Can it be bypassed by staff making an error? • Will the software record the exact exposure time an item is in the workspace, or is it just a single recording? • Will the software recognise another patient's material if it enters the workspace after the first witnessing check?
Procedure on detection of error?	• Does the laboratory have a clear policy on immediate ceasing of the process, and detection of the cause of error? • If using an electronic system, are there predetermined codes to identify the type of error to type into software? • Does the laboratory have a guaranteed "authority to stop" so all staff (regardless of seniority) are encouraged to voice a concern if sample identity is involved?		

Several companies (TESTO, Planer, LabGuard, Comark) have developed monitoring systems to enable simple, long-life, discrete, wireless monitoring of these liquid nitrogen tanks. These systems each have their strengths and weaknesses, and as we have mentioned earlier in this chapter, sometimes there is no factory support for some of these systems in various parts of the world, so risk assessing the equipment is very important.

It is always an interesting risk assessment exercise when dealing with a tank loss event that may only be as rare as a 1:20 year event, however the contents of each tank may be irreplaceable, and the terrible job of having to contact each patient involved in a tank that was lost, should make it an easy risk minimisation decision to instigate.

There are two main methods for monitoring these ubiquitous small 35–50 litre tanks electronically:

(a) To determine the depth of the liquid nitrogen, or
(b) To determine the internal temperature of the tank

Monitoring the depth of liquid nitrogen often requires a probe that draws a large current, so batteries in wireless transmitters do not have a long life. Often these depth alarms are hardwired, meaning there are cables all over the tanks and into side-walls of laboratories. The benefit of this system though, is that you can set a depth of liquid nitrogen that the system will alarm at. Monitoring the temperature at a defined area of the tank is the other method, and the probe is normally placed under the inside of the tank neck. The temperature that the alarm should be set at is important because if liquid nitrogen level drops there will still be liquid and vapour phase above the liquid inside the tank which keeps the tank cold, until the liquid level drops quite low and the temperature rises.

There are benefits for each recording method, so this will form part of your laboratory equipment risk assessment, which could include the frequency of the temperature recording, the method of alarm notification, how user-friendly the software is, whether the system allows internet capability to link multiple laboratories together, will it use a multipath alarm system (i.e. Ethernet and SMS capability), and how robust the system is. One wireless monitoring system is shown in Fig. 7.7.

Either way you look at it, if a patient has gametes or embryos inside a tank that is failing, the two questions they will ask are:

• "What temperature did the tank get to?" and
• "Did my embryos thaw out accidentally?"

You can only answer those questions with a temperature probe placed inside the tank and with a constant electronic monitoring system and software.

As part of low-risk laboratory management, a good process is to take your oldest tank (remove the gametes and embryos and place into a new tank), and now damage this old, empty tank so it fails and log the internal temperature and video the process. This gives fantastic information, and an understanding of how much any external tank condensation is related to humidity and what you can expect in your area of the world, determining where sensors should be placed, and whether it is worth recording the outside temperature of the tank. Only then can you see what you need to record and how you need to act, and the time you have to react.

In one tank destruction test I have done in Sydney, there was no external tank condensation for over 2 h and the tank lost 10 cm of liquid nitrogen depth per hour. However, a different tank with a different failure cause also had no external condensation, but took 10 h to warm up from the normal liquid nitrogen temperature to −50 °C. This information is crucial to helping you choose which system is best for your needs, setting your alarm points, setting your monitoring alarm pathway, working out how many people need to receive the alarm, and working out your safety process to enter a room that may have higher levels of atmospheric nitrogen than normal, and what to do if the oxygen alarm is also sounding when you arrive at the laboratory.

Having electronic monitoring of all tanks is surprisingly cheap, and really is a requirement for modern low-risk laboratory management.

Embryo Culture and the Benefits of Low Risk Strategies

Whilst it is not in the scope of this chapter to discuss all the mechanisms of human embryo culture, there are some very simple items where data analysis has shown to be helpful to remove or adjust standard laboratory processes. More importantly, they tie in nicely with some low-risk laboratory management processes covered in this chapter. They show how simple low-risk processes can be extended into a human culture lab, with beneficial results.

We shall look at just a few of these laboratory processes, as an indication that by just changing one item during a period can result in eliminating a sub-standard culture practice, showing that prospective laboratory management decisions, staff believing in the change and performing it, and subsequent data analysis can provide positive outcomes.

Reducing Incubator Openings

One aim of laboratory management is to have enough incubators to ensure culture conditions are not affected by having to continually open the incubators, and disrupt the culture environment.

Data shown in Fig. 7.8a is obtained from bench-top incubators (MINC, COOK, Australia), and shows that there can be a large variation in incubator openings, based on their location to workstations and position on the bench. Figure 7.8b then uses the number of incubator openings as the X-Axis, and implies that there is also a large increase in ongoing pregnancy rate from a 40 % average in the incubators opened >8 times/day, to a 60 % average for the patients cultured in the incubators that are opened less frequently (5–8 times/day).

Laboratories can use simple experiments such as this to plan on the number of incubators needed. As part of low risk management, they can plan on not opening an incubator more than five times a day, and then determine how many incubators

a

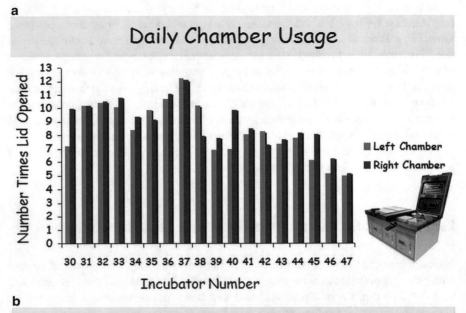

b

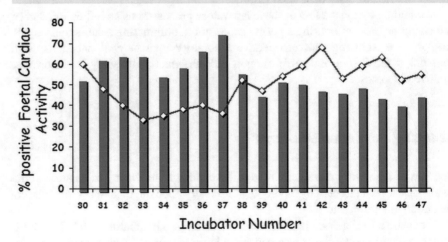

Fig. 7.8 (**a, b**) With a reduced number of incubator openings, the embryo culture conditions are kept constant, and patients have a higher ongoing pregnancy rate, expressed as percent positive Foetal Cardiac Activity (unpublished data courtesy of Dr Matthew VerMilyea)

are needed to be purchased to process the patients in the laboratory. The purchase price of incubators is a very small cost over the 7–10 year life of the incubator, and having risk-associated logic to determine the number of incubators for a laboratory, is a positive management process.

Be Clear on Reasons for Touching Gametes or Embryos

As we have covered earlier in this chapter, there is a risk associated with every time you move or view embryos.

It can be a risk of dropping the dish, cooling the dish, changing the pH or, if you change the dish type or the culture media, it comes with a potential identity mistake risk that you have to cover.

For this reason, managers wanting to run low-risk laboratories need to set rules and clear boundaries on the reasons they have for moving gametes or embryos, and be clear in their interpretation in laboratory policies and documents.

A good start is to ensure:

- Every movement of a gamete or embryo is completely necessary, and can't be overcome. Many separate stages (e.g. media holding dishes used on certain days of culture, etc.) can immediately be eliminated, along with the risks mentioned above.
- Every movement of embryos is associated with a solid scientific reason. For example, why would a blastocyst unit need to assess an embryo on Day 2 or Day 4? There is no need to remove an embryo from an incubator just to check that it is a 4-cell or a morula, when that information is rarely used in selecting a blastocyst on Day 5.
- Can all movements and assessment of embryos be limited only to the stages when you may already be handling the embryos to change culture media formulations? You may also assess whether there is any need to use stage-specific media as they require a Day 3 media handling process that could be eliminated.

Keep the culture system as simple as possible, and try and perform minimal handling. If handling has to happen, move the contents as small a distance as possible and use temperature and pH supporting equipment, as you would have already purchased this laboratory equipment to reduce risk, as explained earlier in this chapter.

Leave Embryos Alone and Reduce Heating of Media

One experiment performed was to ensure we were reducing unnecessary handling of embryos grown to blastocyst stage (i.e. eliminating the grading of embryos on Day 2 and Day 4), and then ensuring that we were using media that had a maximum equilibration time of 48 h. This was in an attempt to reduce breakdown of media ingredients to ammonium that can happen under prolonged heating. Many units may equilibrate their blastocyst media dishes from the afternoon of Day 2. Whilst the embryos may only be in the dish for 48 h, the media exposure to heat has now been 48 h + equilibration time that may be another 18 h = 66 h.

Table 7.5 Data from two laboratory process changes determined by setting low-risk laboratory strategies (unpublished data courtesy of IVFAustralia)

All patient ages, Day 5 culture	Before changes (2011)	After changes (2012)	Significance
Blastulation rate (%)	48 %	53 %	$X^2 = 17, P < 0.0001$
	5 % more blastulation on almost 20,000 fertilised oocytes		
Extra blastocysts grown		990	
Utilisation rate (%)	35 %	46 %	$X^2 > 100, P < 0.0001$
Extra vitrified blastocysts		450	

If pre-gassed culture oil is used as an overlay, then small 20 or 50 µl droplets of culture media stabilise their pH extremely rapidly, so dishes can be easily prepared on the day of use, and can be used after an hour.

Whilst there are two linked items in the data expressed in Table 7.5 (i.e. reducing exposure of culture media to heat, and, leaving the embryos alone on Day 2 and Day 4), together they have a very positive benefit, and they are both low-risk laboratory management principles that fit nicely with this chapter.

Service, Maintenance and Fit-for-Purpose Testing

Frequency of Laboratory Quality Control

Laboratory QC can be one area that it is very difficult to get sensible and helpful service frequencies to follow for IVF laboratories.

Whilst an international quality standard such as ISO9001 will say that you have to perform periodic QC on laboratory equipment, there is no definition on the frequency and content of what "periodic" means. Standards that are used in diagnostic pathology laboratories (such as ISO15189) that involve technical competence assessment also have no definitions on frequency of QC.

As a result, international bodies such as the World Health Organisation or National Association of Testing Authorities (NATA) have come up with Maintenance Manuals [17] or a General Equipment Calibration and Checks document [18] to instruct the laboratory on the expected frequency for some common equipment checks.

These manuals and documents may be perfect for diagnostic pathology laboratories, however an IVF laboratory has a lot of equipment that is not covered by these basic pathology maintenance frequencies.

As part of laboratory management systems, it is very helpful for the Laboratory Director to take the best of all existing systems as your start point. For standard laboratory equipment (i.e: centrifuges, fridges-freezers, pipettes, biological safety cabinets, balances, microscopes, etc.) follow documented QC frequencies for pathology laboratories. A fantastic and thorough document to start with, is the simple equipment list such as the NATA General Equipment Calibration and Checks document [18]. You can never do "too much" QC, and meeting a pre-existing standard requirement is always the best process.

With that as your background level of QC for simple equipment, the specialist laboratory items that are not covered by these existing documents (i.e. culture incubators, gas manifold systems, UPS systems, incubator gas monitoring systems, gas alarm sensors), will require a risk analysis or knowledge of manufacturer's recommendations, that will result in a defined service and calibration frequency for all equipment in the laboratory.

Whilst service and calibration are QC items to consider, the laboratory also needs to ensure that items are working correctly each day of use, BEFORE they are used for culture. In an IVF laboratory, it is not acceptable to leave a warmed surface for 6 months without validation by the user. So this then brings a new terminology into the laboratory operations of "fit-for-purpose" testing. All your work surfaces and tube warmers used each day are then tested before use to ensure the temperature is correct prior to use that day are added.

As an example, a full equipment QC schedule for a standard IVF laboratory may take the appearance of Table 7.6.

Methodology of Laboratory Quality Control

Once the laboratory has determined the equipment to check/service/calibrate, and the frequency of these actions, they now need to determine the methodology that also explains any mathematics used to eliminate error and increase accuracy. Again, it is always sensible to use existing proven methodology wherever possible. Some existing documents [17] or published Technical Bulletins/Technical Notes [19] are easy to locate, have covered the errors, and are often endorsed by the national measurement institutes of their country.

This will then only leave specialist equipment that is serviced by external service providers and these service frequencies will be guided by national standards (i.e. for gas manifolds or sensors), or internal electrical requirements (i.e. UPS systems), and the lab will have minimal need to understand the methodology for these externally provided services.

Whilst the laboratory doesn't need to know exactly how the electrics are serviced, they can request different service frequencies and increase the service aims performed. For example, whilst a yearly inspection is all that is required on a UPS, your risk assessment may determine that since your UPS system will power your incubators which are critical equipment to you, then you may decide that a 6-monthly service is better risk management. You may also decide that the UPS battery life needs to be calculated before the service starts, using the incubators that are currently running on the UPS. This will ensure at each service the exact UPS battery life is known, and is written on the report the provider gives you.

Table 7.6 QC checks performed on IVF laboratory equipment

Item	QC frequency	Who performs
User check calibration and fit-for-purpose testing		
Viewing of all electronic temperature-probe systems	Daily	Staff in-house
Recording of temperature	Daily	Staff in-house
Daily fit-for-purpose test of all warmed surfaces using calibrated thermometer + thermocouple	Daily	Staff in-house
Liquid nitrogen depth checking of all tanks	Daily to fortnightly	Staff in-house
Replace-refill humidity water in incubators	Weekly to monthly	Staff in-house
Replace any humidity flasks in incubators	Monthly to 3 monthly	Staff in-house
Culture incubator back-to-base alarm circuit test	Monthly	Staff in-house
Oxygen and CO_2 alarm sensor activation check	Monthly	Staff in-house
Balance single point check	Monthly	Staff in-house
Balance repeatability check	3 monthly	Staff in-house
Displacement pipettes	3 monthly	Staff in-house
Timer check (against accurate national clock)	6 monthly	Staff in-house
Warmed surface or thermometer calibration (against calibrated thermometer + thermocouple)	6 monthly	Staff in-house
Gas analysers for testing Incubator CO_2-O_2 % (tested against known gas concentrations)	6 monthly	Staff in-house
Planned calibration by external service providers		
Air conditioning and filters checked-cleaned	3 monthly	External
Gas manifolds supplying gas to incubators	6 monthly	External
Servicing-testing of all O_2 and CO_2 alarm sensors	6 monthly	External
Structure integrity check for any large LN2 tanks (i.e. >100 l)	6 monthly	External
UPS load testing and battery testing (see if it meets designed run time with current load)	6 monthly	External
Embryo slow-freeze machinery with any moving solenoids	6 monthly	External
Calibration of culture incubators	Yearly	External
Calibration of balance	Yearly	External
Calibration of centrifuge speeds	Yearly	External
Professional clean of operating microscopes	Yearly	External
Laminar and Class II cabinets tested	Yearly	External
Filters + UV lights on VOC removing fans	Yearly	External
Recertification by a certified reference lab of the calibrated thermometer + thermocouple	Yearly	External
Testing as needed when fails user-check calibration		
Pipettes	When fail	External
Warmed surfaces	When fail	External
Analysis machinery (Gas analysers, VOC testing machines, particle counters, etc.)	When fail	External

This covers the frequency of check and who should perform it

The Work Instruction/SOP or Policy that dictates how this is to be done in the laboratory (or which external company performs the QC), could be added as a final column

Recording and Documenting Laboratory Quality Control

If there is no worksheet or report, assume that there is no proof that you have performed the test/check/calibration or service.

With QC that is performed by your laboratory staff in-house, ensure that your worksheets or calibration reports have clear acceptance or pass/fail levels documented on them, and any temperature offsets that need to be applied to thermometer values before they are recorded on your daily worksheets. There is no point checking something unless all staff are actually aware at what stage the equipment is out of range or needs recalibration, factory servicing or indeed discard and replacement.

For the services/calibrations performed by external service providers, ensure that you choose a provider wherever possible, that carries national certification of a testing authority. In many areas of the world, they will be accredited to the international standard ISO17025, which is your safety to ensure they are testing according to a set process or standard, and they also get assessed on their methodology and processes.

Staff are human, and can miss or ignore certain calibration tolerances during equipment checks. Staff can also suffer from involuntary automaticity that we discussed earlier in the identity witnessing section. By this, I mean that if they are expecting that equipment will pass the service/check, then sometimes they fail to notice obvious data that displays the equipment has actually failed its testing. For this reason, having a second person review and countersign QC that is performed on equipment that has acceptance or pass/fail levels, is a good low-risk laboratory management process. It helps overcome simple human error, and can remove equipment from service before any problems are allocated to that equipment.

If this countersigning person is also the Lab Supervisor, or even a specifically tasked Senior Scientist, it then makes the Laboratory Management aware of the strengths and weaknesses of equipment that is in service at any given time. It also shows that there is good management control of the laboratory.

Reducing Laboratory Risk Using Laboratory Performance Measures

All the items we have covered in this chapter cover safe design, safe ergonomic equipment, safe staffing, safe identity checking, safe embryo management and safe QC to follow. However having a safe lab WITH a high pregnancy rate is the ultimate outcome.

Having data that is easily accessible, obtained as agreed, graphed to visually highlight problems, performed regularly, and involves more than one person in the management pathway, is one of the most important aspects of being able to manage a laboratory (or a series of laboratories) in a low-risk manner.

This takes three interlinked stages:

1. Determining which Laboratory Performance Measure (LPM) markers you want to collect, and the frequency of this data collection
2. Having warning levels known and graphed for each LPM, including pregnancy outcome
3. Having a defined action plan process to follow when a defined number of lab results fall below the warning levels

If data is not known, then the laboratory is not a controlled environment, problems will arise without anyone being aware of the warning signs, and the Laboratory Management will then become reactive, instead of proactive. Having an uncontrolled system is high-risk management (not low-risk management).

What is a "Laboratory Performance Measure"?

A LPM is a defined data set that has been determined to help you manage the laboratory. The terminology can be similar to Key Performance Indicators (KPI's), however KPI's are sometimes linked to financial decisions (i.e. numbers of cycles or tests performed, number of patients treated, profit per cycle, etc.).

A LPM is a pure data expression of what is happening inside the laboratory, so it is nice to use the acronym LPM, to keep the laboratory terminology clear, and separate from financial or business indicators.

LPM's are designed to show an expected development stage or output. They are designed to be different to yearly laboratory data (i.e. total pregnancy rates, breakdowns for IVF or ICSI). These are specific data on a defined group of patients that cover certain boundaries and are normally collected regularly, on a specific group of patients to eliminate data errors caused by patients that may be expected to have different parameters.

For example, they cover different LPM categories:

(a) Quality markers on entry to the laboratory

- Such as: Oocyte maturity, oocyte morphology, average egg numbers

(b) Gross toxicity markers

- Such as: 2PN cleavage rates

(c) Culture quality markers

- Such as: Blastulation rate, utilisation rate, percentage of embryos at a defined grade, survival rate of thawed embryos

(d) Technical markers

- Such as: Fertilisation rate, ICSI necrosis rate

(e) Success markers

  • Such as: Pregnancy rate, pregnancy rate per embryo transferred

So, using this LPM logic, a laboratory may choose a selection of data that covers the processes in that laboratory. For example, they could select five that cover a range of activities, such as:

• Oocyte maturity
• Cleavage rate
• Blastulation rate
• Embryo thaw survival rate, and a very sensitive marker such as
• Pregnancy rate per embryo transferred

If you have multiple laboratories, comparing these LPM's against each laboratory over the same period is called benchmarking.

What are the "Achievement Level" the "Warning Level" and the "Action Level"?

Now that laboratories have selected the type of LPM's they want to measure, they have to now decide what the Achievement Level is that they want their laboratory to maintain.

This can come from existing data from that laboratory, or historical data, but could start as being your average data. That way, the data is not unexpectedly high or low or unachievable. Having a laboratory with a quality system means you can achieve a level, and then when you achieve it consistently, you increase that level and alter laboratory processes to improve. No-one benefits from having achievement levels that are set so high, they are unachievable.

The Warning Level is the value you don't want your laboratory to drop below. Sometimes these are set using the standard deviation (SD) from the average data you used to determine your achievement level. Be careful here to use very small SD's. It is supposed to be a sensitive marker, so use a half-SD.

The Action Level is best described as "how many times do you want the laboratory to be lower than the warning level, before you take action". This is a function of how frequent the data is obtained and how significant the numbers comprising each achievement level are. As an example, if the laboratory is performing at least 250 cycles a year, that would allow the laboratory to be able to get enough cycles per week so the LPM data could be collected weekly. The laboratory could then define their Action Level set as requiring a lab review process if there are two or three LPM's below the Warning Level.

How Often do You Collect Pregnancy Marker Data?

Because LPM development markers are often per egg or per embryo, getting numbers as frequently as weekly is quite easy.

Pregnancy is per patient though, so often several weeks' data needs to be combined to ensure the cycle numbers are not too low. Having LPM or Pregnancy Marker data that is too small will give errors in interpretation, so it becomes unhelpful. These frequencies can be reviewed when your data starts being collected and graphed and the laboratory starts to review its own data with the expected frequency.

How is the Data Reviewed?

In general, the toxicity and quality LPM markers will start dropping well before the pregnancy rate will. If the toxicity and quality markers are obtained and reviewed correctly and the Achievement, Warning and Action Levels are set realistically, then the laboratory will show negative data and the Laboratory Management can begin corrective action before there are several low Pregnancy Markers (as it takes longer to obtain the pregnancy data). That is now efficient low-risk laboratory management in operation, using frequent, consistent data from your own laboratories.

If the Action Level is reached that indicates a laboratory review should start, it is terribly important that the Laboratory Management spends some time checking the rest of the data from cycles in the time period where the LPM's indicated there may be a problem. This is because the laboratory does not want to chase "potential" problems that are only occurring because the laboratory is generating data that is too small to interpret correctly.

During this period, look at other cycle data such as:

- Sample size
- Compare to LPM data from other labs you manage
- Number of first cycle patients (versus repeat cycle patients)
- Average number of eggs collected
- If looking at pregnancy data:

  - Are transfers all the same type (Cleavage versus Blastocyst)
  - Are insemination methods similar (i.e. all ICSI)

- Are "best" clinicians involved, or are they on holidays
- Did laboratory staff do different tasks in that time (i.e. is a new staff member doing embryo transfers now)

  As a result of this data checking, the laboratory will have determined that either:

(a) They believe there is a problem they should review, or
(b) That the data is too small and to re-review when the next LPM data is generated

What to Cover During a Laboratory Review?

If a Laboratory Review is indicated, there must be a standard, logical, structured investigation process. Often these take the form of checklists to ensure nothing is forgotten. This review now looks at the operation, the equipment and the technical processes in the laboratory. Some examples may be:

- Temperatures of all stages, warmers, surfaces in lab and in the egg collection area.
- Incubator surfaces.
- Egg collection suction pressures.
- Media/oil batch numbers, cold chain delivery proof. Discard oil if confused.
- Change/test gas cylinders (send back to supplier for retesting of contents and percentages/mixtures).
- Check culture plastic-ware.
- Change/test humidity water/bottles in incubators.
- Check lab environment (VOC's).

Sometimes, even after viewing the LPM data, re-checking the cycle data, performing a laboratory review, there may be nothing that you can identify as causing the drop in LPM data. You may be faced with having to accept that the data may simply be too small to make a decision on, and to support your laboratory processes and re-review the system after the next few LPM results.

Having a laboratory that is well managed and in control, means that at every stage, for every laboratory, you know what the raw material, toxicity, quality and pregnancy markers are. In that way, there should be no surprises, and you are acting proactively, not reactively.

This means that all the low-risk laboratory management items we have covered in this chapter are now in operation. It is very rare for a well-managed, low-risk laboratory to experience a significant and unknown pregnancy rate reduction over a large number of patients.

References

1. Code of Practice for Assisted Reproductive Technology Units (2014). Reproductive Technology Accreditation Committee; Fertility Society of Australia. ISBN 978-0-947285-03-6.
2. Human Fertility and Embryology Authority Code of Practice 8th ed. (2013). http://www.hfea.gov.uk/docs/Code_of_Practice_8_-_October_2013.PDF.
3. Directive 2004/23/EC of the European Parliament and of the Council of 31 March 2004 on Setting standards of quality and safety for the donation, procurement, testing, processing, preservation, storage and distribution of human tissues and cells. http://eur-lex.europa.eu/LexUriServ/LexUriServ.do?uri=CELEX:32004L0023:EN:NOT.
4. International Standards Organisation. ISO9001:2008. Quality management systems—requirements. http://www.iso.org/iso/home/standards/management-standards/iso_9000.htm.
5. International Standards Organisation. ISO15189:2012. Medical laboratories—requirements for quality and competence. http://www.iso.org/iso/home/store/catalogue_tc/catalogue_detail.htm?csnumber=56115.

6. Requirements for the supervision of pathology laboratories (2007 edition). National Pathology Accreditation Advisory Council; Australian Government Department of Health and Ageing. ISBN 1-74186-509-3.
7. Mortimer D, Mortimer S. Quality and risk management in the IVF laboratory. Cambridge, UK: Cambridge University Press; 2005. p. 48. ISBN 0-521-84349-9.
8. Fair Work Ombudsman. Australian Commonwealth Government (2014). https://www.fwc. gov.au/awards-and-agreements/agreements/find-agreement.
9. Cooper GE, White MD, Lauber JK (editors). Resource management on the flightdeck. Proceedings of a NASA/Industry Workshop (NASA CP-2120); 1980.
10. Civil Aviation Safety Authority. Australian Commonwealth Government. (2014). http://www. casa.gov.au/scripts/nc.dll?WCMS:STANDARD::pc=PC_100994.
11. Helmreich RL, Merritt AC. Culture at work: national, organizational and professional influences. Aldershot, UK: Ashgate; 1998.
12. AS/NZS 2982:2010. Laboratory design and construction. https://infostore.saiglobal.com.
13. ISO 14644.1-7. Cleanrooms and associated controlled environments. https://infostore. saiglobal.com.
14. Model protocols for witnessing the identification of samples and patients/donors. (2009). http://www.hfea.gov.uk/docs/witnessing-protocols.pdf.
15. Fertility Society of Australia. RTAC Technical Bulletin #4. http://www.fertilitysociety.com.au/ wp-content/uploads/20120924-RTAC-Technical-Bulletin-4.pdf.
16. Singapore Licensing Terms and Conditions on Assisted Reproductive Services. (2011). https:// www.moh.gov.sg/content/moh_web/home/Publications/guidelines/private_healthcare_institutions/2011/licensing_terms_and_conditions_on_assisted_reproduction_services_ (1.09MB)_(Issued_on_26_Apr_2011).html.
17. Maintenance manual for laboratory equipment, 2nd ed. (2008). World Health Organisation. ISBN 978 92 4 159635 0. http://whqlibdoc.who.int/publications/2008/9789241596350_eng_ low.pdf?ua=1.
18. Medical testing field application document—general equipment calibration and checks. July 2014. National Association of Testing Authorities. http://www.nata.com.au/nata/phocadownload/publications/Guidance_information/equipment/General-Equipment-table.pdf.
19. Technical Note 13, User checks and maintenance of laboratory balances. March 2014. National Association of Testing Authorities. http://www.nata.com.au/nata/phocadownload/publications/Guidance_information/tech-notes-information-papers/technical-note-13.pdf.

Chapter 8
Cryobank Management

John P. Ryan

Introduction

When discussed in the context of reproductive science, a cryobank is a place of storage that uses very low temperatures to preserve gametes, embryos or other reproductive tissues. Cryobanks have essentially been in existence for as long as techniques to successfully store such biological material have been developed. Unlike some more recent advances in reproductive science, the establishment and management of cryobanks is a branch of science where considerable experience had been obtained with gametes and embryos from a wide variety of animal species prior to systems being developed for humans [1].

The first human pregnancy resulting from cryopreserved human sperm was reported in 1953 [1]. There was then a comparatively long period before the birth of the first child from a frozen human embryo reported in 1984 [2], followed soon after in 1986 by a report that a child from a frozen oocyte was born [3]. The successful cryopreservation of ovarian tissue presented a greater challenge due primarily to the mass of tissue to be frozen. The first birth resulting from the transplantation of thawed tissue was reported by Donnez et al. in 2004 [4].

The basic principles of how cryobanks are managed have not changed greatly over this time but rather have been modified to keep pace with changing technology. The introduction of computers for example has greatly increased the efficiency of cryobank management. The aim of this chapter is to provide reproductive clinicians and scientists a checklist of issues to address when setting up a cryobank.

J.P. Ryan, BScAgr, MScAgr, PhD (✉)
Fertility Specialists of Western Australia and School of Women's and Infants' Health,
University of Western Australia, 25 Queenslea Drive, Claremont, WA 6010, Australia
e-mail: johnryan@fertilitywa.com.au

© Springer Science+Business Media New York 2016
S.D. Fleming, A.C. Varghese (eds.), *Organization and Management of IVF Units*, DOI 10.1007/978-3-319-29373-8_8

Establishing a Cryostorage Facility

Legislative Requirements

A cryobank needs to be set up and managed according to the legislation and accreditation requirements of the state and country in which it exists. Such requirements may influence the length of time samples can be kept in storage, how containers must be labelled and security measures that must be instigated.

In Australia, the Reproductive Technology Accreditation Committee (RTAC) code of practice states that an organisation must ensure the safe management of cryopreserved gametes, embryos and tissues. The code states that an organisation must provide evidence of implementation and review of policies/procedures relating to the identification, retrieval and maintenance of cryopreserved material. Policies should also address limiting the time of storage and managing the disposal of cryopreserved material [5]. In the UK, the Human Fertilisation and Embryology Authority (HFEA) sets mandatory requirements and guidelines for fertility units storing gametes and embryos [6].

Material to Be Cryopreserved

Sperm and Testicular Tissue

A number of cryobanks have been established for the specific purpose of storing donated sperm. Patients have been able to select from a range of anonymous sperm donors on the basis of physical and background characteristics. Such characteristics include height, eye colour, hair colour, hair texture, build/weight, ethnic origin, ancestry, religion, donor occupation and education level. Depending upon the country or state there may also be criteria related to the willingness of the donor's information to be made available to recipients or offspring.

Generally, donors are accepted on the basis of sperm quality and infectious disease risk. Sperm donors are routinely screened for various infectious diseases and genetic traits prior to the release of sperm for reproductive treatments. Routine blood tests used to assess the suitability of men to donate sperm include chlamydia, cytomegalovirus, gonorrhoea, Hepatitis B and C, HIV, HTLV-1/11 and syphilis. Additional tests include a karyotype, blood group, rhesus antibodies as well as genetic tests for conditions such as cystic fibrosis and sickle cell disease. Donor sperm is quarantined for a period of 3–6 months and only released for clinical use if negative blood screens for Hepatitis B and C, HIV, HTLV-1/11 and syphilis are obtained. It is important to note that the exact panel of tests employed may differ between countries and may be governed by legislation.

The cryostorage of sperm is also required in a variety of fertility preservation situations: prior to undergoing chemotherapy or radiotherapy, prior to a vasectomy and prior to prostate or testicular surgery. Sperm cryopreservation is also utilised as part of assisted reproduction procedures. It is sometimes required to ensure availability of sperm in situations where men have difficulty producing samples or when men are not present due to work commitments. It is particularly useful when the concentration of samples is very low or semen quality is deteriorating with time. Likewise, cryostorage of testicular or epididymal sperm is important in optimising treatment options for patients undergoing fertility treatment.

Oocytes, Embryos, Ovarian Tissue

Oocytes are collected from gonadotrophin-stimulated ovaries from women undergoing fertility treatment. They are generally stripped of surrounding cumulus cells and assessed for maturation status. Although oocytes can be stored at the germinal vesicle stage of development it is more common for oocytes at metaphase II of the second meiotic division to be cryopreserved. Oocyte cryopreservation is becoming a routine procedure in many countries and has similar storage requirements as for embryos.

Embryos can be frozen at any time during the preimplantation stage of development, from the pronucleate or zygote stage through to the hatched blastocyst stage. Depending on the number of embryos transferred in a fresh cycle, 40–70 % of patients undergoing IVF treatment would be expected to have embryos available for cryopreservation. The most common stages would be when the embryos are either at the 2–8 cell cleavage stages, 2–3 days post-insemination, or the blastocyst stage, 5 or 6 days after insemination.

For a number of years, oocytes and embryos were exposed to a cryoprotectant agent such as glycerol, dimethyl sulphoxide, ethylene glycol or propanediol before being slow frozen in programmable cryopreservation machines which controlled the rate at which embryos were taken from room temperature to intermediate sub-zero temperatures (−30 to −80 °C) before plunging into liquid nitrogen (−196 °C). Intracellular ice formation, which is detrimental to survival, can be avoided if cooling is slow enough to permit sufficient water to leave the cells of the embryo as the freeze solution surrounding the embryo progressively freezes.

An alternate technique for the cryopreservation of oocytes and embryos, called vitrification, has been adopted over the last 15 years. Vitrification relies on the use of higher concentrations of cryoprotectants to alter the viscosity of cells and very rapid cooling to allow a glass or solid liquid to form thus eliminating the formation of intracellular ice [7]. The technique requires relatively brief exposure to the high levels of the cryoprotectants to avoid toxicity.

Ovarian tissue cryopreservation, still considered to be experimental compared to embryo and oocyte cryopreservation, is generally confined to specialist clinics. Although vitrification protocols have been used [8], greater success has generally been achieved with slow freeze protocols requiring the use of programmable cryopreservation machines [9, 10].

Cryostorage Facility

Design and Location Requirements

A cryostorage facility requires three main areas: (1) an area to keep bulk liquid nitrogen tanks, (2) an area to accommodate liquid nitrogen storage tanks and (3) a work area to facilitate the handling of samples and associated documentation.

Bulk liquid nitrogen tanks range in size from approximately 10 to more than 1000 l capacities. They are used as a source of liquid nitrogen to top up storage tanks or provide liquid nitrogen for freezing, warming and auditing procedures. Non-pressurised bulk tanks are normally less than 100 l though they can be used with pressurised decanting devices. The larger capacity bulk tanks are self-pressurised and although available with a castor base are more suited to a permanent location. Tanks that are greater than 70–80 l capacity would generally be kept in a well-ventilated area, possibly external to the main laboratory area or external to the building, to allow easy access by liquid nitrogen delivery contractors. Lesser amounts of bulk liquid nitrogen may be kept in the same area as storage tanks.

Specific liquid nitrogen vacuum lines can be utilised in some situations to connect external bulk tanks with an outlet within the cryostorage facility or directly to liquid or vapour phase storage tanks. The suitability of this delivery approach is influenced by the cost of installation, the distance that the liquid nitrogen needs to be transported and the time required to deliver a requested volume, as lines often need to be primed before use.

Bulk liquid nitrogen deliveries require ready access to the tanks. As such, positioning of tanks adjacent to delivery docks or areas accessible by trucks or with ground floor access is desirable. The frequency of deliveries is dependent upon the volume capacity and the rate at which the liquid nitrogen is used.

Liquid nitrogen storage tanks should be kept on the floor and arranged to allow easy access. The material used for the floor of the storage area, or at least the area where liquid nitrogen might spill, needs to be resistant to the effects of liquid nitrogen. Liquid nitrogen will cause significant damage to most laboratory floors. The use of roller bases with lockable wheels is highly recommended when tanks are required to be movable. A full standard sized 35–40 l storage tank weighs approximately 50 kg. Tipping devices are also available from suppliers to allow individuals to safely decant small volumes of liquid nitrogen (Fig. 8.1). A standard configuration in small to moderate sized laboratories is to have a number of storage tanks positioned under benches around the outside walls of a storage room. If possible, such benches should be attached to the walls without support legs intruding on the space occupied by the tanks.

Safety Considerations

Liquid nitrogen boils at −196 °C producing nitrogen gas at an expansion ratio of 790× that is capable of displacing oxygen from the air if it occurs in a confined or poorly ventilated area. Thus, the odourless and colourless nitrogen gas has the

Fig. 8.1 Tipping device used to dispense bulk liquid nitrogen

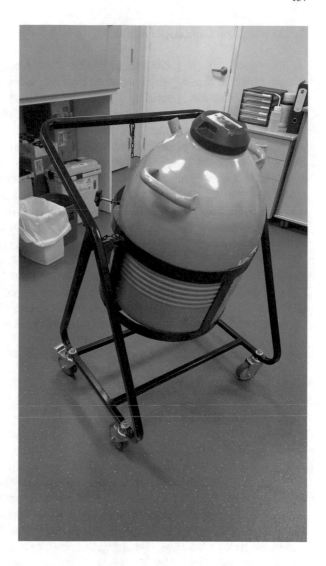

potential to lead to asphyxiation. Also, the extremely cold temperature of liquid nitrogen and cold vapour has the potential to initiate cold burns or frostbite upon contact with unprotected skin. It is essential that oxygen depletion alarms with visual and audible alerts are installed in all cryostorage facilities. Appropriate instructions as to what to do in the case of an alarm condition should also be prominently displayed. Extraction fans should also be installed in cryostorage rooms linked to the oxygen depletion alarms to facilitate evacuation of the nitrogen gas in the case of a significant spill event. A safety audit conducted by appropriately qualified personnel prior to setting up a cryostorage facility is highly recommended.

Laboratory and Sample Security

Access to a cryostorage facility should be limited to laboratory staff. Ideally, storage rooms should be located within an already secure laboratory without direct access from a non-secure area, providing a double layer of security. Laboratories should be securely locked and externally alarmed with swipe card or coded access required during normal operating hours.

Sample security is of utmost importance. To minimise access by inappropriate personnel individual storage tanks can be locked. Indeed, in the UK, the HFEA stipulates that storage tanks must be locked [6]. Temperature and level devices are available for liquid nitrogen storage tanks of all sizes. Such devices provide both real-time and stored temperature histories and will alarm should the level of liquid nitrogen fall below a specified level or the temperature should rise. It is important to note that they may rely on battery power and need to be calibrated annually. Such alarm conditions should be connected to a building management system or external alarm system to notify staff so problems can be quickly identified and rectified. Simpler measuring rod/ruler estimates of liquid nitrogen levels may be effective in detecting slowly failing tanks if performed and recorded on a daily basis though may not prevent damage from a dramatic loss of vacuum.

Cryopreservation Equipment

Liquid Nitrogen Tanks

Bulk Liquid Nitrogen Tanks

Although it is possible to produce liquid nitrogen on-site, the most common scenario is for ART laboratories to have liquid nitrogen delivered by tankers and transferred to either pressurised or non-pressurised vacuum-insulated bulk tanks. Pressurised tanks use natural heat transference or heater units to build up pressure within the tank to facilitate dispensing into smaller containers or to provide liquid nitrogen for auto-fill devices. Automatic systems allow venting of excess pressure. For safety, tank pressure release valves and rupture discs are provided. The capacity of pressurised bulk tanks found most commonly in ART laboratories is in the range 100–250 l (Fig. 8.2). Non-pressurised tanks are generally 25–100 l with static holding times of 130–180 days. Specific details of available tanks can be obtained from manufacturers such as Taylor-Wharton and Air Liquide.

Liquid Nitrogen Storage Tanks

Liquid nitrogen storage tanks are similar in basic design to non-pressurised bulk tanks with the added facility of an inventory system to store samples, generally containing straws or cryovials. They are made from either high strength aluminium

Fig. 8.2 Pressurised bulk
liquid nitrogen tank

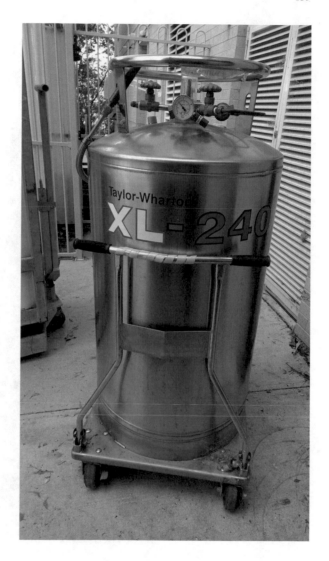

or stainless steel with an insulated vacuumed outer layer to minimise evaporation of
liquid nitrogen. They range in size from 2 to 1000 l, with most IVF laboratories opting for multiple 35–40 l tanks in preference to large capacity tanks that hold in
excess of 500 l (Fig. 8.3). Tanks are designed with indexed neck holders to accommodate stainless steel or plastic canisters, and should have lockable lids. The choice
of the type and size of storage tanks required is dependent upon the available space
for housing the tanks and the intended use.

Fig. 8.3 Liquid nitrogen
storage tank on roller base

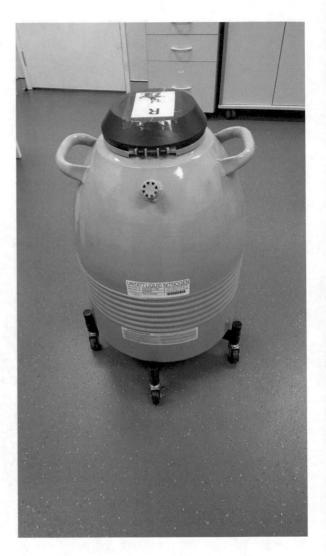

Nitrogen Vapour Phase Storage Tanks

Vapour phase storage vessels have a minimal amount of liquid nitrogen in the bottom or an outer layer of the units, the level in the bottom of which is normally set at or just below the base of the inventory storage system, which is maintained by automatic fill devices with monitors to record and control the internal temperature of the vessel. Such vessels are also equipped with a battery backup facility to maintain operations in the event of a power outage and to allow alarm systems to function. Vapour phase systems should eliminate the risk of liquid nitrogen leaking into cryovials and are also thought to minimise the risk of sample cross contamination compared with liquid storage systems.

Number of Tanks Required

The total number of storage tanks required is dependent upon the range of materials cryopreserved and the size or capacity of the tanks purchased. It is good practice to have a spare fully operational tank that could be utilised immediately when the integrity of a tank in use is compromised. Additional tanks may also be required if samples are quarantined, awaiting the results of viral disease testing, before being transferred to permanent storage tanks.

It is normal practice for sperm to be stored separately to oocytes and embryos. This has generally been due to a greater perceived risk of cross contamination with sperm. Indeed, if samples were contaminated, the viral load of a processed sperm sample would be expected to be considerably greater than that associated with a single oocyte or embryo.

A laboratory should also have a policy of tank replacement which can be developed in conjunction with the tank manufacturer, as the frequency of replacement will be influenced by the materials from which the tank is made and the environment in which it is used.

Inspection and Maintenance Schedule of Storage Tanks

Both liquid and vapour phase storage tanks need to be inspected regularly, irrespective of whether manual or automated processes are employed. Laboratories should have protocols for the checking and filling of tanks. These checks can be implemented daily or at least on a regular basis such as three times a week (for example Monday, Thursday and Saturday). Liquid nitrogen level checks need to be incorporated into daily laboratory checklists completed first thing in the morning or just before leaving the laboratory of an evening. Checklists should list the upper and lower acceptable limits for individual tanks and steps to be taken should a level fall outside the acceptable range. A monthly review of checklists should be carried out to check for an increased rate of liquid nitrogen usage suggesting a need for the tank to be checked by a qualified serviceman or to be replaced. In such a situation samples should be relocated to alternate tanks without delay.

If manual filling of tanks occurs, a level well above the acceptable lower limit should be established to prompt staff to fill the tank. A visual check of the outsides of the tanks should be made at the same time as measuring the level as condensation or ice can form on the outside of some tanks indicating that the integrity of the tank has been compromised. If automatic alarm systems are to be used to monitor liquid nitrogen levels then a check that the alarm is fully operational needs to be carried out at regular intervals (usually monthly). Likewise, the use of battery-operated components requires a protocol whereby batteries are checked and replaced at regular intervals.

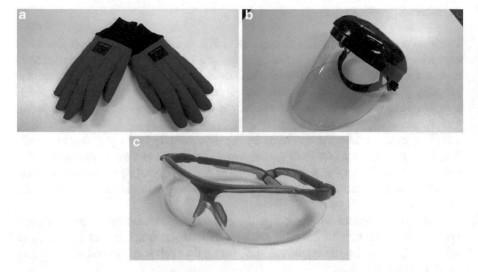

Fig. 8.4 (**a–c**) Personal safety equipment. (**a**) Cryogenic gloves, (**b**) face shield, (**c**) safety goggles

Personal Safety Equipment

Cryostorage facilities should be fully equipped with appropriate safety equipment. There should be sufficient sets of items for use by the number of staff operating in the facility at any given time. Safety equipment includes:

1. Cryogenic Gloves (possibly in small and large sizes) (Fig. 8.4a)
2. Face shield (Fig. 8.4b)
3. Safety glasses or safety goggles (Fig. 8.4c)
4. Protective apron
5. Fully enclosed foot ware, long sleeves

Staff Education

Staff education as to the hazards associated with working with liquid nitrogen must be undertaken. Many laboratories conduct such training internally and often covered as part of an orientation process. Other laboratories take advantage of courses run externally by qualified personnel.

It is important for staff to understand that they could suffer cold burns and severe tissue damage from exposure to liquid nitrogen. Also, that liquid nitrogen can seep into straws and cryovials during storage and that the containers can explode upon warming due to the rapidly expanding nitrogen gas. There is also an infection risk when such containers explode due to the biological material contained within. Only containers certified by a manufacturer to be stored in liquid nitrogen should be stored in such tanks. Manufacturers propose the use of CryoFlex™ tubing for cryovials stored in liquid nitrogen. Internally threaded cryovials with a silicone gasket, stored in vapour phase are considered optimum for the storage of biological samples in cryovials.

Choice of Storage Container

The choice of container to use is largely dependent upon the biological material to be cryopreserved. The container type then dictates the inventory system required to provide a safe efficient cryostorage system.

Sperm Storage

Semen has been stored in plastic straws of various volume capacities, cryovials and glass ampoules. The use of glass ampoules is not routinely practised currently but many clinics around the world still might have such material in storage. Glass ampoules are considered dangerous due to sealing problems and a propensity to leak liquid nitrogen that expands rapidly causing the glass to explode upon thawing.

The plastic straw system developed by Cryo Bio Systems (CBS™) has been adopted widely for human semen cryopreservation and utilises a number of features desirable in a clinically applicable system. The main features include (1) being made from an ionomeric resin that is chemically inert and biocompatible, (2) that can be thermally sealed at both ends to eliminate possibility of cross-contamination to the sample or its environment, (3) is guaranteed leak-proof and shatter-proof at liquid nitrogen temperatures, (4) allows outside printing on the straw, (5) has a tamperproof labelled rod to insert inside the straw, (6) compatible with use of bar codes and (7) uses filling nozzles for efficient and clean manual filling.

Cryovials have also been used extensively and successfully to cryopreserve spermatozoa. Cryovials manufactured to store sperm are made from polypropylene with a silicone seal for an internally threaded cap to ensure they do not leak at cryogenic temperatures. Manufacturers advise that they should be used in nitrogen vapour storage tanks. CryoFlex™ tubing has been developed to encase cryovials giving them an extra layer of protection from leaking nitrogen, though some users have indicated that it can affect freezing and warming rates [11]. They can be sterilised by gamma radiation. A white marking area on the side of the cryovials allows efficient labelling and making them an ideal vessel for bar coding systems.

The storage of testicular tissue, tubules following testicular biopsy or processed testicular sperm has its own challenges. A variety of techniques have been developed utilising containers such as semen straws, flexipets and embryo vitrification devices.

Oocytes and Embryos

Slow Freeze Devices

Plastic straws and cryovials, similar to those used for sperm have been used for the slow freezing of oocytes and embryos. A 0.25 ml polyvinyl chloride (PVC) straw (IMV Technologies) was used for many years but was replaced by a polyethylene terephthalate glycol (PETG) version which can be readily sterilised by irradiation [12]. It is routine to load the oocytes or embryos in the middle of three columns of cryoprotectant medium separated by air bubbles. This isolates the material from the ends of the straws which requiring sealing before cryopreservation. Various methods have been used to seal plastic straws including polyvinyl alcohol (PVA) powder, haematocrit sealant, plastic or nylon plugs, steel ball bearings, ultrasonic sealers and thermal sealing devices.

Vitrification Devices

There is a greater range of storage containers available for the vitrification of oocytes and embryos than developed for slow freezing methodologies. This has come about by the desire to minimise the volume of fluid in which embryos are held to obtain very high rates of cooling to prevent ice formation, often obtained by direct exposure to liquid nitrogen.

The use of an "open" system of vitrification whereby samples are directly exposed to liquid nitrogen, either during the cryopreservation process or whilst in storage, is considered a greater risk of allowing cross contamination with viruses than sealed containers. The open system of vitrification is the basis of the EM grid [13], Cryotop [14], Cryoloop [15, 16], Cryoleaf and hemi-straw [17] methodologies, all of which have been used successfully to vitrify human oocytes and embryos.

However, numerous studies have demonstrated that adequate rates of freezing can be obtained with a sealed system as evidenced by high rates of oocyte and embryo survival upon warming and pregnancies following transfer. Examples of closed vitrification systems include the high security vitrification straws from CBS [18], the Cryotip [19] and Rapid-I device [20].

Contamination Considerations

The issue of contamination of straws or cryovials with pathogenic viruses has been addressed in some detail. Indeed, it has been experimentally demonstrated that cross contamination between liquid nitrogen and embryos may occur if embryos come into contact with contaminated liquid nitrogen [21]. However, there has been no evidence that contamination has occurred in a clinical setting from either liquid nitrogen into sample containers or from containers into liquid nitrogen [21–23].

The use of quarantine tanks, where samples are held awaiting the outcome of viral testing, is often used to manage the risk of exposing cryopreserved samples to various viral diseases. It is however conceivable for cross contamination to occur by moving samples from a quarantine tank that had previously held contaminated samples. The need to often freeze semen samples urgently for oncology patients before any testing can take place can potentially put other samples within the same storage tanks at risk. Many laboratories employ a system whereby they store samples of known contamination (e.g. HIV, Hepatitis B, Hepatitis C) in dedicated tanks and adopt universal precautions with all other samples [11].

Ehrsam has identified a number sources whereby contamination of liquid nitrogen could occur [12]: from biological material contaminating the outside of containers such as straws, from containers already contaminated breaking whilst in storage, from contamination by staff handling samples, from liquid nitrogen from a previously contaminated tank or during the manufacture of the liquid nitrogen. There are a number of precautionary steps an ART laboratory can take to minimise the risk of the cross contamination of samples. As mentioned above, use an appropriately sealed storage vessel; closed vitrification devices are preferred. Disinfecting the outsides of slow frozen vessels upon thawing with an agent such as hypochlorite followed by sterile water can be performed but is not suitable for vitrification devices due to the methods used to quickly transfer material from the storage vessels into the warming solutions. Only sterilised scissors or cutting devices should be used to open straws. Staff should not transfer liquid nitrogen between storage containers, only source nitrogen from bulk supply containers. Likewise, a periodic disinfection of storage tanks should be undertaken to reduce the potential for cross contamination.

Storage Container Labelling Considerations

Hand writing information with standard marker pens or printing directly on storage containers with automated printing devices are common methods of labelling. It is important to confirm that the ink or solvent base of the ink does not create toxic conditions by penetrating the material of the container or releasing volatile compounds in the laboratory work areas. Likewise, it is necessary for hand writing to be legible and unable to be inadvertently rubbed off. Adhesive labels, such as those made by Brady Systems, can be produced with patient details via a computer interface and are manufactured to remain intact and legible at liquid nitrogen temperature. They are commonly used either internally on inserted ID rods or externally around the straws or cryovials.

Bar codes and radio-frequency identification devices (RFID) are used as part of electronic witnessing systems that verify or match patient details on tubes and culture vessels before critical processes are undertaken. Labelling of cryostorage containers with such systems has been suggested to offer a greater level of security by reducing human error. It should be noted that the use of RFID for sperm and embryo vessels at liquid nitrogen temperature is still considered to be under development. However, it has also been suggested that they should not be used at the exclusion of information that can be read by humans due to the risk of machine reading devices not working at critical times [12]. Irrespective of the labelling system utilised, it is strongly recommended to test it thoroughly prior to introducing it into clinical use.

Inventory System

Choice of Inventory System

An inventory system consists of a combination of canisters, goblets of various sizes, visotubes, metal canes or racks to facilitate the safe and efficient storage of samples in liquid or vapour phase tanks (Fig. 8.5). The choice of inventory system is determined by the type of storage tank in use, the containers in which samples are stored, the labelling or sample tracking system employed and personal preference of the scientist. In theory, straws or cryovials associated with a given patient could be stored at multiple sites within a storage tank provided they were labelled with appropriate identifying information. In practice, for ease of location and management, samples are stored together in one location. It is not uncommon for one or two straws to be stored in a single location capable of holding up to 12 straws. This results in a significant amount of storage space that is not utilised but reduces the risk of sample misidentification.

An appropriate inventory system should allow:

1. Continual safe storage of samples at liquid nitrogen temperature (−196 °C)
2. Ease of access to specific samples at known locations
3. Ready identification of samples
4. Removal of samples with no or minimal risk to disturbing other samples
5. Efficient use of available storage space

Comparison of Two Inventory Systems

The use of 35–40 l storage tanks on roller bases is common in ART laboratories. Such tanks have the capacity to hold 6–10 canisters. Table 8.1 compares two commonly used ten canister storage tank systems with one patient's straws only per cane or visotube.

The advantages and disadvantages associated with each system are listed in Table 8.2.

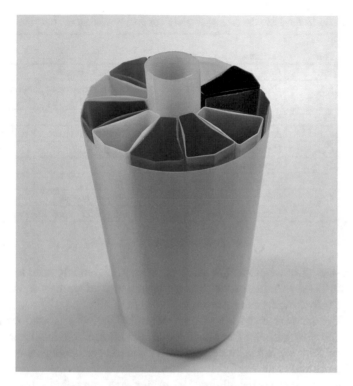

Fig. 8.5 An example of visotubes arranged in a maxi-goblet for storage of cryopreservation straws

Table 8.1 Comparative capacities of two commonly used storage systems

System	Primary level storage unit per canister	Secondary level storage unit	Straws per secondary unit	Straws per primary unit	Straws per canister
1	25 metal canes	2 × 9 mm goblets per cane	5 × CBS straws per 9 mm goblet	10 CBS straws per cane	250 CBS straws per canister
2	2 maxi-goblets	12 visotubes per maxi-goblet	12 × CBS straws per visotube	144 CBS straws per maxi-goblet	288 CBS straws per canister

Record Keeping

Sample Identification

In Australia, current guidelines issued by the RTAC of the Fertility Society of Australia state that both patient and sample identification must normally include three identifiers, at least one of which must be unique to a patient or couple [5]. A patient's

Table 8.2 Issues to consider when comparing two commonly used storage systems

System	Pro or con	Advantage/disadvantage
1	Pro	Relatively easy access to a given patient's straws
	Pro	Empty canes can be stored outside tank and used as a record of empty slots
	Con	Reduced total number of straws can be stored
	Con	Need to remove straw completely from goblet to check details
	Con	Goblets can come loose from cane
2	Pro	Greater total straw storage capacity
	Pro	Easier access to straws during audit
	Con	Need to remove the whole maxi goblet to access
	Con	Potential need to remove upper maxi goblet to access lower level

full name, date of birth and unique clinic number is commonly used to satisfy this requirement. These identifiers should be used on associated worksheet documents, in cryostorage records and database records.

The guidelines permit the use of two identifiers for vessels used for less than seven days providing one of them is a unique identifier. Three identifiers are however required for vessels used for cryopreservation of sperm, oocytes, embryos and reproductive tissue.

It should be noted that an additional identifier such as a unique straw number or embryo number needs to be used when genetically tested embryos are frozen. This allows the correct identification of specific embryos of a known genetic constitution. Embryos are often frozen post biopsy awaiting the outcome of genetic testing. The process of correctly labelling storage vessels, loading the appropriate embryo in the correct vessel and matching subsequent genetic results is an area requiring considerable diligence and should be double witnessed.

An example of the minimum sample identification information that should be recorded on a freeze container (cryovial or straw) would be:

1. Patient full name	e.g. John Frost
2. Patient date of birth	e.g. 25/04/1980
3. Unique patient identification number	e.g. # 12345
4. Straw number	e.g. # 05
5. Date of freeze	e.g. 20/03/2015

The contents of each straw can then be matched with details in the patient's file and electronic or hard copy storage details. Accessible information could include full semen analysis details, embryonic cell stage and grade or genetic testing result.

Database Considerations

Database Cryostorage Details

Below is a list of cryostorage details that should be recorded in a hardcopy book/file or electronic database that is common to sperm, oocytes, embryos and reproductive tissue:

1. Assume full patient and partner identification (Full name, DOB, address, unique identification number) and related semen analysis or embryology details
2. Date of Freeze
3. Method of Freeze
4. Straw number/ID and Colour
5. Storage location details (e.g. Tank/Canister Number/Maxi Goblet Number, Level or Colour/Visotube Number or Colour)
6. Scientist performing the freeze
7. Comments

Additional details specific to the cryopreservation of sperm samples might include:

1. Source of spermatozoa (partner or donor)
2. Total number of straws or cryovials frozen
3. Post thaw result of test sample

Additional details specific to the cryopreservation of oocytes and embryos might include:

1. Source of oocytes (patient's own oocytes or donated—donor details recorded)
2. Developmental cell stage
3. Morphological grade
4. Genetic test result

Allowance in a database also needs to be made to accommodate material that is imported from other clinics. In such cases it is necessary to be provided with all relevant information and aligned with the new storage location details. It should be noted that imported material may be stored in containers that are different to what is routinely used in the receiving laboratory, frozen by methodologies which staff are not familiar with and could be labelled differently.

Search and Report Functions

A database should accommodate search functions to efficiently review cryostorage information. The most common function would be to search for the total number of straws or cryovials a patient still has in storage. Likewise, it might be desirable to search by date of freeze, method of cryopreservation or specific storage location. It is imperative that a database is always kept up to date. Laboratory work procedures should allow data entry to occur at the time samples are frozen or removed from cryostorage or at least within a short period of the task being accomplished.

A database should be able to generate reports of storage details on a patient basis. Furthermore, it should be possible to generate lists of cryovials or straws stored in individual canisters or tanks. Such a function is integral to good auditing procedures. More sophisticated systems are also integrated with patient demographic and contact information, administration and invoicing systems and highlight samples approaching maximum storage times. Whereas a basic spreadsheet can be used to record storage information, the benefits listed above are generally associated with a comprehensive relational database system and makes it a better long-term solution to a laboratory's cryostorage administrative needs.

Patient Communication

A study of embryo cryopreservation in Australia showed that 78 % of stored embryos were subsequently used for treatment; however, 20 % of the women stored their embryos for more than 5 years [24]. Not surprisingly, having a live-birth prolonged the duration of storage. It is not uncommon therefore for a laboratory to maintain storage of gametes and embryos for a considerable period of time. An integral part of an efficient cryostorage system is the communication established between the laboratory and patients. Such communication is generally by way of a letter sent annually to a patient's last known address. An effective communication system is required to:

1. Ascertain whether patients wish to continue storage, donate to other infertile couples or donate to research
2. Allow invoicing for ongoing storage
3. Initiate the disposal of cryopreserved material
4. Confirm that correct contact information is maintained

Advice to continue storage generally initiates a storage invoice, whereas a couple's indication to donate their gametes or embryos to another couple or research would require further consultation and documentation. These processes in turn can be affected by legislation or guidelines specific to each country. The disposal of cryopreserved material can be due to either a decision made by the couple or because a legislated maximum storage period has been reached.

A protocol for the disposal of embryos should also include what to do in circumstances where (a) couples are divorced, (b) where a couple disagree with the fate of the stored material, (c) where one or both partners are deceased or (d) where one or both partners are lost to contact. Options as to the fate of gametes or embryos in the case of death should be considered when consent to freeze the gametes or embryos was originally given by patients. Protocols should also address steps to be taken should contact with patients be lost. These steps are essential and provide evidence should the fate of material become the focus of litigation proceedings.

Risk Assessment and Cryostorage

Potential Areas of Concern

The issue of risk assessment associated with cryostorage of gametes and embryos has been addressed in detail by Tomlinson [25]. A risk assessment is a systematic review to identify potential hazards, weighing up the chances of an event occurring against the consequences of the event occurring. Ultimately it is used as a prompt to implement systems to eliminate or minimise the chance of an adverse event occurring. The areas of concern identified by Tomlinson [25] are (1) physical security of vessels and specimens, (2) liquid nitrogen supply and staff safety, (3) the relative safety of the containment system (vials or straws), (4) the type of nitrogen storage (liquid vs. vapour phase), (5) the suitability of equipment to do the job, (6) witnessing and security of labelling, (7) screening of patients for infectious diseases prior to storage, (8) sample processing in order to lessen the risk of disease transmission, and (9) early warning and monitoring systems.

Misidentification of patients or samples deserves special mention due to the implications encountered should gametes or embryos be mixed up. Indeed, current RTAC guidelines in Australia require clinics to have hazard control plans to identify and mitigate factors known to increase the chance of misidentification. The guidelines discuss the need to address issues such as staff workloads, maximum hours worked without a break, maximum hours worked in a day, the number of consecutive days worked, interruptions to work, changes to scheduling procedures and other factors likely to affect a scientist's concentration.

The major areas of concern, such as identification of patients and samples, should be subject to regular internal audits. Erroneous findings from the planned audits or incident reports related to laboratory activities must be recorded and analysed to determine the cause of the problem and then an appropriate corrective action must be undertaken to prevent a reoccurrence of the problem.

Auditing Storage Facilities

Process of Storage Tank Audits

Audits or storage reviews of the contents of storage tanks should be carried out at regular intervals. The frequency of audits is influenced by accreditation requirements and the assessment of the level of risk in completing the task. In the UK for example, the HFEA suggests that reviews of stored gametes and embryos are done at least once every 2 years [6]. Such reviews are carried out to reconcile the clinic's records with material in storage; to review the purpose and duration of storage and identify any action needed [5].

A full audit involves checking the details on sample containers (e.g. straws or cryovials) against clinic records which could be stored in an electronic database, as hard copies in the form of a book/ledger, file or cards, or both. This procedure generally involves two staff members and is very time consuming. Risks involved include partial thawing/warming of samples, damage to sample containers and risks associated with handling liquid nitrogen. The risk associated with checking details of vitrified samples is thought to be greater than with slow frozen samples due to the reduced volumes of cryopreservation media containing the specimens.

The final step in the audit process is to correct all records to ensure they accurately reflect the details of the biological material in storage. Any changes should be flagged and referenced to the audit performed. In some situations a comment explaining discrepancies needs to be recorded with the storage details to prevent future confusion. This is particularly useful in situations where a physical alteration of the details cannot be made such as a change to the labelling on straws or cryovials.

Common Discrepancies

Audits of storage details may identify situations where samples exist in storage but no or incorrect details are recorded or where records indicate samples are in storage but no or the incorrect numbers of samples are located in storage. Common discrepancies derive from situations such as transcribing incorrect patient details, recording incorrect storage locations, recording an incorrect number of straws or cryovials initially frozen, failure to accurately record use of samples and loss of samples from their storage goblets into the tank. The majority of causes would be avoided if appropriate double witnessing checks were used at appropriate stages of the cryopreservation and thawing processes and details of freezes and thaws were immediately recorded.

Rather than carry out full audits every two years, a more efficient strategy might be to conduct partial audits more frequently, 25 % of the total number of tanks every six months for example. As part of a quality management system, the results of an audit are required to be reviewed to ascertain the underlying causes of the observed discrepancies. Laboratory protocols governing the cryopreservation process might need to be modified, for example, to prevent a reoccurrence of observed discrepancies. Indeed, an investigation of any discrepancies that arise at the time of removing samples from cryostorage in the course of normal clinical activities is a form of auditing which is considered a more time saving method that doesn't expose samples to inadvertent warming.

Computer databases can also be adapted to automatically detect discrepancies in storage details. For instance, if more than one patient's name is linked to a specific storage location or if the total number of straws in a location exceeds the maximum number that could be stored. Such functions are not likely to cover all possible errors but may aid in the identification of a proportion of transcription-based errors.

Transportation of Gametes and Embryos

Transport Coordination

The transportation of gametes and embryos between ART laboratories has become a routine practice for most laboratories around the world. Transportation may be of a short duration between laboratories of the same clinic or internationally requiring a number of days in transit. Indeed, the frequency of transportation cases is such that in most laboratories, the role of coordinating the import and export of gametes and embryos is taken on by one or two scientists familiar with the processes involved. The Transportation Coordinator's role involves liaising with patients, other IVF laboratories, courier companies, government agencies, airlines and administration services.

Use of Dry Shippers

Transportation is carried out in special purpose nitrogen tanks called dry shippers (Fig. 8.6). They are designed to create an internal temperature of close to −196 °C in nitrogen vapour. Dry shippers are similar in design to small standard liquid nitrogen tanks except they have an internal absorbent material packaged around the core that absorbs liquid nitrogen. Excess liquid is removed after the dry shipper is primed allowing gametes and embryos to be transported in nitrogen vapour. The dry shippers, if appropriately stored in an upright position, can maintain temperature for 5–12 days. Dry shippers are generally encased in a sturdy foam lined carry case made from either hard plastic or cardboard to minimise the risk of damage to the dry shipper during transport. The International Air Transport Association (IATA) has regulations governing the suitability of dry shippers to be used for air transport.

Priming of dry shippers should be performed prior to each transportation event. This is achieved by filling the shipper completely with liquid nitrogen, then topping it up periodically as the liquid is absorbed, until the level remains stable. The weight of a fully primed dry shipper should be recorded when the shipper is first used for transportation. This enables a quick weight check of the dry shipper to be performed prior to each subsequent transportation event and is an effective way to ensure adequate priming of the dry shipper. This weight could then be recorded on the dry shipper's usage log sheet and other transportation documentation as evidence that appropriate priming had taken place.

Robust temperature loggers are now available for routine use with dry shippers. This enables tracking over an extended time period and can be checked as evidence that an appropriate temperature was maintained at all times throughout the period of transportation.

Fig. 8.6 Dry shipper used
for the transportation of
gametes and embryos

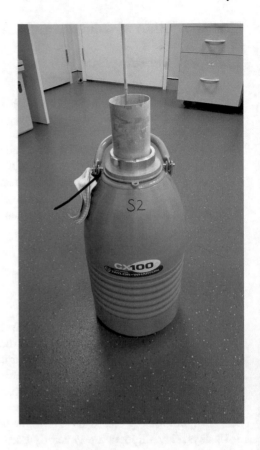

Logistics of Transportation

It is generally accepted that the responsibility for maintaining the integrity of cryostorage vessels and the perceived quality of the enclosed biological material lies with the sending laboratory up until the time the samples leave the laboratory. That responsibility passes to the receiving laboratory once the samples have been appropriately checked and placed in permanent storage. The laboratories do not normally accept responsibility during the period of transportation irrespective of how or by whom the actual transportation is accomplished. Good communication between all parties involved is paramount to the overall success of the process. Although the exact process to enable transportation of biological samples between ART laboratories will be different for each laboratory, the following is an example of the steps required to achieve a successful outcome:

1. Notification by patients that they wish to import or export biological material
2. Patients to complete consent forms at both sending and receiving laboratories to allow transport
3. Completion of government agency documentation if required
4. Organisation of an appropriate courier familiar with dry shipper transportation
5. Prime the dry shipper
6. Schedule collection of the dry shipper
7. Prepare documentation to accompany dry shipper, including sample description and identification, process used for cryopreservation and recommended method for thawing/warming
8. Prepare samples for transport including identification check with witnessing
9. Courier companies to provide details to allow tracking of the dry shipper during transport
10. Sending laboratory to notify patients of transport details
11. Receiving laboratory to notify patients and sending laboratory on receipt of samples
12. Identification of received samples to be checked, witnessed and stored in a storage tank
13. Storage database and patient files at both sending and receiving laboratories updated

Conclusions

The cryopreservation of sperm, oocytes, embryos and reproductive tissue has become standard practice in clinics all around the world that offer infertility treatment. The importance of cryopreservation to the IVF industry is best demonstrated by the fact that between one-third and one-half of all pregnancies established nowadays result from the transfer of frozen-thawed embryos.

Cryobank management is integral to the cryopreservation process and the success of assisted reproductive technologies. It involves continually reassessing available resources and processes to ensure the safe and effective storage of the biological specimens being stored. The design of the laboratory facility and the choice of cryostorage equipment, specimen container and inventory system make up the physical resources that need to be appropriately managed. The record keeping processes involved in storage and transportation, the assessment of risk and the auditing of cryostored material are management components that need to be constantly addressed and adapted to changing needs of the clinic. Appropriately educated staff that have an attention to detail and which diligently follow the established laboratory protocols and accurately record all facets of gamete and embryo storage are also essential to the overall success of a cryopreservation facility.

References

1. Foote RH. The history of artificial insemination: selected notes and notables. J Anim Sci. 2002;80:1–10.
2. Trounson A, Mohr L. Human pregnancy following cryopreservation, thawing and transfer of an eight-cell embryo. Nature. 1983;305:707–9.
3. Chen C. Pregnancy after human oocyte cryopreservation. Lancet. 1986;1(8486):884–6.
4. Donnez J, Dolmans MM, Demylle D, Jadoul P, Pirard C, Squifflet J, et al. Livebirth after orthotopic transplantation of cryopreserved ovarian tissue. Lancet. 2004;364(9443):1405–10.
5. Code of Practice for Assisted Reproductive Technology Units. March 2014 ed. Fertility Society of Australia, Reproductive Accreditation Committee; 2014.
6. Human Fertilisation and Embryology Authority (HFEA). 8th Code of Practice. Edition 8.0 2013.
7. Rall WF, Fahy GM. Ice free cryopreservation of mouse embryos at −196 °C by vitrification. Nature. 1985;313:573–5.
8. Amorim CA, Dolmans MM, David A, Jaeger J, Vanacker J, Camboni A, et al. Vitrification and xenografting of human ovarian tissue. Fertil Steril. 2012;98(5):1291–8.
9. Donnez J, Dolmans MM. Fertility preservation in women. Nat Rev Endocrinol. 2013;9(12): 735–49.
10. Donnez J, Dolmans MM, Pellicer A, Diaz-Garcia C, Sanchez Serrano M, Schmidt KT, et al. Restoration of ovarian activity and pregnancy after transplantation of cryopreserved ovarian tissue: a review of 60 cases of reimplantation. Fertil Steril. 2013;99(6):1503–13.
11. Mortimer D. Current and future concepts and practices in human sperm cryobanking. Reprod Biomed Online. 2004;9(2):134–51.
12. Ehrsam A. Chapter-19 Safe cryobanking. Manual of assisted reproductive technologies and clinical embryology. New Delhi: Jaypee Brothers Medical Publishers Pty Ltd; 2012.
13. Son WY, Yoon SH, Yoon HJ, Lee SM, Lim JH. Pregnancy outcome following transfer of human blastocysts vitrified on electron microscopy grids after induced collapse of the blastocoele. Hum Reprod (Oxf, Engl). 2003;18:137–9.
14. Katayama KP, Stehlik J, Kuwayama M, Kato O, Stehlik E. High survival rate of vitrified human oocytes results in clinical pregnancy. Fertil Steril. 2003;80(1):223–4.
15. Lane MS, Schoolcraft WB, Gardner DK. Vitrification of mouse and human blastocysts using a novel cryoloop container-less technique. Fertil Steril. 1999;72:1073–8.
16. Mukaida T, Nakamura S, Tomiyama T, Wada S, Kasai M, Takahashi K. Successful birth after transfer of vitrified human blastocysts with use of a cryoloop containerless technique. Fertil Steril. 2001;76:618–20.
17. Vanderzwalmen P, Bertin G, Debauche C, Standaert V, Bollen N, van Roosendaal E, Vandervorst M, Schoysman R, Zech N. Vitrification of human blastocysts with the Hemi-Straw carrier: application of assisted hatching after thawing. Hum Reprod (Oxf, Engl). 2003;18:1504–11.
18. Van Landuyt L, Stoop D, Verheyen G, Verpoest W, Camus M, Van de Velde H, et al. Outcome of closed blastocyst vitrification in relation to blastocyst quality: evaluation of 759 warming cycles in a single-embryo transfer policy. Hum Reprod (Oxf, Engl). 2011;26(3):527–34.
19. Kuwayama M, Vajta G, Ieda S, Kato O. Comparison of open and closed methods for vitrification of human embryos and the elimination of potential contamination. Reprod Biomed Online. 2005;11(5):608–14.
20. Hashimoto S, Amo A, Hama S, Ohsumi K, Nakaoka Y, Morimoto Y. A closed system supports the developmental competence of human embryos after vitrification: closed vitrification of human embryos. J Assist Reprod Genet. 2013;30(3):371–6.
21. Bielanski A, Nadin-Davis S, Sapp T, Lutze-Wallace C. Viral contamination of embryos cryopreserved in liquid nitrogen. Cryobiology. 2000;40(2):110–6.
22. Bielanski A. A review of the risk of contamination of semen and embryos during cryopreservation and measures to limit cross-contamination during banking to prevent disease transmission in ET practices. Theriogenology. 2012;77(3):467–82.

23. Bielanski A, Bergeron H, Lau PC, Devenish J. Microbial contamination of embryos and semen during long term banking in liquid nitrogen. Cryobiology. 2003;46(2):146–52.
24. Sullivan E, Dean J, Illingworth P, Chapman M, Ryan JP. A clinical perspective on how long patients stored their cryopreserved embryos and how patients use them. R Aust N Z J Obstet Gynaecol. 2009;49:40.
25. Tomlinson M. Managing risk associated with cryopreservation. Hum Reprod (Oxf, Engl). 2005;20(7):1751–6.

Chapter 9
Management of a Preimplantation Genetic Diagnosis and Screening Service

Steven D. Fleming, Jane Fleming, and Joyce Harper

Introduction

Preimplantation genetic diagnosis (PGD) of embryos was pioneered in the early 1990's and represents one of the major breakthroughs in the alleviation of inherited genetic disorders [1]. It is an alternative to prenatal diagnosis in that it prevents pregnancies that would have resulted in affected offspring from occurring, by identifying non-affected embryos for transfer to the uterus. In recent years, methods of analysis have evolved rapidly, from fluorescence in situ hybridisation (FISH) to comparative genomic hybridisation (CGH) and next generation sequencing (NGS) via whole genome amplification (WGA) [2]. In addition to identifying single-gene defects and chromosome abnormalities, PGD is also used for non-disease diagnoses such as HLA matching and sex selection for family balancing and other medicosocial reasons. Since it is known that the majority of embryos resulting from assisted reproduction technology (ART) display aneuploidy or mosaicism [3, 4], preimplantation genetic screening (PGS) was developed with the aim of increasing delivery rates for patients going through IVF by examining chromosomes. PGS represents

S.D. Fleming, BSc (Hons), MSc, PhD (✉)
Discipline of Anatomy and Histology, School of Medical Sciences, University of Sydney, Sydney, NSW 2006, Australia
e-mail: blueyfleming@gmail.com

J. Fleming, BSc, MSc, PhD
Master of Genetic Counselling Program, Royal North Shore Hospital,
Level 7 Kolling Institute, Pacific Highway, St Leonards, Sydney, NSW 2065, Australia
e-mail: jane.fleming@sydney.edu.au

J. Harper, BSc, PhD
Embryology, IVF and Reproductive Genetics Group, Institute for Women's Health,
University College London, 86-96 Chenies Mews, London, UK
e-mail: joyce.harper@ucl.ac.uk

© Springer Science+Business Media New York 2016
S.D. Fleming, A.C. Varghese (eds.), *Organization and Management of IVF Units*, DOI 10.1007/978-3-319-29373-8_9

an opportunity to screen out such embryos that, if transferred to the uterus, would almost certainly result in either implantation failure or early miscarriage. For PGD or PGS, oocyte and/or embryo biopsy is necessary to provide the polar bodies, blastomeres and/or trophectoderm cells required for analysis. It is the management of these biopsy procedures that this chapter is primarily concerned with, rather than the methods of genetic analysis *per se*.

Implementation of a Clinical Service for PGD/PGS

The decision whether or not to establish a clinical service for PGD and PGS needs to be carefully thought through since there are a number of limiting factors to consider including regulatory restrictions, the scientific and clinical expertise required, and access to a facility for molecular genetic analysis.

Legislation and Licencing

The legislation governing the provision of PGD and PGS varies between different countries and states. For example, in Australia the National Health and Medical Research Council (NHMRC) guidelines mandate that PGD should only be used to avoid the inheritance of a serious genetic condition or disease, and that any clinic offering testing must provide access to both a clinical geneticist and genetic counsellor (http://www.nhmrc.gov.au/guidelines-publications/e78).

Genetic Counselling and Patient Consent

ART has been described as a "roller coaster ride" and there have been many reports documenting the psychosocial impact for couples undergoing fertility treatment. These include both physical and emotional effects that may be linked to the possibility of treatment failure, relationship and family stresses, decision-making, financial concerns, anxiety and depression. There may be added costs and a reduced chance of success associated with PGD, and patients undergoing this treatment have reported significant emotional stress [5, 6].

The European Society for Human Reproduction and Embryology (ESHRE) PGD Consortium guidelines recommend genetic counselling (provided by qualified clinical geneticists and genetic counsellors) for patients: before and after an in-vitro fertilisation/PGD cycle; after the laboratory work up; and additional counselling at pre- and post-natal follow-up [7]. The first aim of this genetic counselling is to provide genetic and treatment information regarding the genetic condition or potential chromosomal abnormality in a way that is meaningful for each couple, and to provide support to assist patients to make a decision that is right for them. Genetic counsellors discuss the severity and inheritance pattern for a condition; record the family pedigree and any relevant family data; provide risk assessment and recurrence risk, and treatment and other reproductive options (such as choosing not to have children, adoption, or use of donor gametes or embryos). Counsellors will review the specific genetic test and limitations of testing (including the accuracy of the test, error rates, and what the test can and cannot diagnose); the expected number of oocytes that might be collected; the potential number of unaffected embryos, the number to be transferred, the potential transfer of carrier embryos, and cryopreservation of embryos not transferred. In addition to the benefits and limitations of testing, the cost and timing of the PGD process, and chance of success are also explored. It is going to become more common that PGD/PGS cycles are freeze all as it gives a longer time to perform the diagnosis and allows transport of the biopsied cells to the genetic diagnosis centre.

The second aim of genetic counselling is to counsel individuals contemplating PGD. Using a patient-centred, non-directive and non-judgmental approach, counsellors strive to develop a rapport with clients so that they can support them through the complex decision-making process, providing advice and problem solving or coping strategies. Individuals undergoing PGD make decisions about the number of embryos to transfer, options when there are no unaffected embryos, and the disposal or donation of embryos on completion of a family. PGD patients should also be advised to avoid having unprotected sex since a number of misdiagnoses are believed to have occurred due to this. As there is the small risk of a misdiagnosis and possible birth of an affected child, couples also need to consider pre-natal diagnosis (PND) of a pregnancy to confirm the genotype of the foetus. Hence, consent forms should include acknowledgement of the necessity to avoid unprotected sex and advised PND. Use of ART technologies is also linked to low birth weight, gestational and neonatal problems, and congenital abnormalities. In addition to treatment related decisions, genetic counsellors can also explore unrealistic expectations, concerns, communication with family and friends, and other general health issues, and can refer clients for psychological assessment or further counselling if required. Both the information and counselling aspects of genetic counselling are important to ensure clients feel adequately prepared to provide informed consent for PGD.

As with any medical treatment, there are associated risks with each step of the PGD process and patients need to understand the limitations. The accuracy (specificity and sensitivity) of the genetic test will vary and many tests are developed for the individual case. In addition, embryos may not survive the biopsy or culture process and many early embryos are mosaic, which may lead to a missed diagnosis or misdiagnosis [8–11]. Therefore, if a patient achieves a pregnancy, prenatal testing (which carries a small risk of miscarriage) is recommended to confirm the genotype. New ethical concerns have arisen over the use of PGD in a number of different scenarios: for gender selection for social reasons, to select against embryos carrying susceptibility to late-onset adult conditions (such as inherited forms of breast and ovarian cancer), and the creation of saviour siblings through the use of HLA typing to select embryos as potential donors for children with a severe haematological condition. This highlights the importance of up-to-date guidelines with involvement of professional bodies to ensure new trainees are aware of current recommendations, which will ensure the best outcomes for those undertaking PGD now and in the future. For example, in the UK it is now legally permissible for an infertile carrier for a late onset disease to have an affected embryo transferred should there be no other embryos available.

Equipment and Consumables

Historically, equipment that was considered necessary to establish a PGD clinical service included a micromanipulation rig incorporating a double tool-holder, so that zona-drilling and blastomere biopsy micropipettes could be set up along the same axis and used consecutively. Typically, the zona-drilling pipette would be back-filled prior to use with acidified medium (pH 2.3–2.5) such as Dulbecco's, Earle's or Tyrode's for the purpose of "burning" a hole through the zona pellucida (ZP). Though this arrangement had made it much easier to locate the hole drilled through the ZP, considerable skill was still required to control the size of the hole created using a flow of acid. Furthermore, there remained a real risk of over-exposure of the embryo to acid if the flow was not ceased and reversed immediately following zona-drilling, and it was necessary to rapidly remove the embryo away from the area of the micro-drop of media in which acid had been applied. Therefore, alternative means for zona-drilling were investigated including the use of contact and non-contact lasers, the latter being generally accepted as the preferred method these days by virtue of their relative safety, ease and speed of use. The significant cost of a laser is offset to some extent by the savings made by no longer having to forge or purchase zona-drilling micropipettes.

With the advent of laser-assisted oocyte and embryo biopsy, the choice of micro-manipulation rig is simplified by a high quality double tool-holder no longer being a deciding factor. Hence, any inverted microscope that can accommodate a laser and micromanipulation rig should be fit for purpose including those available from Leica, Leitz, Nikon and Olympus. Likewise, any micromanipulation rig that can be adapted to one or more inverted microscopes should be suitable including those available from Eppendorf, Narishige and Research Instruments (RI). The choice of laser system is less straightforward since their design features and associated image analysis software are more variable. Nevertheless, infrared (1.46–1.48 μm) non-contact laser systems are available from a number of reputable manufacturers including Hamilton Thorne, Medical Technology Vertriebs-Gmbh (MTG) and RI. The choice of micro-injector is largely determined by end-user preference over air injectors versus oil injectors, and a combination of both types may be used for holding the oocyte/ embryo in position and aspiration of the biopsied cell(s). Again, any micro-injectors that can be adapted to the tool holders of one or more micromanipulators are suitable, including those available from Eppendorf, Narishige and RI.

Consumables necessary for establishing a clinical service for PGD and PGS include powder-free gloves, DNA detergents, biopsy media, biopsy micropipettes, non-stick wash and transport buffer, DNA-free pipette tips, and UV-irradiated PCR tubes for collection and transport of cells.

Table 9.1 Example of a generic biopsy worksheet

Embryo stage and number	Embryo grade	Number of cells biopsied	Biopsied cell integrity	Visibility of nucleus
D3/1	8CG1	1	Intact	Visible
D3/2	8CG2	1	Intact	Visible
D3/3	6CG2	1	Intact	Visible
D3/4	6CG3	1	Intact	Not visible
D3/5	10CG2	1	Intact	Visible
D3/6	10CG3	2	Lysed/intact	Visible
D3/7	10CG4	0	N/A	N/A
D3/8	7CG2	1	Intact	Visible
D3/9	9CG2	2	Lysed/intact	Not visible
D3/10	4CG4	0	N/A	N/A

Labelling, Records and Database Entry

Accurate and thorough labelling and records of each oocyte and/or embryo biopsy dispatched for analysis are absolutely critical, both to avoid unnecessarily discarding a perfectly healthy embryo and the unwitting transfer of an affected embryo. Consequently, individual oocyte/embryo culture and double-witnessing of biopsies and biopsy tubing should be incorporated into the process to markedly reduce the risk of errors occurring. Furthermore, the double-witnessing of each biopsy should be documented using a biopsy worksheet (Table 9.1).

Depending upon the number of mature oocytes and/or embryos a patient has available for biopsy, several culture dishes may be required since it is essential to culture each embryo within an individual well so as to avoid any possibility of coalescence of media micro-drops resulting in potential uncertainty over the identity of two or more embryos. In this respect, 4-well plates are probably preferable to Petri dishes since only one 4-well plate is required to culture up to four embryos individually. Each culture dish and each well of each culture dish should be clearly labelled to avoid any confusion over the location of each and every embryo. Likewise, each biopsy dish and each micro-drop of biopsy media within each biopsy dish should be clearly labelled to concur with the labelling of each culture well to avoid any confusion over the identity and location of each and every biopsied cell. Every removal and replacement of an embryo in culture prior to and following biopsy should be double-witnessed and documented. Similarly, every removal of a biopsied cell from a biopsy dish should be double-witnessed and documented, as should the washing and tubing of those cells. The labelling of the PCR tubes into which the biopsied cells are placed should also be double-witnessed.

Provision of a Clinical Service for PGD/PGS

The effective provision of a clinical service for PGD and PGS requires considerable forward planning and organisation of resources, especially the availability of adequate staffing, equipment and consumables. Biopsies may be performed on the oocyte, zygote, cleavage stage embryo, morula or blastocyst but are typically carried out on days 0, 1, 3 and/or 5 of development. Therefore, only polar body, blastomere and trophectoderm biopsies will be discussed in this chapter. The ESHRE PGD consortium guidelines for the biopsy of oocytes and embryos have been proposed previously [12].

Scheduling and Planning of Patient Treatment

Since biopsy and tubing is extremely time-consuming and requires the undivided attention of at least two staff members, it is wise to plan well in advance precisely which are the optimal days of the week on which to perform oocyte and/or embryo biopsy. Once determined, it is then simply a matter of working back through the calendar to decide when to commence pituitary down-regulation and controlled ovarian hyper-stimulation (COH). It is also sensible not to overload staff with more PGD/PGS patients than they can properly cope with during any given period of time. Naturally, it will be necessary for all patients to have their oocytes inseminated via intra-cytoplasmic sperm injection (ICSI). In all cases it is vital that all cumulus cells, including the corona radiata, are removed from the ZP prior to biopsy in order to reduce the risk of a misdiagnosis.

Preparation of Biopsy Media and Consumables

Once a patient has begun COH it is advisable to check stocks of all media and consumables necessary to perform biopsy and tubing. Most centres offering genetic analysis will prefer to provide their own specimen collection buffer and UV irradiated PCR tubes. However, it is also necessary to have ready in place adequate supplies of biopsy media, dishes and micropipettes. Therefore, it is good practice to perform a monthly inventory of all relevant biopsy media and consumables to ensure adequate supplies are available as and when required. However, it is important to maintain the sterility of all consumables when conducting a stock inventory. Hence, any unwrapped items must be handled under laminar flow while wearing powder-free sterile gloves. An absolute minimum list of necessary biopsy media and consumables would be as follows:

Biopsy media
Biopsy micropipettes
Biopsy wash buffer

PCR collection/transport tubes
Permanent marker pens
Biopsy dishes
Pipette tips
Transfer pipettes

Decontamination of Biopsy Equipment and Working Areas

Contamination of biopsy samples can result from intrinsic factors, such as cumulus cells and spermatozoa, and from extrinsic factors, such as somatic cells from staff working within a laboratory. In order to minimise the risk of a misdiagnosis, it is important to ensure that the equipment to be used while handling biopsied material and the working area in which such handling will occur are wiped clean of any residual contaminating DNA. Donning powder-free sterile gloves, a DNA detergent such as DNA-*free*™ can be used along with sterile surgical swabs to wipe down stereo dissecting microscopes, pipettes and laminar flow working surfaces. Naturally, this is best done immediately prior to commencing the biopsy procedure and the gloves themselves should also be wiped over using the DNA detergent.

Sterile Clothing and Aseptic Technique

Contamination of biopsy samples with stray DNA from skin and hair cells can occur. Therefore, it is worthwhile minimising the risk of such contamination by implementing a policy whereby all staff involved in performing and witnessing a biopsy procedure are required to wear sterile clothing and practice aseptic technique. To achieve this, sterile surgical gowns, facemasks, hats and powder-free gloves should be worn at all times. All washing and tubing of biopsied samples should be performed within a laminar flow cabinet and all PCR tubes should remain capped when not in use.

Polar Body Biopsy

Biopsy of the first and second polar bodies is an approach suitable for determination of maternal genetic and chromosomal defects alone. It is essential in all cases of PGD and PGS that the first and second polar body are analysed. These can be biopsied simultaneously or sequentially. Sequentially, this is done by biopsy of the first polar body soon after oocyte retrieval (day 0) and the second polar body soon after fertilisation (day 1). Simultaneous biopsy is done on day 1. The advantages of polar body biopsy include early diagnosis during the treatment cycle, enabling fresh embryo transfer, and minimal impact upon subsequent embryogenesis since the polar bodies do not contribute to the further development of the embryo. The limitations of polar body biopsy are that only the maternal chromosomes are analysed and there is a potential for misdiagnosis due to subsequent post-zygotic aneuploidy. The risk of a misdiagnosis may be minimised in the latter instance by following up second polar body with blastomere and/or trophectoderm biopsy.

Denudation, ICSI and biopsy dishes are prepared and pre-equilibrated to 37°C using a non-CO_2 dependent buffered medium such as MOPS or HEPES. Oocytes are denuded prior to biopsy using cumulase or hyaluronidase, according to the standard operating procedure (SOP) of oocyte preparation for ICSI. Evidently, only those oocytes that have progressed to metaphase II (MII) and have extruded the first polar body are amenable to biopsy. Of the MII oocytes, however, only those possessing an intact polar body should be considered suitable for biopsy since fragmented polar bodies will not yield a valid result following PGD. All MII oocytes with an intact polar body are inseminated via ICSI immediately prior to the biopsy procedure. To perform the biopsy, the injected oocyte is held with its polar body at either the 6 o'clock or 12 o'clock position using a holding micropipette and a non-contact infrared laser is used to drill a hole in the ZP large enough for a polar body biopsy micropipette to pass through. The hole should be drilled at such a position that the biopsy micropipette will meet the polar body when introduced through the ZP along a horizontal axis. In order to keep the polar body intact during the biopsy procedure, it is important to keep the aspiration pressure low so that the polar body is removed very slowly and does not disappear up the biopsy micropipette. Once aspirated from the oocyte, the polar body should be deposited in the biopsy microdrop away from where the oocyte is placed for ease of subsequent handling. Each biopsied oocyte is then transferred from the biopsy dish into a separate well of a clearly labelled 4-well culture dish containing pre-equilibrated fertilisation or early cleavage media, this being double-witnessed and recorded on the biopsy worksheet. Its corresponding polar body is washed in non-stick biopsy buffer and placed into a clearly labelled PCR tube, this also being double-witnessed and recorded on the biopsy worksheet.

Blastomere Biopsy

Biopsy of one or two blastomeres is an approach suitable for determination of post-zygotic genetic defects of both maternal and paternal origin. Blastomere biopsy is typically performed early on day-3 before compaction has begun. The main advantage of blastomere biopsy is early diagnosis during the treatment cycle, enabling fresh embryo transfer. The limitations of blastomere biopsy include loss of embryonic genetic material and misdiagnosis as a consequence of mosaicism, which is most common at this stage. Biopsy of two blastomeres decreases the risk of a misdiagnosis but increases the risk of impairment to subsequent development [13].

Biopsy dishes are prepared and pre-equilibrated to 37°C using a non-CO_2 dependent buffered biopsy medium, such as MOPS or HEPES, devoid of divalent cations

(Ca^{2+}/Mg^{2+} free). Each micro-drop of media within each biopsy dish is clearly labelled to correspond with each cleavage stage embryo to be biopsied. Usually, only those embryos containing at least six clearly defined blastomeres on day-3 are considered suitable for biopsy. Each embryo for biopsy is placed into its corresponding micro-drop of biopsy medium for 10 min to loosen the tight junctions between adjacent blastomeres, this being double-witnessed. To perform the biopsy, the embryo is held in place using a holding micropipette and a non-contact infrared laser is used to drill a hole just large enough for a blastomere to squeeze through but small enough to avoid unintentional loss of further blastomeres during washing of the embryo following biopsy. In order to avoid lysis of the blastomere during the biopsy procedure, it is important to keep the aspiration pressure low so that the blastomere is removed very slowly and does not disappear up the biopsy micropipette. Once aspirated from the embryo, the blastomere should be deposited in the biopsy micro-drop away from where the embryo is placed for ease of subsequent handling. Each biopsied embryo is then transferred from the biopsy dish into a separate well of a clearly labelled 4-well culture dish containing pre-equilibrated blastocyst culture media, this being double-witnessed and recorded on the biopsy worksheet. Its corresponding blastomere is washed in non-stick biopsy buffer and placed into a clearly labelled PCR tube, this also being double-witnessed and recorded on the biopsy worksheet.

Trophectoderm Biopsy

Biopsy of several (2–10) cells from the trophectoderm lining the blastocyst is an approach suitable for determination of post-cleavage genetic defects of both maternal and paternal origin. Trophectoderm biopsy is typically performed on day-5, and occasionally on day-6. The main advantages of trophectoderm biopsy are that it provides more cells for analysis and avoids loss of cells from the inner cell mass, which is the tissue destined to become the foetus. The limitations of trophectoderm biopsy include the inability of all embryos to develop to the blastocyst stage and the risk of misdiagnosis due to chromosomal mosaicism between the trophectoderm and inner cell mass.

One approach to performing trophectoderm biopsy is to drill a hole in the ZP of all day-3 embryos in order to assist subsequent herniation of the trophectoderm by day-5. Early on day-5, the development of all embryos is assessed to determine which of them have reached the blastocyst stage, possess an inner cell mass and display evidence of trophectoderm herniation; it is these embryos which are suitable for trophectoderm biopsy. Alternatively, blastocysts may be zona-drilled at the onset of the biopsy procedure to obtain access to trophectoderm cells. Biopsy dishes are prepared and pre-equilibrated to 37 °C using a non-CO_2 dependent buffered medium such as MOPS or HEPES. Each micro-drop of media in each biopsy dish is clearly labelled to correspond with each blastocyst to be biopsied, transfer of each blastocyst to each biopsy dish being double-witnessed. To perform the biopsy, the blastocyst is held in place using a holding micropipette such that the herniating trophectoderm is visible along the same axis but on the opposite side from the holding micropipette. Using a blastocyst biopsy micropipette, aspirate 2–10 of the herniating trophectoderm cells and pull them far enough away from the remainder of the trophectoderm within the ZP in order to stretch the cells connecting the two. Using a non-contact infrared laser, rupture the cell junctions adjacent to the leading edge of the biopsy micropipette, moving the position of the laser each time it is activated in order to avoid causing the tissue to become tough and fibrous. It is important to control the aspiration pressure immediately following detachment of the herniating trophectoderm cells so that they do not disappear up the biopsy micropipette. Once separated from the blastocyst, the trophectoderm cells should be deposited in the biopsy micro-drop away from where the blastocyst is placed for ease of subsequent handling. Each biopsied blastocyst is then returned to its separate well within each clearly labelled 4-well culture dish containing pre-equilibrated blastocyst culture media, this being double-witnessed and recorded on the biopsy worksheet. Its corresponding trophectoderm cells are washed in non-stick biopsy buffer and placed into a clearly labelled PCR tube, this also being double-witnessed and recorded on the biopsy worksheet.

Preparation, Co-ordination and Dispatch of Biopsied Material

All preparative steps, including washing and tubing of biopsied cells, should be double-witnessed and, therefore, it is necessary for the embryologist performing the procedure to be assisted by another embryologist. To minimise contamination of the biopsied cells from extrinsic factors such as stray DNA, it is important that both embryologists wear non-powdered sterile gloves, surgical gown, facemask and hat, and that all procedures are performed within a laminar flow cabinet. Keeping the PCR tubes capped when not in use also minimises the risk of contamination. To minimise contamination of the biopsied cells from intrinsic factors such as cell material from different biopsies, it is important that pipette tips are replaced with unused sterile tips between all washes with non-stick buffer. Also, it is good practice to rinse each unused sterile tip with three or more loadings/flushings of clean, unused non-stick buffer. Should there be any suspicion that any consumable has been in contact with a potential source of contamination such as a non-sterile surface or exposed skin then it should be replaced with an unused sterile item.

To avoid iatrogenic lysis of biopsied cells, they should be handled as gently as possible during the washing process, which typically involves pipetting them through 3–5 micro-drops of clean, unused non-stick buffer. Polar bodies are particularly fragile and susceptible to lysis, so it is wise to simply place them into just one micro-drop of non-stick buffer before transferring them immediately into a PCR tube. Indeed, in our experience (Steven Fleming and Peter Sprober; personal communication) perfectly good analysis results may be achieved without incorporating potentially hazardous multiple washes of biopsied cells. To achieve efficient washing, it is good practice to rinse and preload the pipette tip with clean, unused non-stick buffer from the micro-drop to which the biopsied cells are to be moved, flooding the biopsied cells with a few microliters of the freshly preloaded buffer before aspirating them into the pipette tip and transferring them to the wash micro-drop.

Following washing, cells are transferred to a PCR tube in a minimal volume (≤ 2 µl) of non-stick buffer so as to prevent excessive dilution of cell lysis and DNA amplification reagents during subsequent analysis. The cells are pipetted directly into the conical bottom of a clearly labelled PCR tube, this being double-witnessed and recorded on the biopsy worksheet, and the PCR tube is immediately recapped. It is important not to introduce any air bubbles while pipetting the cells into the PCR tube so as to avoid bubbles subsequently bursting, which may result in loss of cells further up the PCR tube or cell lysis. Due to the highly transparent nature of the PCR tube walls, it may be possible to visualise the cells within the tube to verify their successful transfer. Should this prove difficult, an alternative approach is to observe the expulsion of the cells onto the sidewall of the PCR tube, a few millimetres above the bottom of the tube. However, it then becomes necessary to microfuge the cells to the bottom of the PCR tube prior to packaging and transport of the biopsy samples.

Once tubing of all biopsies is complete, it is good practice to double-check that the labelling of the PCR tubes matches what has been recorded on the biopsy worksheet in order to verify that each and every biopsy can be accounted for with respect to patient ID and each embryo, whether it be remaining in culture or having been vitrified. The biopsy samples may then be placed into a PCR tube rack with the lid securely fastened down with sticky tape. The rack may then be carefully packed into an appropriate insulated shipping container such as a poly-foam container or small Eski™, and completely surrounded with pre-frozen ice packs or dry ice. It is important to pack the container well enough to prevent unnecessary movement of the PCR tube rack. The container should be securely sealed using packing tape and should be immediately sent to a facility for molecular genetic analysis, along with any necessary paperwork, by courier or via some other form of specially rapid same-day delivery. This is especially important if there is to be any possibility of receiving the results of analysis soon enough in order to perform a fresh embryo transfer of an unaffected embryo. Notification of the delivery should be sent to the analysis facility, along with any available tracking and staff contact information. In this way, the analysis facility will be adequately prepared to perform the analysis immediately upon receipt of the biopsy samples and will be able to email the results through as soon as they are available.

Methods of Analysis and Interpretation of Results

As stated earlier, it is not within the scope of this chapter to delve into the detailed methodology of molecular genetic analysis, so this section is merely a very brief and superficial overview of the methods currently in use and analysis of the results they produce. The chromosomal and genetic make-up of oocytes and preimplantation embryos may be analysed using a variety of methods. Historically, these methods included PCR, metaphase cytogenetics, interphase multiplex FISH, primed in situ labelling, and spectral imaging. More recently, powerful methods with a fast turn-around have been developed including WGA, CGH and NGS.

Fluorescence In Situ Hybridisation

Interphase FISH was used for many years as the main means of PGD for chromosomal aneuploidies, translocations and inversions and PGS [14, 15]. However, FISH methodology was prone to various analysis problems including signal overlapping or splitting, loss of micronuclei during fixation, and hybridisation failure, especially where more than one round of hybridisation was required in order to analyse more chromosomes [16]. Hence, FISH proved not to be a suitable technique for obtaining a complete karyotype from a single cell, which is what provision of a reliable clinical service for PGD and PGS demands.

Comparative Genomic Hybridisation

Complete karyotyping is possible using CGH since it allows the entire genome to be screened for differences in DNA sequence copy number using just a single hybridisation, comparing the patient sample against a DNA sample reference. Furthermore, since CGH analyses the entire length of each chromosome it is also able to detect segmental aneuploidy [17, 18]. Array CGH utilises individual probes spotted onto glass slides and an overnight hybridisation step. Since the patient and reference DNA samples are labelled with different fluorochromes (traditionally, green for the patient and red for the reference), their comparative hybridisation to each probe will result in a green–red ratio of fluorescence that can be rapidly interpreted via fluorescence image analysis. Hence, gains of DNA sequences (e.g. trisomy) in the patient sample are indicated by a ratio >1:1 whereas losses (e.g. monosomy) are indicated by a ratio <1:1.

Combined with WGA of single cells and using DNA libraries specific to the 24 human chromosomes [19], array CGH has proven to be a powerful and reliable method of analysis for PGD and PGS [20, 21]. However, one of the limitations of CGH is that it cannot detect haploidy and polyploidy, though these aberrations are usually observed during fertilisation checks. Furthermore, there remains a very small risk of misdiagnosis and, therefore, ongoing management of patients needs to take such risk into consideration. For this reason, patients are often advised to have PND should they become pregnant following PGD or PGS. CGH is rapidly being replaced by NGS, which is cheaper and gives more information than CGH.

Risk Assessment and Auditing of PGD/PGS

Since PGD and PGS are highly complex, expensive clinical services, it is important to properly assess their relative benefits and risks for patients individually and collectively within any given facility. Equally important, audits of PGD and PGS data should be conducted regularly to determine the quality of the service provided both in terms of the percentage of embryos yielding valid data and the percentage of normal live births eventuating. The latter is particularly relevant in light of recent reports suggesting that PGS does not significantly increase live birth rate.

Summary

ART facilities offering PGD and PGS are now established in many cities around the world. These clinical services offer an effective means of avoiding pregnancies in which the foetus would almost certainly be either aborted or born suffering a serious genetic condition. For the patient, it avoids the trauma of miscarriage, termination, or a lifetime caring for a severely disabled child. For the state, it represents a considerable saving in medical care expenditure, so is a clinical service that should be adequately funded.

References

1. Handyside AH, Kontogianni EH, Hardy K, Winston RML. Pregnancies from biopsied human preimplantation embryos sexed by Y-specific DNA amplification. Nature. 1990;344:768–70.
2. Wells D, Sherlock JK, Handyside AH, Delhanty JD. Detailed chromosomal and molecular genetic analysis of single cells by whole genome amplification and comparative genomic hybridisation. Nucleic Acids Res. 1999;27:1214–8.
3. Zenzes MT, Casper RF. Cytogenetics of human oocytes, zygotes and embryos after in vitro fertilisation. Hum Genet. 1992;88:367–75.
4. Delhanty J, Griffin D, Handyside AH, Harper JC, Atkinson G, Pieters MHEC, Winston RML. Detection of aneuploidy and chromosomal mosaicism in human embryos during preimplantation sex determination by fluorescent in situ hybridisation (FISH). Hum Mol Genet. 1993;2:1183–5.
5. Lavery SA, Aurell R, Turner C, Castellu C, Veiga A, Barri PN, Winston RM. Preimplantation genetic diagnosis: patients' experiences and attitudes. Hum Reprod. 2002;17:2464–7.
6. Karatas JC, Barlow-Stewart K, Strong KA, Meiser B, McMahon C, Roberts C. Women's experience of pre-implantation genetic diagnosis: a qualitative study. Prenat Diagn. 2010;30:771–7.
7. Harton G, Braude P, Lashwood A, Schmutzler A, Traeger-Synodinos J, Wilton L, Harper J. ESHRE PGD consortium best practice guidelines for organization of a PGD centre for PGD/preimplantation genetic screening. Hum Reprod. 2011;26:14–24.
8. Colls P, Escudero T, Cekleniak N, Sadowy S, Cohen J, Munne S. Increased efficiency of preimplantation genetic diagnosis for infertility using "no result rescue". Fertil Steril. 2007;88:53–61.
9. DeUgarte CM, Li M, Surrey M, Danzer H, Hill D, DeCherney AH. Accuracy of FISH analysis in predicting chromosomal status in patients undergoing preimplantation genetic diagnosis. Fertil Steril. 2008;90:1049–54.
10. Hanson C, Hardarson T, Lundin K, Bergh C, Hillensjo T, Stevic J, Westin C, Selleskog U, Rogberg L, Wikland M. Re-analysis of 166 embryos not transferred after PGS with advanced reproductive maternal age as indication. Hum Reprod. 2009;24:2960–4.
11. Wilton L, Thornhill A, Traeger-Synodinos J, Sermon KD, Harper JC. The causes of misdiagnosis and adverse outcomes in PGD. Hum Reprod. 2009;24:1221–8.
12. Harton GL, Magli MC, Lundin K, Montag M, Lemmen J, Harper JC. ESHRE PGD Consortium/Embryology Special Interest Group—best practice guidelines for polar body and embryo biopsy for preimplantation genetic diagnosis/screening (PGD/PGS). Hum Reprod. 2011;26:41–6.
13. Scott Jr RT, Upham KM, Forman EJ, Zhao T, Treff NR. Cleavage-stage biopsy significantly impairs human embryonic implantation potential while blastocyst biopsy does not: a randomized and paired clinical trial. Fertil Steril. 2013;100:624–30.
14. Griffin D, Wilton L, Handyside A, Winston R, Delhanty J. Pregnancies following the diagnosis of sex in preimplantation embryos by fluorescent in situ hybridisation. Br Med J. 1993;306:1382–3.

15. Harper JC, Dawson K, Delhanty JD, Winston RM. The use of fluorescent in-situ hybridization (FISH) for the analysis of in-vitro fertilization embryos: a diagnostic tool for the infertile couple. Hum Reprod. 1995;10:3255–8.
16. Liu J, Tsai Y-L, Zheng X-Z, Yazigi RA, Baramki TA, Compton G, Katz E. Feasibility study of repeated fluorescent in-situ hybridization in the same blastomeres for preimplantation genetic diagnosis. Mol Hum Reprod. 1998;4:972–7.
17. Voullaire L, Wilton L, Slater H, Williamson R. Detection of aneuploidy in single cells using comparative genomic hybridisation. Prenat Diagn. 1999;19:846–51.
18. Voullaire L, Slater H, Williamson R, Wilton L. Chromosome analysis of blastomeres from human embryos by using comparative genomic hybridisation. Hum Genet. 2000;106:210–7.
19. Wells D, Delhanty JD. Comprehensive chromosomal analysis of human preimplantation embryos using whole genome amplification and single cell comparative genomic hybridization. Mol Hum Reprod. 2000;6:1055–62.
20. Wilton L, Williamson R, McBain J, Edgar D, Voullaire L. Birth of a healthy infant after preimplantation confirmation of euploidy by comparative genomic hybridisation. N Engl J Med. 2001;345:1537–41.
21. Hu DG, Webb G, Hussey N. Aneuploidy detection in single cells using DNA array-based comparative genomic hybridisation. Mol Hum Reprod. 2004;10:283–9.

Chapter 10
Data Management in the ART Unit

John P.P. Tyler

Introduction

When I began my career in "fertility" in the early 1970s my first research project involved sorting collected data by pushing a metal rod through holes punched around the outside edge of cards. Each hole represented a data variable and was clipped through to the edge if it applied. Lifting out un-clipped cards left those you wanted to find. If a recent publication [1] reviewing 121,744 records used the same card format it would require a rod almost 5 m long! Thankfully, time, processes, software and the hardware to run it have evolved since the first consumer computers became available in the mid 1970s. Does anyone remember Visicalc software? Suddenly we simple scientists had a tool we could control ourselves rather than rely on tech-heads in the Information Technology (IT) department who frequently did not think like us.

The patient record should of course be considered the central point for managing a single person's care across time at a particular ART clinic. Examples of possible sections and their inclusions are given in Table 10.1, although the list is not exhaustive. The long-term maintenance of complete and accurate medical records is also a requirement of health care providers and is generally enforced as a licensing or certification prerequisite.

Traditionally, medical records have been written on paper and maintained in folders divided into sections (e.g. progress, orders and prescriptions, and test results), with new information being added to each section chronologically. To the next professional talking to that patient the paper file gives an overall feel for what has happened before.

J.P.P. Tyler, PhD (✉)
Next Generation Fertility, 1 Fennell St., Parramatta, NSW 2151, Australia
e-mail: john@tylers.com.au

© Springer Science+Business Media New York 2016
S.D. Fleming, A.C. Varghese (eds.), *Organization and Management of IVF Units*, DOI 10.1007/978-3-319-29373-8_10

Table 10.1 Examples of sections and their inclusions in an ART patient's paper medical record

Sections in a patient's paper file	Examples of inclusions
Identification	The patient's accession number(s). The patient's address. The patient's phone and email contacts. Details of spouse/partner. Links to use of donor tissue.
Consultations	Details of different clinicians and medical specialists previously visited. Details of Counselling sessions. Details of Genetic Counsellor sessions.
Medical history	Detailed general medical history for female and male. Gynaecological and Obstetric history for female. Andrological history for male. Specific history regarding the couple. Genetic histories if relevant. Diagnoses.
Medical management and progress notes	Detailed documentation of a patient's clinical status or achievements during care.
Investigative results	Endocrine reports. Serology reports. Semen analyses reports. Radiology/ultrasound reports. Genetic reports. Operative and surgical reports. Embryology and cryopreservation reports.
Consents and agreements	Informed consent: treatment(s). Informed consent: giving or receiving donated material. Informed consent: cryopreservation. Acknowledgement of privacy laws. Informed consent: release of patient information.
Treatments	Details of each and every treatment undertaken in the unit including outcomes.
Drug administration	Records of all medications given and used including batch numbers, etc.
Correspondence	Patient referral documentation. Copies of all letters sent to referring practitioners. Letters to and from the patient. Copies of all statutory and regulatory submissions.

Paper-based records do however require a significant amount of storage space, have a habit of becoming "lost" when required and maintenance of them, and filing into them, is time consuming and labour intensive. Similarly, while the correct record may be filed in a patients notes finding it easily can often present a challenge. Thus the evolving electronic health record [2, 3] not only reduces the cost of storage (i.e. no compactus systems are required) but also allows quick, simple finding of data. Electronic records are simply a digital record of the traditional patient notes but maintained in a format capable of being used securely and shared simultaneously by numerous staff whether within the same facility or across geographically separate locations.

Finally, each set of notes for an individual (whether paper or electronic) uniquely identifies that person by way of several labels. These include but are not limited to that person's first and last names, their date of birth and their accession or Medical Record number. An electronic database organises this collection of data and, if relational and well designed to "interact" with the user, can use the above identifiers to handle many different ways of displaying content. This is particularly important for infertility patients since, unlike the classic paper patient notes of the past, it is a couple that are being treated and a database easily allows information from each "linked" partner to be reviewed.

While this chapter covers many aspects of data management in a modern day ART clinic particular attention is paid to aspects pertaining to patient management and embryology laboratory data with such features as patient billing and accounts, purchasing and the control of appointments assumed to use standard commercially available systems whether they are integrated or not. This author strongly believes a functional database is a fundamental attribute for the establishment and running of a successful ART Unit.

Current Use of Databases in ART Units

Today, the data management of a patient's treatment should have electronic components even if the ART Unit is not fully paperless. To test this premise a survey has been conducted via EmbryoMail, the moderated discussion group devoted to mammalian embryology (http://www.embryomail.net), using Survey Monkey, a cloud based, anonymous web survey system (https://www.surveymonkey.com). The results have been used to illustrate aspects of this chapter.

The request to participate in the survey was posted at the end of January 2014 and when closed several weeks later 123 replies from multiple countries had been received (Fig. 10.1). Surprisingly, when asked the question "Does your embryology laboratory use a database to record and review patient treatments?" nine ART Clinics (8 %: Fig. 10.2) replied "No" inferring they relied solely on paperwork alone to manage their embryological data. This might suggest that their ability to adequately monitor and review their Unit's performance would be less than adequate. It was also noticeable that most of the replies to the survey came from North America, Europe and Australasia, the initiators of ART, but the few replies from the rapidly growing "markets" of Asia, India, South America and Africa gave very similar responses.

Database vs. Spreadsheet

Most people would be familiar with a spreadsheet (i.e. Microsoft Excel) and as shown in Fig. 10.3 it remains their preferred option to handle ART data. These computer programs organise data in tabular form (i.e. in rows and columns) and

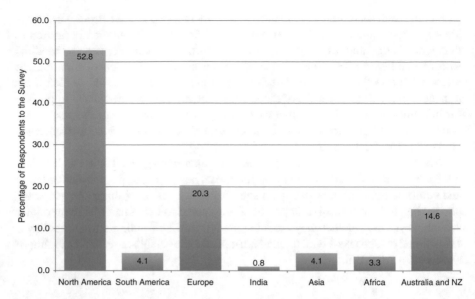

Fig. 10.1 Survey responses to the question "In what Geographic area of the world is your clinic located?"

allow user defined calculations and analysis after "sorts and finds" (filtering) to create a summary in various graphical or chart formats.

However, a spreadsheet has weaknesses for an ART Unit. Firstly, multiple people cannot usually access the data simultaneously and you need to safeguard against erroneous entries and inadvertent corruption by well meaning but perhaps poorly trained staff. Who has not sorted on the last name of a patient, but not included any of the other columns, thereby effectively randomising the data and requiring retrieval of the last backup!

Secondly, if you want the information for long-term storage then data duplication can become an issue. For instance, if the rows of your spreadsheet contain fields like a patient's name and address on each record that information will eventually cause problems. The same patient's address may be different in, say, three of ten treatment cycles or the woman might have changed from using her maiden name to that of her husband, so which one is currently correct (or non offending) for correspondence? A relational database where data tables are related to each other keeps this information in only one place allowing easy update, minimising redundancy and disk storage space.

For the modern ART Unit databases are therefore the best option but they, in turn, are usually limited in their ability to create "good-looking" charts for reports. Thus in most cases, using a combination of a database to store, maintain and summarise patient records with a spreadsheet to analyse selected, exported information for reporting purposes works best.

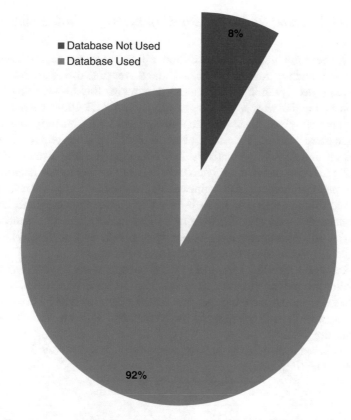

Fig. 10.2 Survey responses to the question "Does your embryology laboratory use a database to record and review patient treatments?"

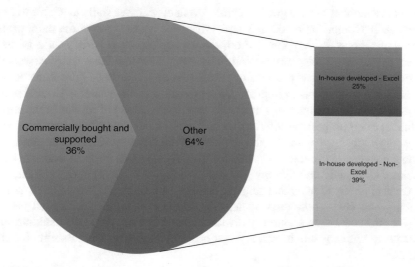

Fig. 10.3 Survey responses to the question "What type of database do you use?"

Commercial Versus In-House Development of a Database

It has always been my premise that an in-house database allows much more flexibility than a commercially purchased package since over time use of an in-house database is equally as dynamic as a patient's treatment. But in-house packages do require constant maintenance. If I were starting a new ART Unit then purchase of a complete commercial package with integrated patient billing and appointments, etc. would make more practical and financial sense especially since you would likely be a stand-alone unit requiring relatively few operating licences usually purchased annually. Similarly because there is no existing data to import the data dictionary for the computer program (which defines each field, the format of the information it contains and relationships, etc.) can be used to create processes and laboratory paper worksheets ensuring collection of required information. In essence you are purchasing a proven, already thought out system with access to assistance from knowledgeable programmers to meet your local conditions.

However, herein also lies a long-term disadvantage of the commercial tactic. In order to tailor the package to your circumstances the underlying software application has to be modified meaning that any future upgrades will involve additional cost and may take time to implement. And remember, software and hardware *will* change over time.

This may be one reason why 64 % of respondents to the survey favoured use of in-house systems (Fig. 10.3).

Commercially Available Systems

There are a number of very good integrated systems commercially available to manage an ART Clinic. Table 10.2 is a non-exhaustive list of some of the more prominent applications and suppliers. From the survey the most widely used of these appear to be Baby Sentry (http://www.babysentry.com) and Ideas (http://www.mellowoodmedical.com) and the developers of these programs have spent considerable time liaising with clients to improve their product over the years. A Google search also shows up other contenders and there was also a spread of replies in the survey including eIVF (http://www.eivf.org), and MediTex IVF (http://www.meditex-software.com). Most run on the Windows platform but if you were an Apple aficionado using a conversion program to "virtually" run Windows on MacOS would not be a problem. Ultimately, as with any program, training of staff is going to be required but the availability of technical help, particularly at installation, would be part of the establishment cost. Those respondents of the survey who used commercial systems did not add comments about any dislike of their system, so when deciding on a package, as with any purchase it is about cost, functionality and suitability for your purposes.

Table 10.2 Examples of commercially available ART Unit Management Databases

Name of software	Company	Country	Website or contact
ARTis	Simplus Software Private Ltd	India	http://www.artisivf.com
Babe IVF System	Cleodora Medical Ltd	Finland	Cleodora.software@gmail.com
BabySentryPro	Medical and Genetics Software Corp	USA	http://www.babysentry.com info@babysentry.com
DynaMed	IMA Systems	Germany	http://ima-systems.com sales@ima-systems.com
eIVF	PacificHwy.com Inc	USA	http://www.eivf.org sales@ practicehwy.com
FertiMorph	Image House Medical	Denmark	http://cellcura.com post@cellcura.com
IDEAS	Mellowood Medical	Canada	http://mellowoodmedical.com info@mellowoodmedical.com
PALASH IVF	Seed Healthcare Solution	India	http://seedhealthcare.com nileshk@seedhealthcare.com
IVF Software	Fertsoft AB	Sweden	http://www.fertsoft.com Martin.bjorkman@fertsoft.com
MeDialog IVF	Armada OAO	Russia	http://www.armadaitgroup.com IR@armd.ru
Ankh Clinic and Laboratory E-SUITE	ANKH Data Systems	USA	http://ankhdatasystems.com
MediTEX	MediTEX GmbH	Germany	http://www.meditex-software.com meditex@critex.de
Carpusoft IVF	Carpusoft d.o.o	Croatia	http://www.carpusoft.hr info@carpusoft.hr
Cloudenvision	Envision	USA	www.cloudenvision.com cloudenvision@gmail.com

In-House Developed Systems

Two-thirds of respondents in the survey used in-house developed ART Databases. This seemed a lot but the sample size of 123 would not be a high proportion of the ART labs in the world, simply those interested in completing a survey hosted via EmbryoMail. It might also suggest that perhaps these were long established Units where in-house development was a necessity before commercial software became available. Similarly, applications used were "standard" software with Microsoft Excel predominating. A spreadsheet accounted for 28/72 (38.9 %) but a similar proportion used databases including Microsoft Access, SQL and FileMaker Pro.

What Data Should Be Collected?

A fundamental question! Scientists will tell you that as time elapses the questions change and thus the amount of data collected may also alter, meaning they usually expand! While commercial packages may allow additional data fields to be added this is certainly an area where in-house developed databases are proficient. The flexibility of being able to add (or hide from view) data fields as treatment options for a couple change (a recent example would be the addition of parameters generated from video recordings of embryo culture e.g. use of an EmbryoScope) or as research projects come and go, requires only a small amount of programming. Similarly should you ever wish to publish from your database and avoid criticism then sufficient well-collected data is required [4].

How Much Data Should Be Collected?

The survey responses again suggest the way ART Units operate. There was a spread of replies from <25 data points to >200 but those Units collecting the least amount of data (~33 % collect <50 fields) would not have a particularly good handle on their performance (Fig. 10.4). To put this into perspective the Australian auditing body overseen by the Reproductive Technology Accreditation Committee (RTAC), feels it prudent to collect 94 fields of data for each individual treatment cycle attempt in order to adequately report on national birth outcomes [5]. The UK's regulatory body, Human Fertilization and Embryology Authority (HFEA), appears to collect less data (approx. 60 fields) but in the USA the Society of Assisted Reproductive Technologies (SART) requires more at 200. These latter regulatory bodies create different reports to that of Australia including identifying individual clinics.

A recent speaker at the annual congress of the Asia Pacific Initiative on Reproduction [6] has also stated that fertility registers should be set up in the "emerging" ART markets of China and Indonesia and that India is attempting to do this by voluntarily asking its clinics to input data over the Internet. While only 26 data points are requested, significantly limiting interpretation, this is a start.

Couple Medical History

Summary of any form of ART data requires basic demographic information to be collected. Obvious parameters include the individual's age (ART outcome such as ovarian stimulation, number of oocytes collected and miscarriage rate is directly related to female age), their height and weight (use of FSH is directly related to BMI), and contacts (address for correspondence, phone number for SMS's and nurse liaison, etc.). These parameters generally remain fixed although sometimes a person's weight reduces as they take advice from their managing clinician!

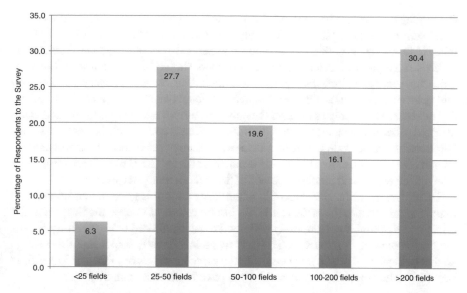

Fig. 10.4 Survey responses to the question "How much data do you collect in each record of an IVF/ICSI treatment cycle?"

Naturally a diagnosis derived from investigative tests and responses to treatment should also be included for both the man and woman since the prognosis, for example, for a woman with only tubo-peritoneal issues will be different to one who has PCO and a partner with a triple defect semen analysis result. Provision should also be made for multiple factors.

The Treatment Plan

Armed with a diagnosis obtained from a competent clinical couple work-up, a plan of treatment recorded in a database allows nursing staff to easily begin and coordinate a couple's treatment cycle. Treatment of course should not only include IVF/ICSI but also allow for less invasive forms of management including ovulation induction with timed coitus and IUI. Similarly administration staff can use the plan to accurately bill couples at reception giving the impression that a clinic is well organised and has good communication. Anything that instils confidence in a couple helps reduce their overall stress levels and may improve their outcome to treatment.

Female Ovarian Stimulation and Oocyte Collection

Data collected on ovarian stimulation are necessary clinical measures. Not only should the amount of medication given to a woman be recorded but also the starting dose, type (i.e. recombinant FSH or urinary products and source, etc.), method of use (i.e. agonist or antagonist approach) and batch/lot numbers so that in the unlikely event of a recall those patients receiving it can be easily identified. A simple form letter to those patients affected can then be generated very quickly from a database.

This same premise also means batch numbers should be recorded for all disposables for embryo culture and other ware including oocyte recovery needles and embryo transfer catheters. Of course with a relational database batch and lot numbers can be entered once only as the date they are first used. Then by a simple relationship affected patients can be identified. This latter approach can reduce data entry for staff particularly if a bar code reader is used. Summarising data by drug type and amount should be a standard clinical Key Performance Indicator (KPI) used to review a clinician's competence and identify risk of OHSS and other adverse events.

Finally, in countries like Australia where drug supply is government funded and is not a direct cost to the patient, it is likely that return of unused medication to the clinic (for disposal not re-supply!) will need to be monitored more carefully from a medical economics perspective. The cost to society of over dispensing these drugs so that patients will not be inconvenienced by having to return to the clinic multiple times to collect more is, in future, likely to have more accountability.

Male Semen Data and Sperm Preparation

For a long time the contribution of the male to ART outcome has been underplayed but as more "mining" of databases occurs unforeseen relationships have been found. Male age is now also seen as a determinant of pregnancy rate outcome and many clinics no longer use ICSI for all couples successfully diagnosing those who only require IVF. This modality also has economic advantages to the clinic requiring less staff time and practical oocyte and sperm preparation. Similarly the attention to detail in sperm preparation pre-insemination long touted by research seminologists is also now apparent. Time to "event" monitoring can also be used as an embryologist KPI.

Fertilisation and Embryo Culture

This is the domain of the embryologist and given their scientific training should be where all data necessary in their interpretation of culture and control of their laboratory should occur. It has been my experience that embryologists always want to improve their work and/or find out why others have perhaps better fertilisation rates or lower post ICSI degeneration rates. Thus all fields in this area of the database, and any summary reports automatically generated, should be available to all scientific staff and not be restricted to management. Openness breeds improvement and transparency. Locking down summary reports to management only access will significantly stifle staff interest and thus the quality improvement processes.

When I have reviewed commercial software systems there are usually multiple windows for embryo data entry and when closed they disappear behind the programmers' structure. Being able to see all data in a single layout may seem too busy to some but embryology is about interpretation, not only of summary data but also of separate pieces of data. For instance a person who has ten oocytes collected but only has one blastocyst for transfer may have had a high rate of GV's or 3PN's initially or a poor blastocyst utilisation rate with perhaps culture ceasing at the morula stage or the creation of poorly formed blastocysts not suitable for cryopreservation. These scenarios provide two different stories to the patient particularly if the database has been programmed to be able to see the culture outcomes of all oocytes ever collected across multiple treatment cycles. It is surprising how repeatable culture of one couple's embryos can be when this is reviewed. Then when the outcome of any thawed frozen embryos is added the picture can become even clearer. Often, as embryologists, we never fully summarise or perhaps even review our embryo culture for patients. Furthermore, as methods for videoing embryos evolve and PGD/PGS gains acceptance, and becomes less expensive as a standard procedure for each embryo, these details also need inclusion in ART databases.

Similarly, reviewing all oocytes collected over a time period, irrespective of the number collected from an individual, allows audit of ovarian stimulation protocols perhaps prompting review of drug use policy.

Embryo Cryopreservation

This is an area where databases totally outperform spreadsheets. When embryos are frozen and thawed it is possible to automatically keep track of those remaining in store and easily create dewar inventories either in location or patient last name order. If a spreadsheet is used unless the user has particular programming skills I usually see the tracking of embryos being maintained manually. This approach is fraught with problems. Similarly, such units frequently do not (or cannot) do a complete annual stocktake of their liquid nitrogen dewars (because of its difficulty) so I suspect it is likely that they are losing considerable income from cryostorage fees as administration loses the ability to interrogate those patients requiring follow-up invoices. While this might seem imprudent and a little unethical to some social minded staff the ability to make a profit from treating patients in an ART Unit is fundamental to its continued existence and allows payment of acceptable salaries and the upkeep and maintenance, plus purchase of new equipment as technology changes. Databases significantly aid management in ensuring profits are made. This is business 101.

An oft-neglected aspect of cryopreservation data is quality control. While thaw rates are easily collected if a simple relationship is established using the date of embryo freeze then no matter when embryos are thawed (and this may be many years apart) visualisation of all patient outcomes can assure the lab that their process of cryopreservation is working well. A relationship can also be established between the scientist performing the cryopreservation process and its outcome, again creating an embryology KPI.

When Should Data Be Added?

The advantage of databases is that data is simultaneously available to all staff logged in to the system. Thus if the progress of a patient's embryo culture in the laboratory is followed by a clinician then adding data as it is collected makes sense. Against this is the view that if multiple staff are collecting data and entering it then how do you ensure that all fields required are actually collected for each patient? An alternative approach is to enter all data once only at the completion of culture and cryo-preservation since it is often the scientists who talk to the patients about progress of embryos in culture and the clinician is informed when they arrive for embryo transfer. This of course depends on the Unit's processes and is not appropriate if the unit is paperless. However whichever approach is taken final validation of the content of a patient record should always be required.

How Should Data Be Organised?

Historically the patient's paper file was divided into organised sections but retrieving information simply and quickly was often problematic. Furthermore, an updated summary of relevant issues and outcomes was never available in the paper format, something well programmed databases easily visualise.

Any database used (either commercially purchased or developed in-house) should have editable features. Figure 10.5 shows that for survey respondents these features were mostly available (approx. 70 % of the time) but the ability to create automatic patient correspondence appeared weak. This programming would only involve a form-style letter with field merges confirming previous verbal communication. Feedback from patients generally confirms their appreciation of this approach and from a legal perspective you can confirm dialogue. It was also marginally worrying that approx. 20 % of respondents had no database security and approx. 35 % were unable to lock out change once data had been entered and validated.

Access and Security

Because databases are simultaneously available to multiple users, access both to the database itself and layouts within it should be restricted according to user privileges. Log-in to the program should always be recorded "behind the scenes" as part of the user's profile and a single user should be barred from logging into more than one computer terminal. Similarly if that terminal remains inactive for a while re-login should be required. This is often seen as an inconvenience by staff but when it is explained that they are responsible for their data entry their thought process changes.

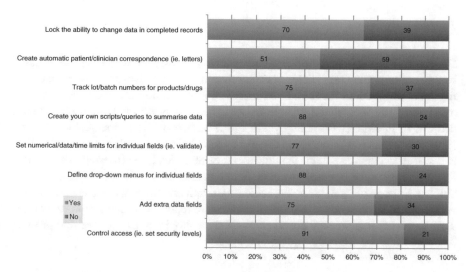

Fig. 10.5 Survey responses (as whole number percentage) to the question "In your database can you easily...?"

A similar development occurred with double witnessing in the embryo lab. In its early days staff would often just countersign an action without observing it but recent cases of embryo mix-up, etc. [7] now means staff have taken on responsibility.

Other aspects of security include embryologists never needing to be in a patient's accounts layout and clinical staff not being able to enter embryological data (only see summaries). I have known some clinicians take umbrage at this because they see it as loss of their authority but the ART Clinic comprises a Team where everybody has skills and contributes to the final result, so this is simply an old fashioned attitude.

At some point in time a record is deemed complete. This may be after the successful birth of a live baby or many months earlier after a negative pregnancy test. Once complete, validated and signed off as such, that record needs some way of being locked to prevent accidental unauthorised change. Changes may need to be made into the future but access to this feature should be limited to management. This is a major weakness of spreadsheets.

With respect to privacy and ownership of medical records this has been defined well in many countries of the world. Thus the data contained within the medical record belongs to the patient whereas the physical form the data takes (paper or electronic) belongs to the entity responsible for maintaining that record. Again different countries have different requirements for how long records need to be kept but the electronic version should always be more easily retrievable. This is another reason why data dictionaries are important since who knows how data will be stored into the future but at least the format of the current database will be known.

Finally some ART accrediting bodies require clinics to have a management plan should they cease business operations. Patient databases must be included in this too.

Field Definitions

Databases have evolved significantly over time. For instance while the use of numbers to define some "text" fields was commonplace a few decades ago so that sorting could easily occur the use of text entry is now commonplace and never hampers data interrogation. Even the American date format (yyyy/mm/dd) that used to be my nemesis in FileMaker Pro many years ago is now easily interchangeable with the European format (dd/mm/yyyy). The use of calculation fields also allows validation and so-called container fields can allow pdf or text files to be inserted. This means that anything can be scanned and entered to a database for reference. While my unit still has some paper patient notes, including treatment consents, it has been useful for the scientists to scan the consent of a patient to regress excess embryos they have cryopreserved. It is an easy observation for a paranoid manager to see due process has been followed when discarding embryos.

Layout and Navigation

To this author this is everything. Naturally if you use a commercial package you will have little control over this aspect of displaying your information but for in-house developers this is where discussions amongst users can lead to brilliant solutions. Great layouts (including choice of font and its size, use of colours, and alert flags) and easy navigation between them will not only improve the user experience but also lead to better and quicker data entry by staff, often with fewer errors. If a lot of data is entered at one time then the tab order is also paramount. Nobody wants their eye to be bouncing all over a screen looking for the next empty field to complete. There also needs to be sequence, and if paper laboratory worksheets are used to initially collect some data then that sequence should match data entry. Let us be honest, computer data entry is a necessary chore so anything that can improve compliance and user friendliness helps.

As with paper documents I have always believed everything should fit on one page. This can sometimes be a challenge but it is when document control as part of a quality system works best. Thus a layout should basically fit within a standard 15-in. computer screen and these days should also be compatible with Tablet format (i.e. iPads, etc) and the user should not need to scroll to be able to see all parts of an open window/layout. This means moving between layouts in a record by the use of buttons contained in a menu bar should be simple and if multiple layouts are required for data entry then the last field on a layout could contain a default option on field-exit to automatically direct the user to the next layout without the necessity of clicking a button.

Import of Data

If your Clinic does not provide all facilities necessary for monitoring a patient's treatment then the ability to import data from "outside" pathology laboratories is likely to be useful. All diagnostic endocrine data, and that from monitoring the stimulation of a patient with FSH, can be imported from other providers' computer systems. This may require a bridging program where formats and links are defined but I have also seen manual entry performed. The latter of course bypasses any issues of security and compatibility but requires considerable staff input. It goes without saying that if import of such data is automatic then strong validation that the correct data goes to the correct person/record is required. Diagnostic imaging reports of ultrasound investigations can also be imported. For a start-up clinic this is again where purchase of a commercial package wins out.

Validation of Data Entry

This can take several forms but usually occurs at the time of data entry with a field being programmed to control this. For instance ranges can be specified for date entry or be controlled by the use of specific pull-down menus. A classic example I used in teaching the use of limiting data entry was for the question "How many times do you have intercourse per week?" Logically, this should be in the range 0–7 with whole number multiples of this, but I once extracted over 200 different number and text replies to this question making any form of statistical analysis or summary report based on this field impossible.

Validation should also take the form of comparison with other fields. For instance if no embryos are available for transfer then transfer information fields (e.g. use of tenaculum or obturator) should remain empty. Similarly any dates of events associated with a patient's course of treatment should be sequential and be flagged if they deviate.

A useful feature to program in-house is to get staff to enter the most important data (perhaps that relating to billing and number of embryos in cryostore, etc.) a second time into a new blank layout. Warning flags appear if the data input is different to that originally entered and printing of any summary data can only occur once that validation has occurred. Similarly if a copy of a report is printed it is useful to automatically state this in the "footer".

Reporting

A good database will allow reporting of whatever data is required and access to these summaries should be available to all staff. There is not likely to be an embryologist anywhere who does not want to check their pregnancy rate based on perhaps the ICSI procedures they have performed or the embryo transfers they have been a part of. Depending upon the number of cases handled monthly reporting of basic data should be mandatory and these reports should be discussed amongst the group as part of their Unit's quality control and management. Obviously the significance of any review also depends upon the number of cases being reviewed so in smaller units the frequency may extend to quarterly. Basic reports will usually include such items as the number of treatment cases (e.g. IVF, ICSI, and involvement of donated tissue), the number of cancelled cycles (i.e. those not progressing to oocyte collection), the number of oocyte collections, the number of embryo transfers and the number of pregnancies. Figure 10.6 gives an example of a summary template from the author's database summarising the types of treatments and various outcomes from each. This same template can be used after performing a find on any number of variables to extract the information you require (e.g. a particular time range, patient age grouping or treatment modality). Thus a number of KPI's can be created from such a summary format. As evidenced by Fig. 10.7 most units replying to the survey summarised their data.

Numbers by Treatments		Rx	Fail Stim	Fail UOR	Fail Fert	Fail Cleav	Cryo all	Fail Thaw	Tx	Preg	Preg %	Preg N/K	Ems Tx	Ems Fz	Pt's with Fz
ART CLASSIC RX	FER	139	0	0	0	2	0	5	132	55	41.7	0	136	0	0
ART CLASSIC RX	ICSI	155	4	3	8	1	5	0	134	50	37.3	0	149	184	67
ART CLASSIC RX	IVF	150	7	1	7	3	9	0	121	53	43.8	0	143	221	75
Grand Total		444	11	4	15	6	14	5	387	158	40.8	0	428	405	142

Fig. 10.6 An example of a database summary "template" for ART

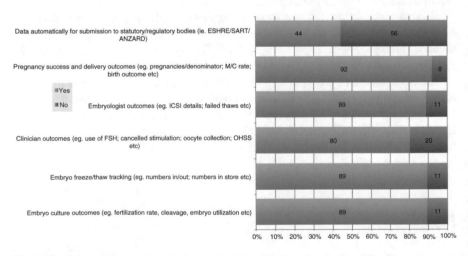

Fig. 10.7 Survey responses (as whole number percentage) to the question "Can the system you use summarise.....?"

Data Backup

If your fertility unit does not have a disaster recovery plan that includes a computer backup policy (i.e. copying and archiving of data) then stop reading this book now and find out how to do it!

The primary purpose of backup is to recover data after its loss, whether by deletion or file corruption. Secondarily it allows recovery of data from an earlier time. Therefore backup of data should be automatic, be at least daily and should also include off-site storage. While use of "Cloud" based technology for backup could also be considered it might be prudent to consider any privacy issues. Most importantly make sure your IT department regularly confirms that systematic backup is occurring and get them to demonstrate their ability to actually recover functional files you can use. Do not take their word for it!

Export of Data

If you cannot export data from a commercially purchased database to a spreadsheet or statistical package do not buy it. There should always be a time when review of data is required whether it be for publication, internal reporting to management, business plan or budget purposes. If in-house developed databases are used then this should mean that any or every field can be moved if required. I have seen some commercial suites control export of data but this significantly limits your flexibility in interrogating your data.

An important part of the regular export of data (or summary within your database) is that it allows outliers to be easily identified. For instance a date of birth or "Rip Van Winkle" age will clearly show itself and allow correction. Occasionally less obvious erroneous entries such as use of large amounts of FSH for stimulating an ovary are discovered because an extra digit is added, and this only becomes apparent when creating reports.

Data Audit and Research

Today, all good fertility units should use a Quality System approach to manage their ART program. This may take the form of ISO 9001 or another Standard specific to your country. In Australia for instance, NATA accredited laboratories have to conform with ISO 15189 and the regulatory body's (RTAC) Code of Practice is also based on ISO principles (http://www.fertilitysociety.com.au/wp-content/uploads/RTAC-COP-2015.pdf). Regular audit of performance is a mandatory part of such systems requiring a schedule to be defined annually to review processes.

Compliance with Regulatory Bodies

Most staff find long-hand preparation of standard reports arduous but this is what computers do uncomplainingly best. There is absolutely no reason why submission of required data to statutory or regulatory bodies should not simply be a matter of defining a date range and pressing a button. Furthermore there is also little need to verify exported data before submission (beyond what your program already does of course) since statutory bodies usually run validation and checking programs that report on inconsistencies. These discrepancies are usually "typos" or missing data and are easily amended for re-submission. According to the survey summary only 44 % of respondents can automatically create data for submission to their governing authority (Fig. 10.7). This would seem low when it is a mandatory component of an ART Unit's registration. However unlike Australia, where there is a 2 year delay in reporting national statistics because data is submitted annually "on bulk" when birth outcomes are known, the Singaporean government requires the on-line submission of more than 200 data points immediately after a patient completes embryo transfer and cryopreservation. While this dynamic approach has merit for the Unit its full potential does not seem to have been utilised and Singaporean Units still rely on their own database system.

The UK has a similar approach with treatment cycle data submitted to the HFEA when a couple register for treatment, at the completion of their treatment cycle and later, following the outcome of any pregnancies. Again any reports generated by the HFEA do not directly aid the clinic in monitoring themselves. Since both the above government bodies also require submission of data over the internet, Units are faced with a double data entry task.

The Database as Part of a Quality System

An ART Unit's database system is capable of handling much more than just patient details and can also include records of equipment including their commissioning and validation, service and maintenance and perhaps scanned (or downloaded from the suppliers website) copies of operational manuals. Stock levels of consumables can be managed and ideally any paper documents can be held for download ensuring Document Control is maintained.

As previously mentioned export of data allows auditing of multiple facets of your system including monitoring of adverse or untoward events which would include the incidence of failure to collect oocytes, failed thaws of cryopreserved embryos, OHSS, multiple pregnancy and miscarriage etc. These audits thus allow all aspects of the treatment of patients to be risk assessed.

Key Performance Indicators (KPI's)

The best ART Unit in the world will occasionally have periods of poor outcomes and the difficulty then is in determining from where the issue (if any) is emanating. Classically the embryology laboratory is the first place to look but given you "can't make a silk purse out of a sow's ear" it is also worth examining ovarian stimulation practice and basic patient history. Also, given that our patients are biological variables we should not be surprised by fluctuations. The question is when is a fluctuation a trend? Applying standard QAP practice using various KPI's can help determine this or at least give confidence that processes have not changed, but patients have. Databases can, and should, be programmed to handle these easily. As examples:

Clinical KPI's can include:

- Incidence of failed ovarian stimulation
- Amount of FSH used
- Incidence of failed oocyte collection
- Oocyte immaturity rate (as an index of time from hCG)
- Freeze all rate (as an index of OHSS risk)
- Multiple pregnancy rate (as an index of number of embryos transferred)

Embryological KPI's can include:

- Oocyte degeneration rate (if ICSI is used)
- Fertilisation and ploidy rate
- Cleavage and blastulation rate
- Embryo utilisation rate and incidence of cryopreservation
- Implantation rate.

Unit KPI's can include:

- Incidence of complaints
- Pregnancy rate
- Miscarriage rate
- Live delivery rate
- Incidence of adverse events.

Staff Competency

No member of an ART Unit Team can treat or manage patients without having been trained. However, previously trained staff can wander from agreed protocols (i.e. cut corners) or become complacent about their ability over time. Competency statements derived from KPI data or extracted for an individual confirm a staff member's continued excellence. This should also be part of clinical credentialing. From a database it is easy to confirm that an embryologist has maintained their skills by competently performing, say, 50 ICSI injections annually or a clinician has adequately managed their patients with low OHSS risk.

Internal Quality Assurance

This can take many different forms and databases allow some interesting embryological data interrogation and presentation of reports. As an example for each ART cycle attempt in the author's laboratory a simple summary is created confirming that the patient, clinician and embryologist has completed processes as required. The report shows salient events throughout the treatment cycle, compares data with the Inter-Quartile range of data for age and treatment matched patients and highlights adverse contributing factors such as age and BMI (Fig. 10.8). Details of all embryo culture outcomes for patients on the same day are shown for cross-reference. A similar format can be used for the thawing of frozen embryos by displaying data for all embryos frozen on the same day as the patient and for all embryos thawed on the same day. This is useful confirmation of a laboratory in control. While not exhaustive this approach has significant merit and could not be produced from a spreadsheet, only a database.

Conclusion and the Future

It should now be obvious that a database for managing patient treatment and embryological data is an integral part of any ART Unit. There is a plethora of choice from fully integrated commercial systems to exceptional software applications that you can tailor to your own needs. However all databases need constant maintenance and update to remain relevant so choose wisely since you do not want to change systems a few years down the track. Vindication of the need for continued evolution of any database used in the ART Unit is that 98 % of labs responding to the questionnaire felt their own database (Fig. 10.9) could be improved upon!

As to the future, technology is likely to lead change. With the growing use of Tablets many programs are already available to the user wherever the Internet is accessible. Tablets also make entry of data relatively easy and while this author has not yet seen it in operation the concept of using a Tablet to collect data beside the microscope rather than using paper worksheets is appealing. It also means that the logged-on person will automatically be registered as the creator of that information. Similarly tab order is irrelevant when a touchscreen is used because a user familiar with a layout will go directly to the relevant field. Similarly, if your security is set sufficiently strongly to limit hacking and maintain privacy, then there is no reason why controlled access for patients to update their personal information and perhaps view the status of their cultured or cryopreserved reproductive tissues could not

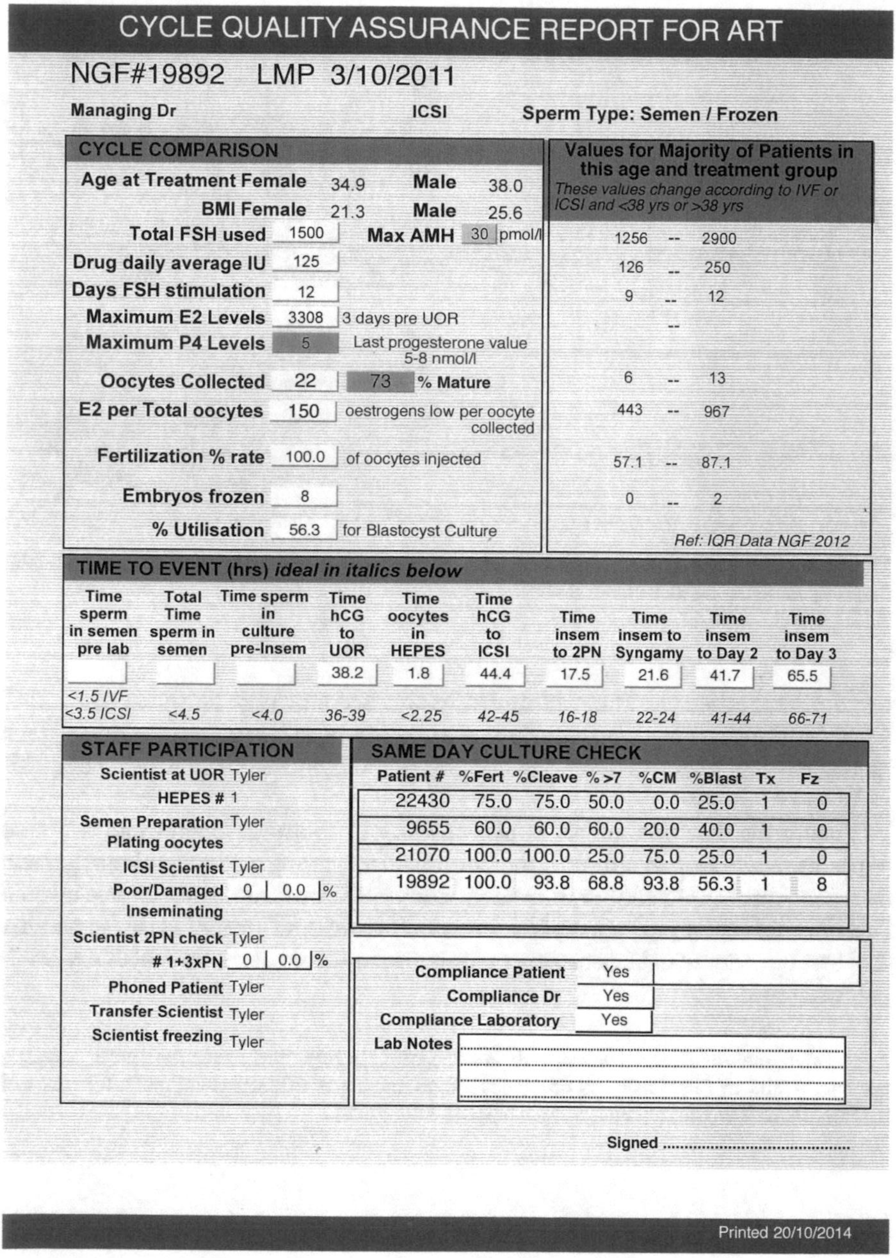

CYCLE QUALITY ASSURANCE REPORT FOR ART

NGF#19892 LMP 3/10/2011

Managing Dr **ICSI** **Sperm Type: Semen / Frozen**

CYCLE COMPARISON

				Values for Majority of Patients in this age and treatment group (*These values change according to IVF or ICSI and <38 yrs or >38 yrs*)
Age at Treatment Female	34.9	**Male**	38.0	
BMI Female	21.3	**Male**	25.6	
Total FSH used	1500	**Max AMH**	30 pmol/l	1256 -- 2900
Drug daily average IU	125			126 -- 250
Days FSH stimulation	12			9 -- 12
Maximum E2 Levels	3308	3 days pre UOR		--
Maximum P4 Levels	5	Last progesterone value 5-8 nmol/l		
Oocytes Collected	22	73 % **Mature**		6 -- 13
E2 per Total oocytes	150	oestrogens low per oocyte collected		443 -- 967
Fertilization % rate	100.0	of oocytes injected		57.1 -- 87.1
Embryos frozen	8			0 -- 2
% Utilisation	56.3	for Blastocyst Culture		*Ref: IQR Data NGF 2012*

TIME TO EVENT (hrs) ***ideal in italics below***

Time sperm in semen pre lab	Total Time sperm in semen	Time sperm in culture pre-Insem	Time hCG to UOR	Time oocytes in HEPES	Time hCG to ICSI	Time insem to 2PN	Time insem to Syngamy	Time insem to Day 2	Time insem to Day 3
			38.2	1.8	44.4	17.5	21.6	41.7	65.5
<1.5 IVF <3.5 ICSI	*<4.5*	*<4.0*	*36-39*	*<2.25*	*42-45*	*16-18*	*22-24*	*41-44*	*66-71*

STAFF PARTICIPATION

Scientist at UOR Tyler
HEPES # 1
Semen Preparation Tyler
Plating oocytes
ICSI Scientist Tyler
Poor/Damaged 0 | 0.0 %
Inseminating
Scientist 2PN check Tyler
 # 1+3xPN 0 | 0.0 %
Phoned Patient Tyler
Transfer Scientist Tyler
Scientist freezing Tyler

SAME DAY CULTURE CHECK

Patient #	%Fert	%Cleave	% >7	%CM	%Blast	Tx	Fz
22430	75.0	75.0	50.0	0.0	25.0	1	0
9655	60.0	60.0	60.0	20.0	40.0	1	0
21070	100.0	100.0	25.0	75.0	25.0	1	0
19892	100.0	93.8	68.8	93.8	56.3	1	8

Compliance Patient Yes
Compliance Dr Yes
Compliance Laboratory Yes
Lab Notes

Signed ....

Printed 20/10/2014

Fig. 10.8 An example of an ART cycle QA report

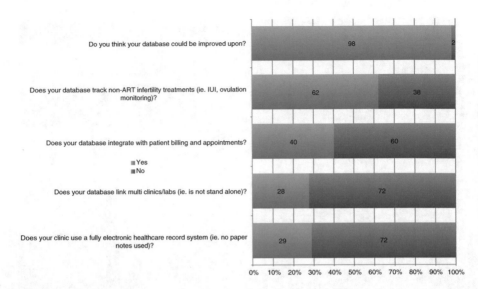

Fig. 10.9 Survey responses (as whole number percentage) to the question "Do you think your database could be improved upon etc?"

occur. Cloud based software will probably also become more prevalent (see http://www.carpusoft.hr) but it is unlikely that any form of universally standardised data management system will be created because of multiple commercial and geographically based factors.

Finally the data you collect is also the key to future developments. A recent paper used a hybrid intelligence method that, integrating a genetic algorithm and decision learning techniques from mining an ART medical database, provided an "accurate and early prediction of the outcome" of an ART treatment [8]. In another 40 years our current data management systems may seem like a version of my original metal rod!

Acknowledgements Special thanks to the readers of EmbryoMail who took the time to complete my survey and to FileMaker Pro developer David Barten of "Dzines Solutionz", for years of patience in dealing with my often simple but difficult requests.

References

1. Bhattacharya S, Maheshwari A, Mollison J. Factors associated with failed treatment: an analysis of 121,744 women embarking on their first IVF cycles. PLoS One. 2013;8(12):e82249. doi:10.1371/journal.pone.0082249.
2. Levine BA, Goldschlag D. An HER primer. Part 1. ContemporyObgGyn.net; 2013a. p. 54–6.
3. Levine BA, Goldschlag D. An HER primer. Part 2. ContemporyObgGyn.net; 2013b. p. 54–6.
4. Craft C, Forman R. Analysis of IVF data. Lancet. 1997;349(9047):284.

5. Macaldowie A, Wang YA, Chambers GM, Sullivan EA. Assisted reproductive technology in Australia and New Zealand 2011. Sydney: National Perinatal Epidemiology and Statistics Unit, the University of New South Wales; 2013.
6. Malhotra N. How to set up a fertility register in emerging markets. ASPIRE Abstract Book; 2014. p. 33.
7. Spriggs M. IVF mixup: White couple have black babies. J Med Ethics. 2003;29:65.
8. Guh RS, Wu TCJ, Weng SP. Integrating genetic algorithm and decision tree learning for assistance in predicting in vitro fertilization outcomes. Expert Syst Appl. 2011;38(4):4437–49.

Chapter 11
Implementation of a Total Quality Management System

James Catt

Introduction

The concept of a quality system is not a new one, manufacturers have been using these systems for the past 70 years to set up, control and monitor their manufacturing processes. Some of the central tenets have been well explained and published by Edwards Deming [1]. Deming's tenets were:

Appreciation of a system: understanding the overall processes involving suppliers, producers and customers (or recipients) of goods and services.
Knowledge of variation: the range and causes of variation in quality, and use of statistical sampling in measurements.
Theory of knowledge: the concepts explaining knowledge and the limits of what can be known.
Knowledge of psychology.

Well, no matter how precious we are about IVF (and it is special), it can still be viewed as a manufacturing process and the quality systems used to control it. In broad terms manufacturing requires source material from suppliers that is suitable for the manufacturing process. These source materials are then used for manufacture so that the product meets expectations and is saleable to customers (product realisation). This is equivalent to the provision of sperm and oocytes suitable for IVF (provision of source material), fertilisation, culture, transfer and cryopreservation of gametes and embryos (manufacture) and the meeting of customer expectations, either pregnancy or ongoing infertility management (product realisation). Once we have managed this mental somersault, then the principles behind TQM become eminently usable in IVF clinics.

J. Catt, PhD (✉)
Optimal IVF, PO Box 4234, Black Rock North, Melbourne, VC 3195, Australia
e-mail: jimc@optimalivf.com.au

© Springer Science+Business Media New York 2016   217
S.D. Fleming, A.C. Varghese (eds.), *Organization and Management of IVF Units*, DOI 10.1007/978-3-319-29373-8_11

The difference between quality assurance and quality control is worth explaining at this point. Quality assurance is setting up the manufacturing process to give the expected result and quality control is the independent monitoring of the process to ensure the product is meeting specification; i.e. can you produce, transfer and cryopreserve embryos and how well do you do it?

Development of a TQMS

The easiest way to develop and implement a TQMS is to have a system in place and design the IVF clinic and processes around this. This is called a "top down" approach. It is most suitable for new IVF clinics (or new satellites, for established clinics) where one is not encumbered by pre-existing processes. However, most of us have come from clinics established some time ago, before TQMS was heard of in IVF and so the development of a system is more difficult, encumbered by pre-existing processes and entrenched staff. How often have we heard the phrase "I have been doing this for the past 15 years without any problems, why would I change now?" A difficult question to answer without being pejorative! In my view the best way to implement a TQMS system into an established IVF unit is to start with the laboratory, for the sole reason that scientists should be evidence driven and most laboratories recognise the need for standardisation and consistency. Once established in the laboratory the TQMS can then be extended into other areas. The key point with developing a TQMS system is to introduce it with stakeholder "buy-in" and "ownership" so that people accept the premises and help with the implementation. The development of a TQMS by directorial management techniques is pejorative, counterproductive and will result in difficulty. Indeed one of the tenets of quality management is to involve staff in both the design and implementation (continuing personal development) of such systems to promote good practice.

A very useful tool used in developing a TQMS is process mapping. In essence, process mapping is the stepwise representation of a process either from a global perspective (e.g. how the managerial set up works with roles and responsibilities) or from a single process perspective (e.g. sperm preparation for conventional IVF). Process mapping outlines how processes interact within an IVF unit and how co-dependent the processes are. We have always found that "group" process mapping involving all those who participate in a procedure to be of most benefit. This approach ensures that everybody can contribute and the result is a consensus of opinion and practicability. Apart from anything else, group process mapping is good fun. Details of different approaches to process mapping in IVF is given by Mortimer and Mortimer [2].

Quality assurance dictates that the processes be designed to manufacture the product. With IVF clinics this starts right from the top; do you have the correct managerial structure in place? Are the facilities suitable for IVF in terms of space, accessibility and clean air (low volatile organic compounds, VOCs)? Is the equipment used suitable and validated? The specifics behind these areas are dealt with in others chapters of this book. My remit is to drill down into more detail behind setting up protocols for conducting the processes in the IVF laboratory and methods used to monitor them along with the personnel involved.

Standard Operating Procedures

A standard operating procedure (SOP) is specified as a series of work instructions that define a particular procedure (e.g. oocyte retrieval, embryo transfer). In the IVF laboratory it is important to realise that work instructions by themselves are not enough. Ideally, the underlying principle behind the procedure should be stated and written so that an informed individual can understand the principle. The principle should ideally be referenced back to the source. The SOP usually contains a list of disposables, equipment to be used and a time frame for setting up and carrying out the procedure. Again the language and detail should be enough that any reasonably informed individual is able to follow the instructions. Just as an aside here, this is precisely the area that an auditor will look at when reviewing the SOP; i.e. can I conduct the procedure using these instructions?

A typical example of a SOP for oocyte retrieval is given in Appendix. As can be seen from this, there are clear instructions on how to conduct oocyte retrieval but what a SOP usually lacks is technique to ensure that the temperature and pH, during recovery, washing and assessment remain as constant as possible. In other words there are basics of oocyte/embryo handling, manipulation and observation that are common to the whole of embryology that are not specified in each SOP. The universalities of maintaining conditions outside of an incubator are central to any good embryology laboratory and considerable time should be spent to ensure conditions are kept constant and that personnel are fully competent in these critical areas.

Competency

There is a temptation in IVF to suggest that competency should be based on the number of procedures performed [3]. Whilst it is reasonable to expect that, the more procedures performed the greater the competency, but what if the procedures are performed poorly? Just because I conducted 200 OPU in the past year does this ensure that they were done properly? This is one of the more common problems found in IVF laboratories and is often described as SOP "slippage", whereby corners are cut by often, experienced embryologists to expedite the procedure. Whilst we are always looking for better ways to conduct our procedures any changes/variations should only be introduced after discussion and authorised by the laboratory manager/scientific director. Unauthorised variations are often detrimental and are one of the sources of variation we see. This is not meant to discourage innovation but there has to be defined ways whereby innovation has to be assessed and introduced.

Competency is defined as the ability to carry out a procedure or a series of procedures to give a quantitative outcome. For example, in our previous OPU example, competency would be attained after a series of conditions are met. The conditions would include: all oocytes are consistently recovered (as checked by the trainer) in a reasonable time frame (as defined by the laboratory manager). For OPU (as indeed any procedure carried out outside of an incubator) great care must be taken to ensure that there is minimal exposure to adverse conditions [4] by either using a controlled environment chamber or specific handling techniques designed to minimise temperature and pH changes (as defined in the laboratory manual).

Competency has two components, attainment of initial competency via training and ongoing maintenance of competency by objectively continuously measuring outcomes. Most IVF units do have adequate training and assessment programmes but are often lacking in ongoing competency. This is discussed below in the staff performance section.

Certification Standards

Certification is the process whereby an organisation (and individuals) meets a series of standards that are recognised as being relevant to the organisation. This is different to accreditation that looks at voluntary compliance with a series of standards or guidelines. Some countries already have compulsory regulations that IVF units must follow (e.g. HFEA in the UK) and it is illegal not to follow them. Other countries (e.g. Australia) have codes of practice or guidelines that IVF units should follow, or clearly demonstrate they are not engaging in risky behaviour, before they become eligible for government support. Some countries (e.g. Japan) have a voluntary code of practice that members adhere to but there is no compulsion for IVF units to join the group. Many countries (such as India) have legislation before government but these have not been ratified as yet. Any scheme whether compulsory or not always gives precedence to regulations or standards that affect the running of medical facilities. This would include running day surgeries, or procedural units that usually fall under government health departments.

International Organisation for Standardisation (ISO) operates out of Geneva and is an internationally recognised organisation that publishes a number of standards to help industrial organisations. Part of their mission statement is "International Standards make things work. They give world-class specifications for products, services and good practice, to ensure quality, safety and efficiency". ISO has been suggested to be useful for IVF units [5].

Perhaps the ISO standard most relevant to IVF units is 9001:2008 [6] and its main provisions are listed below:

Management must have a quality policy linked to the business and customers

All employees must be familiar with the quality policy

Data is collected and used to change the quality system

The quality system is regularly audited to determine its effectiveness

Traceability of all raw materials through to the final product is maintained

Customer requirements/feedback drive the product

Records are kept of all non-conformances and the corrective actions used

As can be seen these are very general requirements meaning that they are suitable to most manufacturing organisations. ISO itself does not accredit organisations but allows third party certification accreditation bodies (CAB) to assess organisations against the standard. Auditing is carried out by professional auditors who are usually aided by a technical expert, who should have extensive knowledge of that industry sector.

Those units who have ISO 9001:2008 will be assessed using the provisions above to see whether they meet the standard. There are several categories of recommendations arising from an audit:

A "must" recommendation means that something has to be done to make the organisation compliant. Usually the organisation must have made changes within a short period of time (usually 15 working days).

A "could" recommendation suggests that significant benefit may be obtained by accepting the recommendation. An organisation usually responds to these within 3 months as to whether they consider the change worthwhile.

An "opportunity for improvement" is a suggestion that something could be done differently that may result in an improvement. The organisation is under no obligation to respond to these.

There is another ISO standard, ISO 15189:2012—Medical Laboratories—requirements for quality and competence [7], which can be used for pathology laboratories (e.g. blood screening tests and semen analysis) associated with IVF units but the emphasis of ISO 15189 is focussed on efficacious testing, reporting and uncertainty of measurement, not about how an organisation works to deliver a final product (patient outcomes).

Internal Quality Assurance (IQA) and External Quality Assurance (EQA) Schemes

Both of these scheme types should be used in IVF units. IQA schemes measure how your processes work, usually related to historical data i.e. how are we doing now compared with last year? They are also of vital importance for continual monitoring of individual process steps, so that if problems occur they can be used for troubleshooting. EQA schemes, on the other hand, look at your performance compared to others; e.g. how are we doing compared to an average clinic? Out of necessity EQA are more limited than IQA schemes because EQA schemes have to recognise a series of parameters that are accepted by all units and hence, in effect, become lowest common denominators representing a minimal standard.

IQA schemes should look at every aspect of the IVF unit and cover all areas laid out in the quality manual, especially as defined by ISO 9001. From a business perspective the areas to be covered would be an annual management review of procedures and policies, stakeholder feedback (both staff and patients) and review of key business parameters (Key Performance Indicators, KPI). KPI should also be set for clinicians, nurses and scientists, as outlined below. For laboratory performance, KPI should be set to measure every area including oocyte quality, embryonic development and outcomes.

There are several EQA schemes commercially available but most of these are centred on Andrology. Two online IVF EQA schemes including embryology and more are available (Fert-Aid [8] and NEQAS [9]) and one sample and video based (EQASRM [10]). The big limitation with these schemes is that there is no consensus on the parameters used for comparison. Perhaps, in the future a scheme can be produced that uses the ALPHA/ESHRE consensus [11] with an emphasis on "time appropriate" embryo development parameters.

Key Performance Indicators

Key performance indicators are used throughout industry as a method of assessing and controlling every aspect of the organisation. IVF units are no exception. A generic diagram of how KPI work to interact between the different areas within IVF is shown in Fig. 11.1. It is clear from this diagram how the areas within an IVF unit interact via the KPI.

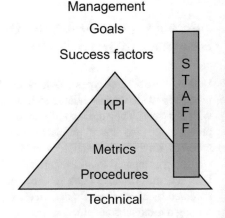

Fig. 11.1 Structure of an organisation; e.g. IVF unit showing how KPI interact with everyone

Business KPI

These define the outputs that have a direct effect on the business. A few examples are listed below; this list is not meant to be comprehensive!

Growth: 5–10 % growth per year in OPU's
Market share: 5 % increase per year
Recruitment: 5–10 % of new patients per year
Costs per cycle: 10 % profit per cycle
Costs per baby: 2 % decrease per year

Obviously many other business factors come into play but it is clear from the above examples that some of these will directly impinge on how the laboratories are run.

Process Controlling KPI

These are defined as the metrics that we use to examine each of our IVF procedures to make sure they are working as expected and can be used to segment the process into important sectors. Perhaps the best example of this is the use of a syngamy check to estimate the quality of oocytes (and hence effectiveness of stimulation). The contention is that syngamy (initial entry into the first cell division) is independent of laboratory/culture conditions but is an inherent property of an oocyte reflecting its overall quality. This is backed by long-standing circumstantial evidence that zygotes going into early syngamy have a greater implantation potential than those that do not [12, 13] and that recognised poor quality oocytes from ageing patients or poor responders have slower syngamy rates. The use of a syngamy KPI enables us to broadly distinguish between stimulation problems and laboratory problems. In terms of embryo development we would advocate the use of the Alpha/ESHRE consensus developmental milestones given in Table 11.1 [11]. The consensus is a very simple one that uses on-time, appropriate development as the best means to assess embryos.

In addition to the consensus KPI we also need to monitor the outputs that help us make embryos in the first place. A list of KPI follows that we believe to be useful but, again, this list is not meant to be comprehensive! The list is meant to cover most areas of IVF that the consensus does not cover. Reporting from these KPI is usually stratified according to patient age, the most useful group being aged 39 or less to reflect most of the patient population whilst excluding the obvious serious effect of patient age.

Percent of follicles greater than 15 mm diameter yielding oocytes
Percent of recovered oocytes at metaphase II
Percent of normal fertilisation with conventional IVF

Table 11.1 Alpha/ESHRE consensus on the timing of observation of fertilised oocytes and embryos and expected stage of development at each time point

Type of observation	Timing (hours post insemination)	Expected stage of development
Fertilisation check	17 ± 1	Pronuclear stage
Syngamy check	23 ± 1	Expect 50 % to be in syngamy (up to 20 % may be at the 2-cell stage)
Early cleavage Check	27 ± 1	2-cell stage
Day-2 embryo assessment	44 ± 1	4-cell stage
Day-3 embryo assessment	68 ± 1	8-cell stage
Day-4 embryo assessment	92 ± 2	Morula
Day-5 embryo assessment	116 ± 2	Blastocyst

Percent of injected oocytes normally fertilised by ICSI

Percent of injected oocytes degenerate after ICSI

Percentage of zygotes that were transferred or frozen (utilisation rate)

Percentage of transferred embryos (fresh and frozen) that form a foetal heart

Cumulative pregnancy rate per cycle; Defined as pregnancy rate after both fresh and
    frozen embryos (from that stimulated cycle) have been transferred

Percentage of patients achieving a take home baby

Staff Performance KPI

All staff, including nurses, clinicians and scientists, are assessed annually and a KPI system is usually used to determine performance. In broad terms this defines the ongoing competence of staff after they have been trained. It should be obvious from the above KPI lists that some of these KPI, as well as reporting the IVF procedures as a whole, can also be used for individuals. To derive individual KPI is relatively easy; we compare an individual result against the average for all those involved in the procedure. We usually suggest that a minimum of 20 procedures per year be conducted before an assessment is made. Any individual with results outside two standard deviations from the average warrants further investigation. A typical example of individual results is given in Fig. 11.2, reflecting results from ICSI. A further chapter in this book details the statistical analysis of process control using KPI in more detail.

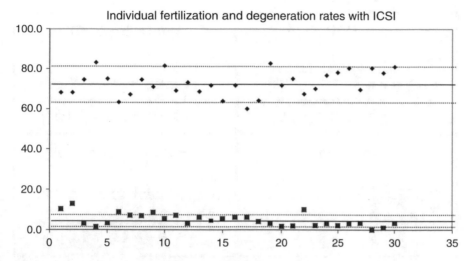

Fig. 11.2 Example of using KPI for individual assessment. Individual results are plotted against the average (±2 SD) for normal fertilisation and degeneration rates. The X axis is the individual scientists and the Y axis is the percent of total oocytes injected

KPI Dashboards [14]

The plethora of data available from our databases needs managing properly to avoid data overload. One of the best ways of coping with this data is to graphically represent it in a series of dashboards, with each dashboard showing a particular set of data pertinent to those viewing it. There are large numbers of programmes both commercial and free that can aid with setting up of these dashboards, but most people familiar with excel can produce their own. The key elements to a dashboard are to have a database with the KPI being entered and these are automatically graphed into the pictorial dashboard to illustrate the data. Perfect for managers with short attention spans!

A couple of examples are given below: a managerial one illustrating OPU numbers, new patient recruitment, pregnancy rates and overall profit and loss statements (Fig. 11.3). A laboratory one could be implantation rates for fresh and frozen transferred embryos, percent of patients having blastocyst transfer and percent of patients having embryos frozen (Fig. 11.4). The details of the dashboards do not matter; the important thing is that, if the data is collected, it can be presented in a logical fashion and help drive the organisation to its goals.

Peer Review

The definition of peer review is an assessment of a process by a person or people who have similar qualifications and experience of those processes they are assessing. Whilst this sounds like a good idea there are inherent problems. People with similar

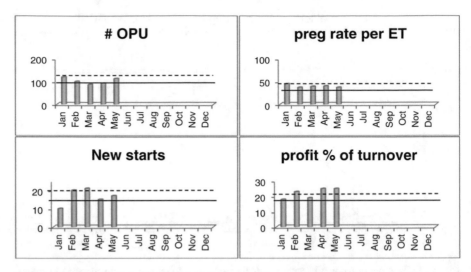

Fig. 11.3 Hypothetical dashboard for business KPI. The *solid lines* represent last year's data and the *dashed lines* represent targets

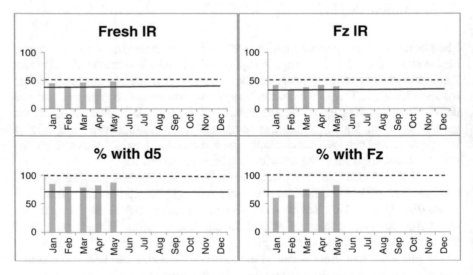

Fig. 11.4 Hypothetical dashboard for laboratory KPI. The *solid lines* represent last year's data and the *dashed lines* represent targets

qualifications and experience are usually employed in the industry and so conflicts of interest arise. One method of peer review used to be using a professional whose business was elsewhere in the country but with the commercialisation of IVF resulting in many units in many parts of the country, peer review became very difficult. However, commercialisation has resulted in a number of similar professionals within an organisation, geographically and institutionally disparate, that can act as peer reviewers. However, the results of these reviews are not available outside of the organisation and are therefore of limited use to others.

Finally there has been a spate of independent consultation companies formed, usually with experienced personnel "retiring" from mainstream laboratories that do offer an independent peer review service. The value of this type of service is unknown and unregulated making it difficult to assess.

Conclusions

The benefits of implementing a TQMS far outweigh any problems found during the implementation. This chapter was designed to indicate that a TQMS can be used to control and monitor all aspects of an IVF unit from administration and management, through nursing and laboratories to deliver the best possible outcome for our patients. Once a TQMS has been implemented it should be more or less self-running and ensure that key areas are under control and reporting correctly. Just a reminder to finish with; quality is about rejecting the status quo and is a journey, not an end.

Appendix: Typical Standard Operating Procedure (SOP) for Oocyte Retrieval

Standard Operating Procedure for Oocyte Recovery (SOP 001.3)

Principle

36–40 h post trigger (administration of human chorionic gonadotrophin) the oocytes should be mature enough to be recovered by transvaginal ultrasound. The clinician aspirates the mature follicles and the recovered follicular fluid is kept at 37 °C until the fluid can be searched. Cumulus oocyte complexes (COC) are identified, washed and placed in an incubator until insemination.

Day-1 Set-Up for OPU

Consumables

Falcon 2057 14 ml tubes
4-well dishes (one for every six oocytes expected)
Fertilisation medium (FM)
Flush buffer (B)
Gamete buffer (GB)

Cleavage medium (CM)

1. Label 1× Falcon 2057 tube per patient with "GB" and add 10 ml GB.
2. Place in heating block overnight.
3. Label 4-well dishes (one per every six oocytes expected) with patient's full name, IVF number and date of birth. Label dish OPU.
4. Aliquot 0.7 ml FM into OPU dish. Overlay all wells with 0.2 ml oil. Place dishes in incubator and leave overnight.
5. Aliquot 10 ml of B into a Falcon 2057 tube and label as "FLUSH". Tightly cap and place in warm oven overnight.

Day-0 OPU

Consumables

Warmed GB in Falcon 2057 tubes
Pasteur pipettes
Falcon 3037 centre well dishes
Falcon 3002 Petri dishes
B in Falcon 14 ml tube
Patient lab-notes and history

1. Check lab notes to confirm that consents are complete.
2. Aliquot approximately 2 ml of warmed GB into the outer well of the 3037 dish, 1 ml into the centre and place on warming tray.
3. Place Falcon 3003 Petri dishes on warming trays for searching.
4. Confirm patient's consent then check patient into theatre by confirming patent details, full name and date of birth both verbally by asking the patient their full name and DOB, and confirming this with the paperwork/ID bracelet/hospital sticker.
5. The follicular aspirates are passed to the embryologist as obtained.
6. The fluid should be poured carefully into a 6 or 10 cm Falcon Petri dish and the contents observed under a stereomicroscope.
7. Search the dish to identify the cellular material that is likely to contain oocytes. Identify the putative COC, remove using a Pasteur and wash in the outer well of the 3037 dish. Transfer to centre well and confirm presence of COC.
8. Repeat these steps until all the follicular aspirate tubes have been examined for the presence of oocytes.
9. Once the oocyte collection is complete, transfer the COC from the centre well into well #4 of the OPU dish and then distribute amongst wells 1–3.
10. Place in CO_2 incubator until insemination.
11. Clean up the work area discarding all used dishes, pipettes and tubes.
12. Wipe all surfaces with water followed by QAC and water again.
13. Note the total number of oocytes collected on the lab notes and complete data entry.

References

1. Edwards Deming W. Quality, productivity and competitive position. Cambridge, MA: Massachusetts Inst Technology; 1982. ISBN 0911379002.
2. Mortimer D, Mortimer S. Quality and risk management in the IVF laboratory. Cambridge, UK: Cambridge University Press; 2005. ISBN 0521843499.
3. RTAC Code of Practice. Fertility Society of Australia; 2014. ISBN 978-0-947285-03-6.
4. Swain JE. Optimizing the culture environment in the IVF laboratory: impact of pH and buffer capacity on gamete and embryo quality. Reprod Biomed Online. 2010;2:6–16.
5. Alper MM, International Standards Organization. Experience with ISO quality control in assisted reproductive technology. Fertil Steril. 2013;100:1503–8.
6. ISO 9001:2008. Quality management systems—requirements. ISO; 2008.
7. ISO 15189:2012. Medical laboratories—medical laboratories—requirements for quality and competence. ISO; 2012.
8. FertAid. www.FertAid.com.
9. NEQAS. www.ukneqas.org.uk.
10. EQASRM. www.eqasrm.com.au.
11. Alpha Scientists in Reproductive Medicine and ESHRE Special Interest Group of Embryology. The Istanbul consensus workshop on embryo assessment: proceedings of an expert meeting. Reprod BioMed Online. 2011;22:632–46.
12. Shoukir Y, Campana A, Farley T, Sakkas D. Early cleavage of in-vitro fertilized human embryos to the 2-cell stage: a novel indicator of embryo quality and viability. Hum Reprod. 1997;12:1531–6.
13. Lechniak D, Pers-Kamczyc E, Pawlak P. Timing of the first zygotic cleavage as a marker of developmental potential of mammalian embryos. Reprod Biol. 2008;8:23–42.
14. Kaplan R, Norton D. The balanced scorecard. Boston, MA: Harvard Business Review Press; 1996. ISBN 9780875846514.

Chapter 12
Optimization of Treatment Outcomes for Assisted Reproductive Technologies

Shahryar K. Kavoussi and Thomas B. Pool

Clinical

Ovarian Factor

AMH

Antimüllerian Hormone (AMH) has rapidly gained acceptance as a very important ovarian reserve test that may predict IVF outcomes and, based on results, may carry the potential to prompt the application of specific stimulation protocols. AMH has been demonstrated to be a strong, directly proportionate predictor of ovarian response [1–3]. Although some studies have found that AMH levels weakly predict pregnancy [4, 5], others have demonstrated that AMH does indeed predict this ultimate outcome although there is not an established cut-off for the lowest AMH level at which pregnancies and live births can be expected [6]. A recent, large study showed that AMH levels positively correlate with the number of oocytes retrieved and that this correlation is not affected by time interval between AMH level measurement and the ovarian stimulation [7].

S.K. Kavoussi, MD, MPH (✉)
Austin Fertility and Reproductive Medicine/Westlake IVF,
300 Beardsley Lane, Bldg B, Suite 200, Austin, TX 78746, USA
e-mail: skavoussi@msn.com

T.B. Pool, PhD, HCLD
Austin Fertility & Reproductive Medicine/Westlake IVF,
300 Beardsley Lane, Bldg B, Suite 200, Austin, TX 78746, USA

Fertility Center of San Antonio,
4499 Medical Drive, Suite 200, San Antonio, TX 78229, USA
e-mail: rpool@fertilitysa.com

© Springer Science+Business Media New York 2016   231
S.D. Fleming, A.C. Varghese (eds.), *Organization and Management of IVF Units*, DOI 10.1007/978-3-319-29373-8_12

Endometriomas

The effect of ovarian endometriomas (OE) on IVF outcomes has been a controversial issue. In recent years, there has been a shift towards not removing asymptomatic endometriomas in women who undergo IVF. Two meta-analyses have shown that surgical intervention, whether it is cystectomy or cyst aspiration, has not been shown to improve IVF success when compared with expectant management prior to controlled ovarian stimulation (COS) [8, 9]. Moreover, although drainage of OE has not been shown to be detrimental to ovarian response to gonadotropins for IVF, there has been evidence that there is a decrease in ovarian response after ovarian cystectomy for OE [9] as well as diminished ovarian reserve following removal of OE, particularly in cases of bilateral cystectomy [10–13].

Tubal Factor

Hydrosalpinges

It has been well-established that hydrosalpinges are detrimental to reproductive efficiency. Hydrosalpinges are associated with an effect on embryo implantation to the extent that, among IVF patients, pregnancy and implantation rates are decreased by approximately 50 % [14, 15] and spontaneous miscarriage rates are increased [16]. The fluid within the hydrosalpinx can enter the uterine cavity and the proposed mechanism of actions of the hydrosalpinx fluid's deleterious effects include embryotoxicity [17], a wash-out effect on embryos, and adverse effects on markers of endometrial receptivity, including decreased expression of $\alpha V \beta 3$ [18] and HOXA10 [19].

The interruption of the leakage of hydrosalpingeal fluid into the uterine cavity is the basis for surgical intervention [20]. Removal of hydrosalpinges by salpingectomy restores IVF pregnancy rates [20] and decreases miscarriage rates as well. In particular, hydrosalpinges that are sonographically visible are recommended to be removed [14, 21]. In certain cases where pelvic adhesive disease to the extent that salpingectomy is not possible or may be precarious to attempt, proximal occlusion of hydrosalpinges from the laparoscopic [22, 23] or hysteroscopic routes is an alternative that has been found to be efficacious. The surgical treatment of hydrosalpinges has been shown to restore $\alpha V \beta 3$ [18, 24] and HOXA10 [19] expression in the eutopic endometrium.

In IVF patients with contraindications to laparoscopy and/or salpingectomy, hysteroscopic occlusion with Essure device is an option [25, 26]. A recent systematic review and pooled analysis was conducted on the safety and efficacy of pre-IVF placement of Essure for tubal occlusion in cases of hydrosalpinx. Although randomized controlled trials (RCTs) are needed, Essure seems effective, in terms of successful placement to occlude hydrosalpinges and is efficacious with regard to subsequent IVF pregnancy rate (PR), live birth rate (LBR), and combined ongoing pregnancy rate (OPR) and LBR per embryo transfer [27].

A theoretical advantage of Adiana over Essure is keeping the uterine cavity free of all foreign matter. A case report on occlusion of unilateral hydrosalpinx prior to IVF resulted in pregnancy [28].

Uterine Factor

Hysteroscopy

Uterine cavity evaluation has been a mainstay of the workup prior to the first IVF cycle. There are data on the prevalence of intrauterine pathology at office hysteroscopy prior to IVF as well as in patients with RIF who then undergo hysteroscopy to reevaluate the uterine cavity. Such pathology includes endometrial polyps, submucous uterine fibroids, intrauterine adhesions, and uterine septae. A study of 678 asymptomatic first-time IVF/intracytoplasmic sperm injection (ICSI) patients who had normal endometrial findings at transvaginal sonography (TVS) reported an 11 % prevalence of unanticipated intrauterine pathology by office hysteroscopy [29]. In a prospective study of 2500 consecutive infertile patients who underwent office hysteroscopy prior to IVF, 22.9 % were found to have intrauterine pathology [30]. A systematic review and meta-analysis of a total of 3179 asymptomatic women undergoing office hysteroscopy prior to a first IVF cycle included one RCT and five non-randomized controlled studies. The patients were either in a hysteroscopy group ($n = 1277$) or a no hysteroscopy group ($n = 1902$), and there was a significantly higher clinical pregnancy rate (CPR) (NNT = 10) and LBR (NNT = 11) in the hysteroscopy group [31].

There was a higher prevalence of abnormal uterine cavity findings (44.9 %) in a retrospective study of 157 patients with a history of two or more IVF failures, suggesting that reevaluation of the uterine cavity would be recommended in patients with RIF [32]. In a study by Demirol et al., 421 patients with two or more failed IVF cycles were randomized to office hysteroscopy or no hysteroscopy. The hysteroscopy group was further subdivided into those with normal (74 % of the group) or abnormal (26 %) findings. Those with normal hysteroscopic findings had a significantly increased CPR than those without undergoing hysteroscopy. Those with hysteroscopy who had intrauterine pathology corrected had a significantly increased CPR than those who did not undergo hysteroscopy [33]. Similar findings were found in another study as well [34]. In addition, in the study by Demirol et al., there was no difference in CPR between those who had normal findings and those with abnormal findings that were corrected, suggesting that the hysteroscopy itself may have a beneficial effect on CPR [33], which was demonstrated in other studies as well [35–38]. Moreover, there is additional recent data that shows improved pregnancy rates when hysteroscopy is performed in the menstrual cycle before ovarian stimulation in fresh cycles as well as before endometrial preparation in frozen embryo transfer (FET) cycles in those with RIF [39].

Endometrial Polyps

It has been suggested that endometrial polyps, the most common type of intrauterine lesion [40], are associated with lower implantation rates and higher rates of miscarriage. There is not a consensus regarding the management of endometrial polyps diagnosed before or during ovarian stimulation for IVF. A retrospective study investigated such scenarios and reported that endometrial polyps <1.5 cm that are found before or during IVF/ICSI cycles did not have an effect on implantation rate (IR) and PR [41]. A similar conclusion regarding PR was made in another study of endometrial polyps <2 cm that were detected during IVF cycles; however, there was a trend towards higher miscarriage rates, suggesting that a freeze-all of embryos with later FET may be beneficial in such cases [42]. A large, retrospective study showed that endometrial polyps <1.4 cm that were found during ovarian stimulation did not have an effect on PR, miscarriage rates, and live-birth rates [43]. Further studies are necessary in order to determine the most appropriate management of endometrial polyps in IVF cycles.

In cases of hysteroscopic polypectomy prior to an IVF cycle, it seems that there is no difference in IVF outcomes if the time interval between polypectomy and initiation of an IVF cycle was <6 months or ≥6 months [44]. A study of effects of endometrial polyps on pregnancy rates and miscarriage rates was conducted with 83 subjects who had endometrial polyps less than 2 cm in diameter suspected by TVS before egg retrieval. The authors found that endometrial polyps of this size did not decrease the PR; however, there was a trend towards an increased miscarriage rate unless a freeze-all was performed with FET a few months later [42]. A small study of nine patients with polyps less than 1.5 cm diagnosed by TVS showed that pregnancy is possible as five patients did become pregnant. These patients had undergone hysteroscopic polypectomy 2–16 days prior to embryo transfer (ET) [45].

Uterine Fibroids

Submucosal uterine fibroids and those with an intramural portion as well as a portion that compresses the uterine cavity, also called submucosal type II myomas, significantly decrease IVF pregnancy rates. Pregnancy rates are improved and miscarriage rates are decreased after these types of uterine fibroids are surgically removed by hysteroscopy or abdominal myomectomy prior to the ART cycle. Although the adverse effects of submucosal fibroids on ART outcomes and the lack of such effects of subserosal fibroids [46] on such outcomes have been well-established, there is controversy regarding the effects of intramural fibroids on IVF. Some studies have shown that intramural fibroids do not have an adverse effect on ART outcomes [47], whereas others have demonstrated that intramural fibroids are indeed associated with adverse reproductive outcomes among IVF patients [48, 49]. In addition, intramural fibroids greater than a threshold size may be associated with adverse IVF outcomes in terms of pregnancy rates if myoma size is greater than 4 cm [50] or decreased LBR if myoma size is greater than 2.85 cm [51].

Although there is some data to suggest that myomectomy for intramural fibroids does increase cumulative delivery rates in ART cases, there is no clear evidence that myomectomy for intramural fibroids improves the compromised ART outcomes [49]. A meta-analysis of 19 observational studies totaling 6087 IVF cycles showed a significant decrease in CPR and LBR among women with intramural fibroids when compared to controls without fibroids [52].

Uterine Septum

Although there is a lack of RCTs regarding the effect of uterine septum resection prior to IVF, several studies have suggested that this practice may be efficacious. A retrospective matched-control study investigated ART outcome after 289 ET before and 538 ET after hysteroscopic uterine septum resection and compared results to two consecutive ETs in the control group. In cases of a large septum, LBRs before surgery, after surgery, and in the control group were 2.7 %, 15.6 %, and 20.9 %, respectively. In those with a small septum, the rates before surgery, after surgery, and in the control group were 2.8 %, 18.6 %, and 21.9 %, respectively [53]. A retrospective matched control study compared spontaneous abortion/pregnancy rate of singleton IVF/ICSI gestations between women with small partial or large uterine septae to those with a normal uterus. Prior to metroplasty, those with small partial or large uterine septae had significantly higher abortion rates than those with a normal uterus. After metroplasty for small partial or large septae, the abortion rates were similar to those with a normal uterus [54]. Another retrospective study showed improved CPR and pregnancy loss outcomes that, after hysteroscopic uterine septum resection, were not different to control patients with a normal uterine cavity [55].

Endometrial Injury

Since it has been hypothesized that a local inflammatory response may enhance endometrial receptivity and facilitate embryo implantation [56, 57], endometrial injury (EI) has been proposed as an adjunct to improve IVF-ET outcomes, particularly in cases of RIF. There has been considerable heterogeneity in studies apart from study design, including differences in the timing of endometrial injury as well as the type and number of EIs employed.

A recent systematic review and meta-analysis included seven controlled studies of EI, described as endometrial biopsy/scratch or hysteroscopy in the cycle preceding ovarian stimulation, among women with RIF undergoing IVF/ICSI. The authors found that the evidence from these studies, four of which were randomized and three of which were non-randomized, demonstrated a beneficial effect of EI as the pooled risk ratio (RR) for CPR showed a 71 % increase in likelihood of clinical pregnancy when compared with no intervention [58].

A Cochrane Review of RCTs comparing any kind of intentional endometrial injury prior to ET with either no intervention or with mock procedure that did not injure the endometrium included five trials for a total of 591 women. Since clinical pregnancy per woman showed substantial heterogeneity, a planned subgroup analysis was performed. Four trials in the subgroup with EI in the cycle prior to ovarian stimulation showed a significant increase in LBR in two of the trials and in CPR in all four of the trials. One trial in the subgroup with EI on the day of oocyte retrieval showed a reduction in CPR and ongoing PR (so not advisable to perform on day of oocyte retrieval). Insufficient data on multiple pregnancy or spontaneous abortion (SAB) rates [59].

A more recent randomized trial showed a significantly higher CPR and LBR among women who had endometrial scratch performed as compared to controls. In this study, the endometrial scratch was performed during oral contraceptive pill (OCP) pretreatment, 7–14 days before stimulation medications were started [60]. In addition, a prospective, nonrandomized, controlled study showed that luteal phase office hysteroscopy and concurrent endometrial biopsy significantly improved IR and IVF outcome [61], and a study of single endometrial biopsy in the proliferative phase of the cycle preceding IVF showed benefit as well [62].

Although the currently available data favors endometrial injury in the cycle preceding the IVF cycle, questions remain as to patient selection as well as the ideal method, timing, and number of EIs performed. EI has shown promise in improving outcomes in RIF patients; however, large RCTs and/or a consensus are required before EI can be considered for routine practice.

Heparin

It has been suggested that heparin may modulate physiologic processes that are involved in the implantation process via its anticoagulant and immunomodulatory properties. There has been controversy as to whether or not heparin, or low molecular weight heparin (LMWH) is efficacious in improving LBRs, and there have been some promising data, particularly in those with RIF. A systematic review and meta-analysis of ten relevant studies included five observational studies with a combined total of 1217 cycles and five randomized with a combined total of 732 cycles. The meta-analysis of the randomized studies showed no difference in CPR, LBR, IR, and SAB rate when comparing heparin treatment during IVF to placebo. The meta-analysis of the observational studies showed a significant increase in CPR and LBR with heparin. Because there were small numbers of women and high methodological heterogeneity in the randomized studies, adequately powered randomized studies are needed for a further evaluation of the potential role of heparin in IVF cycles [63]. A prospective, quasi-randomized, controlled trial of 334 cycles in women with one or two previously unexplained, failed ICSI attempts compared standard IVF treatment to standard IVF treatment with the combination of LMWH 1 mg/kg/day and Prednisolone 20 mg/day. There was a significant difference in PR and IR between groups, favoring the study group, indicating that such adjunct treatment may have a significant effect in unexplained, failed implantation [64].

A recent systematic review and meta-analysis evaluated the effect of LMWH on IR and LBR in women with RIF who are undergoing IVF. Studies included compared LMWH vs control/placebo in women with RIF. Two RCTs and one quasi-randomized trial were included. One study included women with at least one thrombophilia [65] and two studies [66, 67] included women with unexplained RIF. The authors concluded that in women with ≥3 failed implantations (RIF), LMWH significantly improves LBR by 79 % compared with the control group; however, due to the small overall sample size, similar evidence from adequately powered RCTs are required prior to the recommendation of LMWH for routine clinical use [68].

Subclinical hypothyroidism: There has been evidence that subclinical hypothyroidism (SCH), either defined as a Thyroid Stimulating Hormone (TSH) >4.0 or TSH >2.5 with normal Thyroxine (T4) levels and the absence of clinical symptoms of hypothyroidism, may be associated with RPL [69]. Several studies have investigated if the treatment of SCH optimizes IVF outcomes. A randomized study compared a study group of levothyroxine 50 mcg to control in 64 women who underwent IVF/ICSI. Although there was no difference in CPR per cycle between groups, there was a significant decrease in pregnancy loss in the levothyroxine group. In addition, embryo quality, IR, and LBR were significantly improved in the study group as well [70]. A retrospective study of 627 women with SCH with a TSH threshold of 4–5 mIU/L and/or thyroid autoimmunity who underwent IVF found that LBR and miscarriage rates were not impaired in these patients [71].

Male Factor

Sperm DNA fragmentation may be associated with an increased risk of miscarriage [72, 73]; however, an association with RIF has not yet been shown. Although earlier studies suggested that a DNA fragmentation index (DFI) of >27 % may be associated with unsuccessful IVF [74, 75], recent data do not support testing [76–78]. A retrospective study by Dar et al. showed that ICSI in men with a high DFI of >50 % resulted in similar PR compared with ICSI among controls with a normal DFI; there was a trend toward higher miscarriage in the high DFI group [79]. Furthermore, sperm DNA fragmentation is not associated with CPR, biochemical pregnancy, and miscarriage rates after FET with cleavage-stage embryos or blastocysts [80]. Unless future, large studies suggest otherwise, sperm DNA integrity testing should only be in the realm of RIF research at this time.

The potential impact of varicocele repair on ART outcome has been investigated in several small studies. In a study of 242 ICSI cases in men with clinical varicocele, 80 subjects underwent varicocelectomy and 162 were not surgically treated. Total motile sperm counts were increased and sperm defect scores were lower in the varicocelectomy group. CPR as well as LBR was significantly higher and the miscarriage rate was lower in the varicocelectomy group [81]. There is also data that suggests that varicocelectomy significantly increases the sperm retrieval rate in men with clinical varicocele and nonobstructive azoospermia (NOA) although the fertilization rates and CPRs were similar between the study group ($n=66$) and the control group ($n=30$) with untreated varicocele and NOA [82]. Larger studies are necessary to further elucidate the impact of varicocele and varicocelectomy on ART outcomes.

Parental Karyotypes

In couples with RIF, 2.5 % are found to have abnormal karyotypes [83]. This is higher than the rate of karyotypic abnormalities within the general population. Particularly in RPL cases, parental karyotypes may reveal genetic conditions such as balanced translocations, which constitute the majority of parental chromosomal abnormalities and carry the potential to result in an unbalanced translocation in a fetus.

Laboratory

ICSI

Since its advent in 1992 [84], ICSI has become used routinely in the vast majority of IVF units and has been found to be a safe and effective means of treating male factor infertility [85]. ICSI has proven to be a powerful tool in overcoming severe male factor cases which, prior to ICSI, could only be treated with donor sperm. Although there has been conflicting data regarding the efficacy of ICSI in preventing or minimizing total fertilization failure (TFF) in couples with unexplained infertility [86, 87], there have been data to support its use in cases where standard insemination has resulted in lower fertilization than expected or failed fertilization [85]. The application of ICSI has been successfully extended to ART cases that involve sperm retrieval for either obstructive azoospermia or NOA [88]. ICSI is also recommended in order to fertilize cryopreserved-thawed oocytes [85]. Furthermore, ICSI is preferred in cases of preimplantation genetic screening/preimplantation genetic diagnosis (PGS/PGD) in order to eliminate the risk of polyspermy that otherwise may affect the genetic make-up of the resultant embryo [88, 89].

Rescue ICSI

In some cases of TFF after conventional IVF, "rescue ICSI" has been performed in an attempt to salvage the current IVF cycle. Rescue ICSI was first described in 1993 [90] and is a resort taken when ICSI is performed for cases in which fertilization has not occurred after conventional IVF. The main reasons for TFF include failure of sperm to bind to the zona pellucida (ZP) or to penetrate the egg [91, 92] or failure of fertilization after penetration of the egg by sperm [92]. Recently, a retrospective study of 9858 IVF cycles found that an elevated progesterone level (>1.5 ng/ml) on the day of human chorionic gonadotropin (hCG) trigger is significantly associated with the need for rescue ICSI, suggesting that ICSI may minimize the risk of TFF in patients with elevated progesterone on the day of hCG administration [93].

The disadvantages of rescue ICSI include the potential for chromosomal abnormalities within the unfertilized oocytes and the resultant embryos and lower pregnancy rates. Although data are limited, the existing studies do not indicate an increased rate of malformations among children conceived with rescue ICSI. The neonatal outcomes of children conceived after early rescue ICSI have been shown to be similar to those who were conceived after ICSI [94]. The advantage is the cost-effectiveness of rescue ICSI when compared to discontinuing the cycle and proceeding with a subsequent fresh IVF/ICSI cycle and the possibility, albeit low, of pregnancy with the current cycle. Although rescue ICSI can result in successful pregnancies and live births, the PR is low.

IMSI

Motile sperm organelle morphology examination (MSOME) is a new approach which involves real-time high-magnification assessment of unstained spermatozoa [95], and the application of this technology in conjunction with ICSI is called intracytoplasmic morphologically selected sperm injection (IMSI). When compared with the magnification of ×400 that is typically used for ICSI in order to identify major sperm morphological defects, the magnification of IMSI is in the ×6600 to ×13,000 range [96]. IMSI is thought to facilitate the selection of the best available motile sperm for oocyte injection and allows for assessment of nuclear status of spermatozoa. Although the data from one prospective trial of 255 patients did not support the use of IMSI over ICSI for first ART cycles [97], IMSI has been suggested as an alternative for those with recurrent ICSI failures [98] or increased rates of spermatozoa with DNA fragmentation [99] since IMSI aids in the selection of spermatozoa with nuclei that are free of vacuoles which may be associated with impaired embryonic development. Although studies that have examined the efficacy of IMSI have great heterogeneity leading to conflicting results [100], the literature in general has not shown a difference in fertilization rate between IMSI and ICSI. Some studies have demonstrated improvement in blastocyst formation, PR, and IR with IMSI as compared to ICSI [101], although there has been some controversy about the studies [102]. There is a need for more RCTs in order to further determine the potential role of IMSI in ART.

Physiological Intracytoplasmic Sperm Injection (PICSI)

Hyaluronic acid (HA) has been found to be a significant factor in the process of physiologic sperm selection. In order for mature spermatozoa to be able to penetrate the extracellular matrix (ECM) of the cumulus oophorus and then reach the

ZP and fertilize the oocyte, the spermatozoa must extrude specific receptors in order to bind to and digest HA, which is a component of the ECM. It has been hypothesized that ART treatment outcomes may be improved by the selection of spermatozoa by HA in vitro.

A prospective-randomized study examined the role of HA for the selection of spermatozoa that have normal chromatin content in order to optimize ICSI outcomes in the setting of the injection of a limited number of oocytes according to Italian law at the time of study. HA-bound spermatozoa were found to have a significant reduction in DNA fragmentation, a significant improvement in likelihood of having a normal nucleus, and resulted in significantly improved embryo quality and development. In addition, this process was found to speed up sperm selection during IMSI [103]. The same group conducted a retrospective study of a larger number of patients, 293 couples treated with HA-ICSI compared to 86 couples with polyvinyl pyrrolidone (PVP)-ICSI. Results showed that HA-ICSI significantly improves embryo quality and implantation [104].

There are two ready systems for HA-ICSI, the PICSI (PICSI Sperm Selection Device; MidAtlantic Diagnostic Origio) and Sperm Slow (Sperm Slow; MediCult-Origio). In PICSI, a plastic culture dish with microdots of HA hydrogel at the bottom of the dish is used, and HA-bound spermatozoa appear bound by their heads to the bottom of the dish, with tail motility visualized as spinning with vigor. Sperm Slow employs a viscous medium that contains HA; therefore, the attached sperm appear slowed. A prospective, randomized study was conducted in order to compare the two systems, with 50 subjects in the PICSI group and 50 subjects in the Sperm Slow group. There was no difference between groups with regard to good-quality embryo rate (primary outcome) as well as secondary outcomes such as fertilization, pregnancy, and IR. The difference found was with regard to duration of procedure as PICSI took three more minutes to perform than Sperm Slow [105].

In order to investigate whether or not HA-ICSI improves outcomes in those with unexplained infertility and thus, normal semen parameters, Majmudar et al. conducted a prospective, randomized study of first IVF-ICSI-fresh-ET cycles among 156 patients. Subjects were randomized to a PICSI group or a group of ICSI with visual assessment for sperm selection. PICSI did not appear to benefit couples with unexplained infertility and normal semen parameters since there were no differences between groups in terms of fertilization rates, number of top quality embryos, and CPR. There was a trend towards a higher miscarriage rate in ICSI as compared to PICSI [106].

There was a statistically significant reduction in SAB rates among couples with ≤65 % HA-bound sperm in a large, multicenter, double-blinded RCT of ten private and hospital-based IVF programs. In this same study, although there were trends in terms of improvement of CPR and IR, there was no significant difference in these outcomes when PICSI was performed. Further, larger studies are warranted due to some encouraging results observed with PICSI [107].

Assisted Hatching

Assisted Hatching (AH), is a technique that involves the artificial thinning or breaching of the ZP, which is the glycoprotein layer that surrounds the embryo. AH is used in order to attempt to improve IR and PR. Methods used to create an opening in the ZP include acidified Tyrode's solution, partial zona dissection with glass micromanipulation, laser, or piezo micromanipulator. Thinning of the ZP can be performed with proteolytic enzymes, acidified Tyrode's solution, or laser [108].

Although it has been recommended that AH not be routinely offered for all IVF patients, AH has been shown to slightly improve CPR in poor prognosis patients, including those with prior failed IVF cycles [109, 110]. Due to a small number of studies having reported LBR, there is insufficient data on the effect of AH on LBR [109].

AH seems to be associated with increased risk of multiple gestation; however, there is not enough evidence to show an association with an increased risk of monozygotic twins.

Embryo Glue

Macromolecules in human embryo culture media have gained added attention in recent years as potential mediators for improved implantation rates. HA has been demonstrated to be present in the fallopian tube as well as in uterine fluids and increases as the time of implantation approaches [111]. EmbryoGlue™ is a modified culture medium that contains a higher concentration of HA and a low concentration of recombinant HA (rHA) instead of human serum albumin. The IR with this culture medium has been shown to be higher than a blastocyst culture medium [112].

A prospective, randomized trial of 815 IVF/ICSI patients with day 3 ET compared outcomes between 417 patients in the EmbryoGlue group and 398 patients in the control group. There was an increase in CPR among tubal factor patients and an increased IR in RIF patients as compared with the control group. Furthermore, the LBR and triplet delivery rates were significantly higher in the EmbryoGlue group [113]. Similar conclusions in terms of increased IR, CPR, and multiple gestation rates were made in a study of 243 IVF patients with 129 patients in the EmbryoGlue group and 114 patients in the control group. Interestingly, the ectopic pregnancy rate was significantly lower in the study group [114]. In contrast to the studies above but among women with previous failed IVF cycles, a matched controlled study showed a higher fresh IVF-ET LBR for those who did not use EmbryoGlue when compared to the study group.

A Cochrane Review of adherence compounds in embryo transfer media in ART cycles, which included 16 studies that investigated the use of HA in media, found moderate quality evidence of an increase in PR and LBR. In addition, the multiple gestation rate was increased but may have been a function of using HA and/or the transfer of multiple embryos. Further studies of HA with SET are warranted [115].

Extended Culture

Extended culture to blastocyst stage transfer has been employed widely as of the past decade. There has been some evidence that the potential of blastocyst implantation is high, allowing the transfer of fewer embryos [116–119]. The higher implantation rates may be due to top quality embryo selection as well as a greater degree of synchrony between the embryo and endometrium [120]. Although extended culture to the blastocyst stage has been shown to have benefits, many IVF cycles may not result in blastocyst formation in vitro. Clinical predictors of human blastocyst formation and pregnancy after extended culture include younger female age, increased parity, standard insemination, lower required gonadotropin dose, higher antral follicle counts, and the absence of male factor [121].

A Cochrane review found a small significant improvement in LBR with day 5 or 6 blastocyst transfer when compared to day 2 or 3 transfer [122]. Furthermore, a recent review and meta-analysis of seven trials with a total of 1446 cases suggests that blastocyst transfer is associated with improved live birth as well as other pregnancy outcomes after fresh IVF or IVF/ICSI cycles when compared with cleavage stage transfer [123]. In addition, extended culture for cryopreservation of surplus embryos at the blastocyst stage optimizes clinical outcomes for good candidates when compared to cryopreservation and thaw of cleavage stage embryos [124, 125].

PGS

Preimplantation Genetic Screening (PGS) involves the assessment of the chromosome complement within embryonic cells in order to select embryo(s) for transfer that are presumed to have greater implantation potential and a lesser risk of miscarriage. Obtaining oocyte or embryo DNA via biopsy can be accomplished by polar body biopsy, blastomere biopsy at the cleavage stage, or trophectoderm biopsy at the blastocyst stage. At the cleavage stage, biopsy markedly reduces embryonic implantation potential whereas trophectoderm biopsy appears to have no measurable impact [126]. There has been controversy regarding the efficacy of PGS due to factors such as the patient population, technical aspects such as the embryo biopsy itself and the method by which genetic analysis is performed, and mosaicism within the embryo; however, recent data suggests that outcomes may be improved in cases of trophectoderm biopsy and the use of newer technologies for chromosomal analysis such as comparative genomic hybridization (CGH), polymerase chain reaction (PCR), and next generation sequencing. The optimal time to perform biopsy for PGS/PGD has been found to be at the blastocyst stage [127]. Importantly, trophectoderm biopsy is associated with a lesser likelihood of mosaicism as well as an increased amount of DNA available for testing of 24 chromosomes [128].

The main indications for PGS are advanced maternal age (AMA), RIF, and RPL [128]. PGS with fluorescence in situ hybridization (FISH) has been shown to be beneficial for AMA [129]. Several studies have shown that PGS does not increase IR in women with RIF; however, PGS was carried out with FISH and day 3 blasto-mere biopsy was performed in these studies [129–131]. More recent studies have suggested that PGS with comprehensive chromosomal screening (CCS) may be associated with improved ART outcomes. A RCT of blastocyst biopsy with CCS and fresh ET showed an increase in implantation and delivery rates among the study group when compared with the control group of routine care [132]. Next generation sequencing is a newer application for PGS in which there is great interest and may hold promise. A recent systematic review concludes that even with trophectoderm biopsy and techniques that allow for aneuploidy assessments of all 24 chromosomes, the current state of PGS still needs to be proven and is considered experimental until further evidence suggests otherwise [133].

Multiple Embryo Transfer

Multiple embryo transfer has been common practice since the early days of IVF, with the goal of achieving pregnancy for the subfertile couple. Due to advances in culture medium systems, laboratory conditions, cryopreservation-thaw technologies, and stimulation protocols, as well as other factors, ART success rates have improved greatly in the last two decades. Due to the inherent risks that multiple gestation carries for mother and her pregnancy, there have been trends towards elective single embryo transfer (eSET) in good prognosis patients. At the other end of the spectrum, however, are poor prognosis patients who would still benefit from multiple embryo transfer. A recent study found that it is efficacious to perform SET in good prognosis (43 % OPR, 2 % multiple gestation rate) and triple-embryo transfer in poor prognosis patients (18 % OPR, 13 % multiple ges-tation rate); however, ET strategy in those with intermediate prognosis requires further improvement (27 % OPR, 23 % multiple gestation rate) [134]. The American Society of Reproductive Medicine (ASRM) Practice Committee guide-lines for the number of embryos to transfer have been revised over time in order to minimize multiple gestation [135]. A Cochrane Review showed that, in younger women with a good prognosis, SET is associated with a lower LBR than double ET (DET); however, there is no difference in cumulative LBR when comparing a single cycle of DET with either two cycles of fresh SET or one cycle of fresh SET followed by one frozen SET [136].

Cytoplasmic Transfer

The experimental technique known as cytoplasmic transfer involves the introduction of ooplasm from a presumably healthy donor oocyte or zygote into compromised oocytes. Included in this transfer of cytoplasm are mitochondria, mRNAs, and proteins, as well as other factors. A small number of cases have been performed, and although pregnancies have resulted, cytoplasmic transfer is not recommended at this time due to its investigational nature [137].

Summary

In summary, there are various areas in the clinical and laboratory aspects that may be considered when optimizing ART cycles, whether it is a couple's first cycle or after failed IVF cycles. It is critical to maximize the chance of success in ART and, although some of the topics outlined in this chapter are considered standard of care, others require more research in terms of a greater number of, and larger, RCTs prior to determination as to whether they are applicable, safe, and efficacious.

References

1. Broer SL, Mol BW, Hendriks D, Broekmans FJ. The role of antimullerian hormone in prediction of outcome after IVF: comparison with the antral follicle count. Fertil Steril. 2009;91:705–14.
2. Broer SL, Dolleman M, Opmeer BC, Fauser BC, Mol BW, Broekmans FJ. AMH and AFC as predictors of excessive response in controlled ovarian hyperstimulation: a meta-analysis. Hum Reprod Update. 2011;17:46–54.
3. Broer SL, Eijkemans MJ, Scheffer GJ, van Rooij IA, de Vet A, Themmen AP, Laven JS, de Jong FH, Te Velde ER, Fauser BC, et al. Anti-Mullerian hormone predicts menopause: a long-term follow-up study in normoovulatory women. J Clin Endocrinol Metab. 2011;96:2532–253.
4. Bhide P, Gudi A, Shah A, Timms P, Grayson K, Homburg R. Anti-Müllerian hormone as a predictor of pregnancy following IVF. Reprod Biomed Online. 2013;26(3):247–52. doi:10.1016/j.rbmo.2012.11.018. Epub 2012 Dec 8.
5. Broer SL, van Disseldorp J, Broeze KA, Dolleman M, Opmeer BC, Bossuyt P, Eijkemans MJ, Mol BW, Broekmans FJ. Added value of ovarian reserve testing on patient characteristics in the prediction of ovarian response and ongoing pregnancy: an individual patient data approach. Hum Reprod Update. 2013;19:26–36.
6. Reichman DE, Goldschlag D, Rosenwaks Z. Value of antimüllerian hormone as a prognostic indicator of in vitro fertilization outcome. Fertil Steril. 2014;101(4):1012–8.e1. doi:10.1016/j.fertnstert.2013.12.039. Epub 2014 Feb 1.
7. Polyzos NP, Nelson SM, Stoop D, Nwoye M, Humaidan P, Anckaert E, Devroey P, Tournaye H. Does the time interval between antimüllerian hormone serum sampling and initiation of ovarian stimulation affect its predictive ability in in vitro fertilization-intracytoplasmic sperm injection cycles with a gonadotropin-releasing hormone antagonist? A retrospective single-center study. Fertil Steril. 2013;100(2):438–44. doi:10.1016/j.fertnstert.2013.03.031. Epub 2013 Apr 16.
8. Tsoumpou I, Kyrgiou M, Gelbaya TA, Nardo LG. The effect of surgical treatment for endometrioma on in vitro fertilization outcomes: a systematic review and meta-analysis. Fertil Steril. 2009;92(1):75–87. doi:10.1016/j.fertnstert.2008.05.049. Epub 2008 Aug 9.
9. Benschop L, Farquhar C, van der Poel N, Heineman MJ. Interventions for women with endometrioma prior to assisted reproductive technology. Cochrane Database Syst Rev. 2010;11, CD008571. doi:10.1002/14651858.CD008571.pub2.
10. Somigliana E, Berlanda N, Benaglia L, Viganò P, Vercellini P, Fedele L. Surgical excision of endometriomas and ovarian reserve: a systematic review on serum antimüllerian hormone

   level modifications. Fertil Steril. 2012;98(6):1531–8. doi:10.1016/j.fertnstert.2012.08.009. Epub 2012 Sep 10. Review.
11. Uncu G, Kasapoglu I, Ozerkan K, Seyhan A, Oral Yilmaztepe A, Ata B. Prospective assessment of the impact of endometriomas and their removal on ovarian reserve and determinants of the rate of decline in ovarian reserve. Hum Reprod. 2013;28(8):2140–5. doi:10.1093/humrep/det123. Epub 2013 Apr 26.
12. Garcia-Velasco JA, Somigliana E. Management of endometriomas in women requiring IVF: to touch or not to touch. Hum Reprod. 2009;24(3):496–501. doi:10.1093/humrep/den398. Epub 2008 Dec 4.
13. Hirokawa W, Iwase A, Goto M, Takikawa S, Nagatomo Y, Nakahara T, Bayasula B, Nakamura T, Manabe S, Kikkawa F. The post-operative decline in serum anti-Mullerian hormone correlates with the bilaterality and severity of endometriosis. Hum Reprod. 2011;26(4):904–10. doi:10.1093/humrep/der006. Epub 2011 Feb 2.
14. Strandell A, Lindhard A, Waldenström U, Thorburn J, Janson PO, Hamberger L. Hydrosalpinx and IVF outcome: a prospective, randomized multicentre trial in Scandinavia on salpingectomy prior to IVF. Hum Reprod. 1999;14(11):2762–9.
15. Wainer R, Camus E, Camier B, Martin C, Vasseur C, Merlet F. Does hydrosalpinx reduce the pregnancy rate after in vitro fertilization? Fertil Steril. 1997;68(6):1022–6.
16. Camus E, Poncelet C, Goffinet F, Wainer B, Merlet F, Nisand I, Philippe HJ. Pregnancy rates after in-vitro fertilization in cases of tubal infertility with and without hydrosalpinx: a meta-analysis of published comparative studies. Hum Reprod. 1999;14(5):1243–9.
17. Sachdev R, Kemmann E, Bohrer MK, el-Danasouri I. Detrimental effect of hydrosalpinx fluid on the development and blastulation of mouse embryos in vitro. Fertil Steril. 1997;68(3):531–3.
18. Meyer WR, Castelbaum AJ, Somkuti S, Sagoskin AW, Doyle M, Harris JE, Lessey BA. Hydrosalpinges adversely affect markers of endometrial receptivity. Hum Reprod. 1997;12(7):1393–8.
19. Daftary GS, Kayisli U, Seli E, Bukulmez O, Arici A, Taylor HS. Salpingectomy increases peri-implantation endometrial HOXA10 expression in women with hydrosalpinx. Fertil Steril. 2007;87(2):367–72. Epub 2006 Dec 14.
20. Strandell A. Treatment of hydrosalpinx in the patient undergoing assisted reproduction. Curr Opin Obstet Gynecol. 2007;19(4):360–5. Review.
21. Strandell A, Lindhard A. Hydrosalpinx and ART. Salpingectomy prior to IVF can be recommended to a well-defined subgroup of patients. Hum Reprod. 2000;15(10):2072–4.
22. Johnson N, van Voorst S, Sowter MC, Strandell A, Mol BW. Surgical treatment for tubal disease in women due to undergo in vitro fertilisation. Cochrane Database Syst Rev. 2010;1, CD002125. doi:10.1002/14651858.CD002125.pub3. Review.
23. Kontoravdis A, Makrakis E, Pantos K, Botsis D, Deligeoroglou E, Creatsas G. Proximal tubal occlusion and salpingectomy result in similar improvement in in vitro fertilization outcome in patients with hydrosalpinx. Fertil Steril. 2006;86(6):1642–9. Epub 2006 Oct 25.
24. Bildirici I, Bukulmez O, Ensari A, Yarali H, Gurgan T. A prospective evaluation of the effect of salpingectomy on endometrial receptivity in cases of women with communicating hydrosalpinges. Hum Reprod. 2001;16(11):2422–6.
25. Matorras R, Rabanal A, Prieto B, Diez S, Brouard I, Mendoza R, Exposito A. Hysteroscopic hydrosalpinx occlusion with Essure device in IVF patients when salpingectomy or laparoscopy is contraindicated. Eur J Obstet Gynecol Reprod Biol. 2013;169(1):54–9. doi:10.1016/j.ejogrb.2013.02.008. Epub 2013 Apr 2.
26. Sonigo C, Collinet P, Rubod C, Catteau-Jonard S. Current position of Essure(®) micro-insert in the management of hydrosalpinges before in vitro fertilization [article in French]. Gynecol Obstet Fertil. 2013;41(2):133–8. doi:10.1016/j.gyobfe.2012.12.010. Epub 2013 Jan 30.
27. Arora P, Arora RS, Cahill D. Essure(®) for management of hydrosalpinx prior to in vitro fertilisation-a systematic review and pooled analysis. BJOG. 2014;121(5):527–36. doi:10.1111/1471-0528.12533. Epub 2014 Jan 3.
28. Legendre G, Gallot V, Levaillant JM, Capmas P, Fernandez H. Adiana(®) hysteroscopic tubal occlusion device for the treatment of hydrosalpinx prior to in vitro fertilization: a case report [article in French]. J Gynecol Obstet Biol Reprod (Paris). 2013;42(4):401–4. doi:10.1016/j.jgyn.2013.03.008. Epub 2013 Apr 15.

29. Fatemi HM, Kasius JC, Timmermans A, van Disseldorp J, Fauser BC, Devroey P, Broekmans FJ. Prevalence of unsuspected uterine cavity abnormalities diagnosed by office hysteroscopy prior to in vitro fertilization. Hum Reprod. 2010;25(8):1959–65. doi:10.1093/humrep/deq150. Epub 2010 Jun 22.

30. Karayalcin R, Ozcan S, Moraloglu O, Ozyer S, Mollamahmutoglu L, Batıoglu S. Results of 2500 office-based diagnostic hysteroscopies before IVF. Reprod Biomed Online. 2010;20(5):689–93. doi:10.1016/j.rbmo.2009.12.030. Epub 2010 Feb 1.

31. Pundir J, Pundir V, Omanwa K, Khalaf Y, El-Toukhy T. Hysteroscopy prior to the first IVF cycle: a systematic review and meta-analysis. Reprod Biomed Online. 2014;28(2):151–61. doi:10.1016/j.rbmo.2013.09.025. Epub 2013 Oct 5.

32. Cenksoy P, Ficicioglu C, Yıldırım G, Yesiladali M. Hysteroscopic findings in women with recurrent IVF failures and the effect of correction of hysteroscopic findings on subsequent pregnancy rates. Arch Gynecol Obstet. 2013;287(2):357–60. doi:10.1007/s00404-012-2627-5. Epub 2012 Nov 27.

33. Demirol A, Gurgan T. Effect of treatment of intrauterine pathologies with office hysteroscopy in patients with recurrent IVF failure. Reprod Biomed Online. 2004;8(5):590–4.

34. Rama Raju GA, Shashi Kumari G, Krishna KM, Prakash GJ, Madan K. Assessment of uterine cavity by hysteroscopy in assisted reproduction programme and its influence on pregnancy outcome. Arch Gynecol Obstet. 2006;274(3):160–4. Epub 2006 May 10.

35. Bosteels J, Weyers S, Puttemans P, Panayotidis C, Van Herendael B, Gomel V, Mol BW, Mathieu C, D'Hooghe T. The effectiveness of hysteroscopy in improving pregnancy rates in subfertile women without other gynaecological symptoms: a systematic review. Hum Reprod Update. 2010;16(1):1–11. doi:10.1093/humupd/dmp033.Epub. Review.

36. Makrakis E, Pantos K. The outcomes of hysteroscopy in women with implantation failures after in-vitro fertilization: findings and effect on subsequent pregnancy rates. Curr Opin Obstet Gynecol. 2010;22(4):339–43. doi:10.1097/GCO.0b013e32833beaa3.

37. El-Toukhy T, Campo R, Sunkara SK, Khalaf Y, Coomarasamy A. A multi-centre randomised controlled study of pre-IVF outpatient hysteroscopy in women with recurrent IVF implantation failure: Trial of Outpatient Hysteroscopy—[TROPHY] in IVF. Reprod Health. 2009;6:20. doi:10.1186/1742-4755-6-20.

38. Karayalçin R, Ozyer S, Ozcan S, Uzunlar O, Gürlek B, Moraloğlu O, Batioğlu S. Office hysteroscopy improves pregnancy rates following IVF. Reprod Biomed Online. 2012;25(3):261–6. doi:10.1016/j.rbmo.2012.05.013. Epub 2012 Jun 16.

39. Hosseini MA, Ebrahimi N, Mahdavi A, Aleyasin A, Safdarian L, Fallahi P, Esfahani F. Hysteroscopy in patients with repeated implantation failure improves the outcome of assisted reproductive technology in fresh and frozen cycles. J Obstet Gynaecol Res. 2014;40(5):1324–30. doi:10.1111/jog.12315. Epub 2014 Mar 10.

40. Doldi N, Persico P, Di Sebastiano F, Marsiglio E, De Santis L, Rabellotti E, Fusi F, Brigante C, Ferrari A. Pathologic findings in hysteroscopy before in vitro fertilization-embryo transfer (IVF-ET). Gynecol Endocrinol. 2005;21(4):235–7.

41. Isikoglu M, Berkkanoglu M, Senturk Z, Coetzee K, Ozgur K. Endometrial polyps smaller than 1.5 cm do not affect ICSI outcome. Reprod Biomed Online. 2006;12(2):199–204.

42. Lass A, Williams G, Abusheikha N, Brinsden P. The effect of endometrial polyps on outcomes of in vitro fertilization (IVF) cycles. J Assist Reprod Genet. 1999;16(8):410–5.

43. Tiras B, Korucuoglu U, Polat M, Zeyneloglu HB, Saltik A, Yarali H. Management of endometrial polyps diagnosed before or during ICSI cycles. Reprod Biomed Online. 2012;24(1):123–8. doi:10.1016/j.rbmo.2011.09.002. Epub 2011 Sep 16.

44. Eryilmaz OG, Gulerman C, Sarikaya E, Yesilyurt H, Karsli F, Cicek N. Appropriate interval between endometrial polyp resection and the proceeding IVF start. Arch Gynecol Obstet. 2012;285(6):1753–7. doi:10.1007/s00404-012-2238-1.

45. Madani T, Ghaffari F, Kiani K, Hosseini F. Hysteroscopic polypectomy without cycle cancellation in IVF cycles. Reprod Biomed Online. 2009;18(3):412–5.

46. Bernard G, Darai E, Poncelet C, Benifla JL, Madelenat P. Fertility after hysteroscopic myomectomy: effect of intramural myomas associated. Eur J Obstet Gynecol Reprod Biol. 2000;88(1):85–90.

47. Bozdag G, Esinler I, Boynukalin K, Aksu T, Gunalp S, Gurgan T. Single intramural leiomyoma with normal hysteroscopic findings does not affect ICSI-embryo transfer outcome. Reprod Biomed Online. 2009;19(2):276–80.
48. Hart R, Khalaf Y, Yeong CT, Seed P, Taylor A, Braude P. A prospective controlled study of the effect of intramural uterine fibroids on the outcome of assisted conception. Hum Reprod. 2001;16(11):2411–7.
49. Somigliana E, De Benedictis S, Vercellini P, Nicolosi AE, Benaglia L, Scarduelli C, Ragni G, Fedele L. Fibroids not encroaching the endometrial cavity and IVF success rate: a prospective study. Hum Reprod. 2011;26(4):834–9. doi:10.1093/humrep/der015. Epub 2011 Feb 11.
50. Oliveira FG, Abdelmassih VG, Diamond MP, Dozortsev D, Melo NR, Abdelmassih R. Impact of subserosal and intramural uterine fibroids that do not distort the endometrial cavity on the outcome of in vitro fertilization-intracytoplasmic sperm injection. Fertil Steril. 2004;81(3):582–7.
51. Yan L, Ding L, Li C, Wang Y, Tang R, Chen ZJ. Effect of fibroids not distorting the endometrial cavity on the outcome of in vitro fertilization treatment: a retrospective cohort study. Fertil Steril. 2014;101(3):716–21. doi:10.1016/j.fertnstert.2013.11.023. Epub 2014 Jan 11.
52. Sunkara SK, Khairy M, El-Toukhy T, Khalaf Y, Coomarasamy A. The effect of intramural fibroids without uterine cavity involvement on the outcome of IVF treatment: a systematic review and meta-analysis. Hum Reprod. 2010;25(2):418–29. doi:10.1093/humrep/dep396. Epub 2009 Nov 12. Review.
53. Tomaževič T, Ban-Frangež H, Virant-Klun I, Verdenik I, Požlep B, Vrtačnik-Bokal E. Septate, subseptate and arcuate uterus decrease pregnancy and live birth rates in IVF/ICSI. Reprod Biomed Online. 2010;21(5):700–5. doi:10.1016/j.rbmo.2010.06.028. Epub 2010 Jun 25.
54. Ban-Frangez H, Tomazevic T, Virant-Klun I, Verdenik I, Ribic-Pucelj M, Bokal EV. The outcome of singleton pregnancies after IVF/ICSI in women before and after hysteroscopic resection of a uterine septum compared to normal controls. Eur J Obstet Gynecol Reprod Biol. 2009;146(2):184–7. doi:10.1016/j.ejogrb.2008.04.010. Epub 2008 Jun 3.
55. Ozgur K, Isikoglu M, Donmez L, Oehninger S. Is hysteroscopic correction of an incomplete uterine septum justified prior to IVF? Reprod Biomed Online. 2007;14(3):335–40.
56. Granot I, Gnainsky Y, Dekel N. Endometrial inflammation and effect on implantation improvement and pregnancy outcome. Reproduction. 2012;144(6):661–8. doi:10.1530/REP-12-0217. Epub 2012 Oct 1. Review.
57. Siristatidis C, Vrachnis N, Vogiatzi P, Chrelias C, Retamar AQ, Bettocchi S, Glujovsky D. Potential pathophysiological mechanisms of the beneficial role of endometrial injury in in vitro fertilization outcome. Reprod Sci. 2014;21(8):955–65. Epub ahead of print.
58. Potdar N, Gelbaya T, Nardo LG. Endometrial injury to overcome recurrent embryo implantation failure: a systematic review and meta-analysis. Reprod Biomed Online. 2012;25(6):561–71. doi:10.1016/j.rbmo.2012.08.005. Epub 2012 Sep 12.
59. Nastri CO, Gibreel A, Raine-Fenning N, Maheshwari A, Ferriani RA, Bhattacharya S, Martins WP. Endometrial injury in women undergoing assisted reproductive techniques. Cochrane Database Syst Rev. 2012;7, CD009517. doi:10.1002/14651858.CD009517.pub2. Review.
60. Nastri CO, Ferriani RA, Raine-Fenning N, Martins WP. Endometrial scratching performed in the non-transfer cycle and outcome of assisted reproduction: a randomized controlled trial. Ultrasound Obstet Gynecol. 2013;42(4):375–82. doi:10.1002/uog.12539. Epub 2013 Sep 2.
61. Kumbak B, Sahin L, Ozkan S, Atilgan R. Impact of luteal phase hysteroscopy and concurrent endometrial biopsy on subsequent IVF cycle outcome. Arch Gynecol Obstet. 2014;290(2):369–74. Epub ahead of print.
62. Hayashi T, Kitaya K, Tada Y, Taguchi S, Funabiki M, Nakamura Y. Single curettage endometrial biopsy injury in the proliferative phase improves reproductive outcome of subsequent in vitro fertilization-embryo transfer cycle in infertile patients with repeated embryo implantation failure. Clin Exp Obstet Gynecol. 2013;40(3):323–6.
63. Seshadri S, Sunkara SK, Khalaf Y, El-Toukhy T, Hamoda H. Effect of heparin on the outcome of IVF treatment: a systematic review and meta-analysis. Reprod Biomed Online. 2012;25(6):572–84. doi:10.1016/j.rbmo.2012.08.007. Epub 2012 Sep 16. Review.

64. Fawzy M, El-Refaeey AA. Does combined prednisolone and low molecular weight heparin have a role in unexplained implantation failure? Arch Gynecol Obstet. 2014;289(3):677–80. doi:10.1007/s00404-013-3020-8. Epub 2013 Sep 19.
65. Qublan H, Amarin Z, Dabbas M, Farraj AE, Beni-Merei Z, Al-Akash H, Bdoor AN, Nawasreh M, Malkawi S, Diab F, Al-Ahmad N, Balawneh M, Abu-Salim A. Low-molecular-weight heparin in the treatment of recurrent IVF-ET failure and thrombophilia: a prospective randomized placebo-controlled trial. Hum Fertil (Camb). 2008;11(4):246–53. doi:10.1080/14647270801995431.
66. Urman B, Ata B, Yakin K, Alatas C, Aksoy S, Mercan R, Balaban B. Luteal phase empirical low molecular weight heparin administration in patients with failed ICSI embryo transfer cycles: a randomized open-labeled pilot trial. Hum Reprod. 2009;24(7):1640–7. doi:10.1093/humrep/dep086. Epub 2009 Apr 8.
67. Berker B, Taşkin S, Kahraman K, Taşkin EA, Atabekoğlu C, Sönmezer M. The role of low-molecular-weight heparin in recurrent implantation failure: a prospective, quasi-randomized, controlled study. Fertil Steril. 2011;95(8):2499–502. doi:10.1016/j.fertnstert.2010.12.033. Epub 2011 Jan 17.
68. Potdar N, Gelbaya TA, Konje JC, Nardo LG. Adjunct low-molecular-weight heparin to improve live birth rate after recurrent implantation failure: a systematic review and meta-analysis. Hum Reprod Update. 2013;19(6):674–84. doi:10.1093/humupd/dmt032. Epub 2013 Aug 2. Review.
69. Bernardi LA, Cohen RN, Stephenson MD. Impact of subclinical hypothyroidism in women with recurrent early pregnancy loss. Fertil Steril. 2013;100(5):1326–31. doi:10.1016/j.fertnstert.2013.07.1975. Epub 2013 Aug 15.
70. Kim CH, Ahn JW, Kang SP, Kim SH, Chae HD, Kang BM. Effect of levothyroxine treatment on in vitro fertilization and pregnancy outcome in infertile women with subclinical hypothyroidism undergoing in vitro fertilization/intracytoplasmic sperm injection. Fertil Steril. 2011;95(5):1650–4. doi:10.1016/j.fertnstert.2010.12.004. Epub 2010 Dec 30.
71. Chai J, Yeung WY, Lee CY, Li HW, Ho PC, Ng HY. Live birth rates following in vitro fertilization in women with thyroid autoimmunity and/or subclinical hypothyroidism. Clin Endocrinol (Oxf). 2014;80(1):122–7. doi:10.1111/cen.12220. Epub 2013 May 6.
72. Absalan F, Ghannadi A, Kazerooni M, Parifar R, Jamalzadeh F, Amiri S. Value of sperm chromatin dispersion test in couples with unexplained recurrent abortion. J Assist Reprod Genet. 2012;29:11–4.
73. Brahem S, Mehdi M, Landolsi H, Mougou S, Elghezal H, Saad A. Semen parameters and sperm DNA fragmentation as causes of recurrent pregnancy loss. Urology. 2011;78:792–6.
74. Larson KL, DeJonge CJ, Barnes AM, Jost LK, Evenson DP. Sperm chromatin structure assay parameters as predictors of failed pregnancy following assisted reproductive techniques. Hum Reprod. 2000;15:1717–22.
75. Larson-Cook KL, Brannian JD, Hansen KA, Kasperson KM, Aamold ET, Evenson DP. Relationship between the outcomes of assisted reproductive techniques and sperm DNA fragmentation as measured by the sperm chromatin structure assay. Fertil Steril. 2003;80:895–902.
76. Bungum M, Humaidan P, Spano M, Jepson K, Bungum L, Giwercman A. The predictive value of sperm chromatin structure assay (SCSA) parameters for the outcome of intrauterine insemination, IVF and ICSI. Hum Reprod. 2004;19:1401–8.
77. Bungum M, Humaidan P, Axmon A, Spano M, Bungum L, Erenpreiss J, Giwercman A. Sperm DNA integrity assessment in prediction of assisted reproduction technology outcome. Hum Reprod. 2007;22:174–9.
78. Gandini L, Lombardo F, Paoli D, Caruso F, Eleuteri P, Leter G, Ciriminna R, Culasso F, Dondero F, Lenzi A, Spano M. Full-term pregnancies achieved with ICSI despite high levels of sperm chromatin damage. Hum Reprod. 2004;19:1409–17.
79. Dar S, Grover SA, Moskovtsev SI, Swanson S, Baratz A, Librach CL. In vitro fertilization-intracytoplasmic sperm injection outcome in patients with a markedly high DNA fragmentation index (>50%). Fertil Steril. 2013;100(1):75–80. doi:10.1016/j.fertnstert.2013.03.011. Epub 2013 Apr 3.

80. Ni W, Xiao S, Qiu X, Jin J, Pan C, Li Y, Fei Q, Yang X, Zhang L, Huang X. Effect of sperm DNA fragmentation on clinical outcome of frozen-thawed embryo transfer and on blastocyst formation. PLoS One. 2014;9(4):e94956. doi:10.1371/journal.pone.0094956. eCollection 2014.
81. Esteves SC, Oliveira FV, Bertolla RP. Clinical outcome of intracytoplasmic sperm injection in infertile men with treated and untreated clinical varicocele. J Urol. 2010;184(4):1442–6. doi:10.1016/j.juro.2010.06.004. Epub 2010 Aug 19.
82. Inci K, Hascicek M, Kara O, Dikmen AV, Gürgan T, Ergen A. Sperm retrieval and intracytoplasmic sperm injection in men with nonobstructive azoospermia, and treated and untreated varicocele. J Urol. 2009;182(4):1500–5. doi:10.1016/j.juro.2009.06.028. Epub 2009 Aug 15.
83. Stern C, Pertile M, Norris H, Hale L, Baker HW. Chromosome translocations in couples with in-vitro fertilization implantation failure. Hum Reprod. 1999;14:2097–101.
84. Palermo G, Joris H, Devroey P, Van Steirteghem AC. Pregnancies after intracytoplasmic injection of single spermatozoon into an oocyte. Lancet. 1992;340(8810):17–8.
85. Practice Committees of the American Society for Reproductive Medicine and Society for Assisted Reproductive Technology. Intracytoplasmic sperm injection (ICSI) for non-male factor infertility: a committee opinion. Fertil Steril. 2012;98(6):1395–9. doi:10.1016/j.fertnstert.2012.08.026. Epub 2012 Sep 12.
86. Johnson LN, Sasson IE, Sammel MD, Dokras A. Does intracytoplasmic sperm injection improve the fertilization rate and decrease the total fertilization failure rate in couples with well-defined unexplained infertility? A systematic review and meta-analysis. Fertil Steril. 2013;100(3):704–11. doi:10.1016/j.fertnstert.2013.04.038. Epub 2013 Jun 15. Review.
87. Kim JY, Kim JH, Jee BC, Lee JR, Suh CS, Kim SH. Can intracytoplasmic sperm injection prevent total fertilization failure and enhance embryo quality in patients with non-male factor infertility? Eur J Obstet Gynecol Reprod Biol. 2014;178:188–91. doi:10.1016/j.ejogrb.2014.03.044. Epub 2014 Apr 13.
88. Palermo GD, Neri QV, Takeuchi T, Rosenwaks Z. ICSI: where we have been and where we are going. Semin Reprod Med. 2009;27(2):191–201. doi:10.1055/s-0029-1202309. Epub 2009 Feb 26.
89. Palermo GD, Neri QV, Hariprashad JJ, Davis OK, Veeck LL, Rosenwaks Z. ICSI and its outcome. Semin Reprod Med. 2000;18(2):161–9.
90. Nagy ZP, Joris H, Liu J, Staessen C, Devroey P, Van Steirteghem AC. Intracytoplasmic single sperm injection of 1-day-old unfertilized human oocytes. Hum Reprod. 1993;8(12):2180–4.
91. Mahutte NG, Arici A. Failed fertilization: is it predictable? Curr Opin Obstet Gynecol. 2003;15(3):211–8.
92. Rawe VY, Olmedo SB, Nodar FN, Doncel GD, Acosta AA, Vitullo AD. Cytoskeletal organization defects and abortive activation in human oocytes after IVF and ICSI failure. Mol Hum Reprod. 2000;6(6):510–6.
93. Huang B, Li Z, Zhu L, Hu D, Liu Q, Zhu G, Zhang H. Progesterone elevation on the day of HCG administration may affect rescue ICSI. Reprod Biomed Online. 2014;29(1):88–93. doi:10.1016/j.rbmo.2014.03.015. pii: S1472-6483(14)00182-5. Epub ahead of print.
94. Chen L, Xu Z, Zhang N, Wang B, Chen H, Wang S, Sun H. Neonatal outcome of early rescue ICSI and ICSI with ejaculated sperm. J Assist Reprod Genet. 2014;31(7):823–8. Epub ahead of print.
95. Bartoov B, Berkovitz A, Eltes F. Selection of spermatozoa with normal nuclei to improve the pregnancy rate with intracytoplasmic sperm injection. N Engl J Med. 2001;345(14):1067–8.
96. Garolla A, Fortini D, Menegazzo M, De Toni L, Nicoletti V, Moretti A, Selice R, Engl B, Foresta C. High-power microscopy for selecting spermatozoa for ICSI by physiological status. Reprod Biomed Online. 2008;17(5):610–6.
97. Leandri RD, Gachet A, Pfeffer J, Celebi C, Rives N, Carre-Pigeon F, Kulski O, Mitchell V, Parinaud J. Is intracytoplasmic morphologically selected sperm injection (IMSI) beneficial in the first ART cycle? A multicentric randomized controlled trial. Andrology. 2013;1(5):692–7. doi:10.1111/j.2047-2927.2013.00104.x. Epub 2013 Jun 21.
98. Boitrelle F, Guthauser B, Alter L, Bailly M, Bergere M, Wainer R, Vialard F, Albert M, Selva J. High-magnification selection of spermatozoa prior to oocyte injection: confirmed and potential indications. Reprod Biomed Online. 2014;28(1):6–13. doi:10.1016/j.rbmo.2013.09.019. Epub 2013 Sep 28.

99. Hammoud I, Boitrelle F, Ferfouri F, Vialard F, Bergere M, Wainer B, Bailly M, Albert M, Selva J. Selection of normal spermatozoa with a vacuole-free head (x6300) improves selection of spermatozoa with intact DNA in patients with high sperm DNA fragmentation rates. Andrologia. 2013;45(3):163–70. doi:10.1111/j.1439-0272.2012.01328.x. Epub 2012 Jun 26.

100. El Khattabi L, Dupont C, Sermondade N, Hugues JN, Poncelet C, Porcher R, Cedrin-Durnerin I, Lévy R, Sifer C. Is intracytoplasmic morphologically selected sperm injection effective in patients with infertility related to teratozoospermia or repeated implantation failure? Fertil Steril. 2013;100(1):62–8. doi:10.1016/j.fertnstert.2013.02.048. Epub 2013 Mar 30.

101. Lo Monte G, Murisier F, Piva I, Germond M, Marci R. Focus on intracytoplasmic morphologically selected sperm injection (IMSI): a mini-review. Asian J Androl. 2013;15(5):608–15. doi:10.1038/aja.2013.54. Epub 2013 Jul 8.

102. Setti AS, Paes de Almeida Ferreira Braga D, Iaconelli Jr A, Aoki T, Borges Jr E. Twelve years of MSOME and IMSI: a review. Reprod Biomed Online. 2013;27(4):338–52. doi:10.1016/j.rbmo.2013.06.011. Epub 2013 Jun 28. Review.

103. Parmegiani L, Cognigni GE, Bernardi S, Troilo E, Ciampaglia W, Filicori M. "Physiologic ICSI": hyaluronic acid (HA) favors selection of spermatozoa without DNA fragmentation and with normal nucleus, resulting in improvement of embryo quality. Fertil Steril. 2010;93(2):598–604. doi:10.1016/j.fertnstert.2009.03.033. Epub 2009 Apr 25.

104. Parmegiani L, Cognigni GE, Ciampaglia W, Pocognoli P, Marchi F, Filicori M. Efficiency of hyaluronic acid (HA) sperm selection. J Assist Reprod Genet. 2010;27(1):13–6. doi:10.1007/s10815-009-9380-0. Epub 2009 Dec 30.

105. Parmegiani L, Cognigni GE, Bernardi S, Troilo E, Taraborrelli S, Arnone A, Maccarini AM, Filicori M. Comparison of two ready-to-use systems designed for sperm-hyaluronic acid binding selection before intracytoplasmic sperm injection: PICSI vs. Sperm Slow: a prospective, randomized trial. Fertil Steril. 2012;98(3):632–7. doi:10.1016/j.fertnstert.2012.05.043. Epub 2012 Jun 29.

106. Majumdar G, Majumdar A. A prospective randomized study to evaluate the effect of hyaluronic acid sperm selection on the intracytoplasmic sperm injection outcome of patients with unexplained infertility having normal semen parameters. J Assist Reprod Genet. 2013;30(11):1471–5. doi:10.1007/s10815-013-0108-9. Epub 2013 Oct 2.

107. Worrilow KC, Eid S, Woodhouse D, Perloe M, Smith S, Witmyer J, Ivani K, Khoury C, Ball GD, Elliot T, Lieberman J. Use of hyaluronan in the selection of sperm for intracytoplasmic sperm injection (ICSI): significant improvement in clinical outcomes—multicenter, double-blinded and randomized controlled trial. Hum Reprod. 2013;28(2):306–14. doi:10.1093/humrep/des417. Epub 2012 Nov 30.

108. Practice Committee of the American Society for Reproductive Medicine; Practice Committee of the Society for Assisted Reproductive Technology. Electronic address: ASRM@asrm.org. Role of assisted hatching in in vitro fertilization: a guideline. Fertil Steril. 2014. pii: S0015-0282(14)00497-X. doi:10.1016/j.fertnstert.2014.05.034. [Epub ahead of print].

109. Carney SK, Das S, Blake D, Farquhar C, Seif MM, Nelson L. Assisted hatching on assisted conception (in vitro fertilisation (IVF) and intracytoplasmic sperm injection (ICSI). Cochrane Database Syst Rev. 2012;12, CD001894. doi:10.1002/14651858.CD001894.pub5. Review.

110. Martins WP, Rocha IA, Ferriani RA, Nastri CO. Assisted hatching of human embryos: a systematic review and meta-analysis of randomized controlled trials. Hum Reprod Update. 2011;17(4):438–53. doi:10.1093/humupd/dmr012. Epub 2011 Apr 7. Review. Erratum in: Hum Reprod Update. 2012;18(5):600.

111. Carson DD, Dutt A, Tang JP. Glycoconjugate synthesis during early pregnancy: hyaluronate synthesis and function. Dev Biol. 1987;120(1):228–35.

112. Schoolcraft W, Lane M, Stevens J, Gardner DK. Increased hyaluronan concentration in the embryo transfer medium results in a significant increase in human embryo implantation rate. Fertil Steril. 2002;76 Suppl 3:S5.

113. Valojerdi MR, Karimian L, Yazdi PE, Gilani MA, Madani T, Baghestani AR. Efficacy of a human embryo transfer medium: a prospective, randomized clinical trial study. J Assist Reprod Genet. 2006;23(5):207–12. Epub 2006 Jun 20.

114. Wu F, Lü R, Bai XH, Song XR. Influence of EmbryoGlue on the implantation of embryo and pregnancy outcome in vitro fertilization-embryo transfer [article in Chinese]. Zhonghua Fu Chan Ke Za Zhi. 2012;47(2):121–4.
115. Bontekoe S, Heineman MJ, Johnson N, Blake D. Adherence compounds in embryo transfer media for assisted reproductive technologies. Cochrane Database Syst Rev. 2014;2, CD007421. doi:10.1002/14651858.CD007421.pub3.
116. Gardner DK, Lane M, Schoolcraft WB. Culture and transfer of viable blastocysts: a feasible proposition for human IVF. Hum Reprod. 2000;15 Suppl 6:9–23.
117. Gardner DK, Surrey E, Minjarez D, Leitz A, Stevens J, Schoolcraft WB. Single blastocyst transfer: a prospective randomized trial. Fertil Steril. 2004;81(3):551–5.
118. Papanikolaou EG, Kolibianakis EM, Tournaye H, Venetis CA, Fatemi H, Tarlatzis B, Devroey P. Live birth rates after transfer of equal number of blastocysts or cleavage-stage embryos in IVF. A systematic review and meta-analysis. Hum Reprod. 2008;23(1):91–9. Epub 2007 Oct 26. Review.
119. Sepúlveda SJ, Portella JR, Noriega LP, Escudero EL, Noriega LH. Extended culture up to the blastocyst stage: a strategy to avoid multiple pregnancies in assisted reproductive technologies. Biol Res. 2011;44(2):195–9. doi:/S0716-97602011000200012. Epub 2011 Sep 20.
120. Blake DA, Farquhar CM, Johnson N, Proctor M. Cleavage stage versus blastocyst stage embryo transfer in assisted conception. Cochrane Database Syst Rev. 2007 17;(4):CD002118. Review. Update in: Cochrane Database Syst Rev. 2012;7:CD002118
121. Thomas MR, Sparks AE, Ryan GL, Van Voorhis BJ. Clinical predictors of human blastocyst formation and pregnancy after extended embryo culture and transfer. Fertil Steril. 2010;94(2):543–8. doi:10.1016/j.fertnstert.2009.03.051. Epub 2009 May 5.
122. Glujovsky D, Blake D, Farquhar C, Bardach A. Cleavage stage versus blastocyst stage embryo transfer in assisted reproductive technology. Cochrane Database Syst Rev. 2012;7, CD002118. doi:10.1002/14651858.CD002118.pub4. Review.
123. Wang SS, Sun HX. Blastocyst transfer ameliorates live birth rate compared with cleavage-stage embryos transfer in fresh in vitro fertilization or intracytoplasmic sperm injection cycles: reviews and meta-analysis. Yonsei Med J. 2014;55(3):815–25. doi:10.3349/ymj.2014.55.3.815. Epub 2014 Apr 1.
124. Mesut N, Ciray HN, Mesut A, Aksoy T, Bahceci M. Cryopreservation of blastocysts is the most feasible strategy in good responder patients. Fertil Steril. 2011;96(5):1121–5.e1. doi:10.1016/j.fertnstert.2011.08.012. Epub 2011 Sep 3.
125. Zhu L, Xi Q, Zhang H, Li Y, Ai J, Jin L. Blastocyst culture and cryopreservation to optimize clinical outcomes of warming cycles. Reprod Biomed Online. 2013;27(2):154–60. doi:10.1016/j.rbmo.2013.04.006. Epub 2013 Apr 19.
126. Scott Jr RT, Upham KM, Forman EJ, Zhao T, Treff NR. Cleavage-stage biopsy significantly impairs human embryonic implantation potential while blastocyst biopsy does not: a randomized and paired clinical trial. Fertil Steril. 2013;100(3):624–30. doi:10.1016/j.fertnstert.2013.04.039. Epub 2013 Jun 15.
127. Scott KL, Hong KH, Scott Jr RT. Selecting the optimal time to perform biopsy for preimplantation genetic testing. Fertil Steril. 2013;100(3):608–14. doi:10.1016/j.fertnstert.2013.07.004. Review.
128. Ly KD, Agarwal A, Nagy ZP. Preimplantation genetic screening: does it help or hinder IVF treatment and what is the role of the embryo? J Assist Reprod Genet. 2011;28(9):833–49. doi:10.1007/s10815-011-9608-7. Epub 2011 Jul 9.
129. Rubio C, Bellver J, Rodrigo L, Bosch E, Mercader A, Vidal C, De los Santos MJ, Giles J, Labarta E, Domingo J, Crespo J, Remohí J, Pellicer A, Simón C. Preimplantation genetic screening using fluorescence in situ hybridization in patients with repetitive implantation failure and advanced maternal age: two randomized trials. Fertil Steril. 2013;99(5):1400–7. doi:10.1016/j.fertnstert.2012.11.041. Epub 2012 Dec 20.
130. Blockeel C, Schutyser V, De Vos A, Verpoest W, De Vos M, Staessen C, Haentjens P, Van der Elst J, Devroey P. Prospectively randomized controlled trial of PGS in IVF/ICSI patients with poor implantation. Reprod Biomed Online. 2008;17(6):848–54.

131. Yakin K, Ata B, Ercelen N, Balaban B, Urman B. The effect of preimplantation genetic screening on the probability of live birth in young women with recurrent implantation failure; a nonrandomized parallel group trial. Eur J Obstet Gynecol Reprod Biol. 2008;140(2):224–9. doi:10.1016/j.ejogrb.2008.05.005. Epub 2008 Jul 7.
132. Scott Jr RT, Upham KM, Forman EJ, Hong KH, Scott KL, Taylor D, Tao X, Treff NR. Blastocyst biopsy with comprehensive chromosome screening and fresh embryo transfer significantly increases in vitro fertilization implantation and delivery rates: a randomized controlled trial. Fertil Steril. 2013;100(3):697–703. doi:10.1016/j.fertnstert.2013.04.035. Epub 2013 Jun 1.
133. Gleicher N, Kushnir VA, Barad DH. Preimplantation genetic screening (PGS) still in search of a clinical application: a systematic review. Reprod Biol Endocrinol. 2014;12:22. doi:10.1186/1477-7827-12-22.
134. van Loendersloot L, van Wely M, Goddijn M, Repping S, Bossuyt P, van der Veen F. Pregnancy and twinning rates using a tailored embryo transfer policy. Reprod Biomed Online. 2013;26(5):462–9. doi:10.1016/j.rbmo.2013.01.010. Epub 2013 Jan 26.
135. Practice Committee of American Society for Reproductive Medicine; Practice Committee of Society for Assisted Reproductive Technology. Criteria for number of embryos to transfer: a committee opinion. Fertil Steril. 2013;99(1):44–6. doi:10.1016/j.fertnstert.2012.09.038. Epub 2012 Oct 22.
136. Pandian Z, Marjoribanks J, Ozturk O, Serour G, Bhattacharya S. Number of embryos for transfer following in vitro fertilisation or intra-cytoplasmic sperm injection. Cochrane Database Syst Rev. 2013;7, CD003416. doi:10.1002/14651858.CD003416.pub4. Review.
137. Barritt J, Willadsen S, Brenner C, Cohen J. Cytoplasmic transfer in assisted reproduction. Hum Reprod Update. 2001;7(4):428–35. Review.

Chapter 13
Statistical Process Control Analysis to Assess Laboratory Variation as a Means of Quality Control in ART Labs

Alex Steinleitner

Introduction

ART practitioners constantly ask themselves: "Am I producing the best possible outcomes for my patients?" Sadly, it is difficult to provide this assurance to our clients and ourselves. Quality assurance programs can confirm that steps in the ART program are being performed as intended. But quality assurance cannot inform the practitioner whether these steps, when assembled in a system, are producing the best possible quality and patient success.

Clearly this is a question that each ART program needs to ask and affirmatively answer. Review of the 2012 American Society for Assisted Reproductive Technology (SART) data for women aged under 35 demonstrates that a handful of groups produced delivered pregnancy rates that were double that for the median live birth rate (i.e., 41 % per initiated cycle). A substantial number of groups reported success rates better than 50 % above the national average. Clearly these programs are doing something that is entirely different from most centers. We have an ethical obligation to understand these differences and make every effort to raise the quality of the lesser achieving programs to these obtainable standards.

Process stability is a hallmark of a successful enterprise. Whether you are making autos or embryos, the best quality results from an optimized system that consistently performs within tight specifications. Conversely, a chaotic "out of control" process yields highly variable results—both good and bad—and inferior quality on a long-term basis.

A. Steinleitner, MD (✉)
Department of Obstetrics and Gynecology, Sierra Vista Medical Center,
35 Casa Street, #260, San Luis Obispo, CA 93405, USA
e-mail: ccfertility@mac.com

© Springer Science+Business Media New York 2016
S.D. Fleming, A.C. Varghese (eds.), *Organization and Management of IVF Units*, DOI 10.1007/978-3-319-29373-8_13

Industrial engineers have developed mathematical methods known as Statistical Process Control (SPC) to monitor variation within a system and to determine whether a process is stable and "in control." This analysis is routinely employed in manufacturing to assess product quality and to improve the production line process. With the advent of large databases assembled in national registries and electronic medical records systems it is now possible to analyze "big data" to explore the application of SPC analysis for quality improvement in reproductive medicine.

In this chapter we review the fundamental statistical approach to SPC, review a preliminary study of SPC in the IVF setting, and discuss future investigations that we hope will lead to practical tools that will benefit ART practitioners.

Mathematics of Statistical Process Control

Reproductive specialists are very familiar with the common application of the normal distribution in research. The question we ask is: "Are two populations different?" To test this proposition, two large sample sets are assembled, as pictured in Fig. 13.1.

The samples are tested to confirm that each is normally distributed. Then statistical tests are applied to determine whether the sample means are significantly different. This analysis permits the investigator to draw conclusions regarding the sample populations with a level of assurance in the range of 95–99 % (depending on the test). Based on this assessment, the investigator may make statements inferring the cause of the difference (or lack thereof) between the populations.

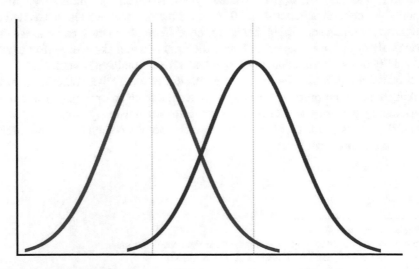

Fig. 13.1 Two large sample sets are assembled

SPC analysis turns this proposition on its head. In medicine we are most often interested to know whether an intervention results in a meaningful change in outcome. That is to say, "Is the treatment group different from the control group?"

In contrast, manufacturers are concerned with consistency. The question that they pose is: "Is every unit within a given population essentially the same?" After all, manufacturing processes are metastable at best. Tools wear out, humans become distracted, and raw materials or the environment may vary. Given that the objective of a manufacturing process is to create a large number of items that are as similar as possible and meet the production specifications, it is essential to constantly monitor the process for emerging variation.

To address this question process control engineers utilize the properties of the normal distribution in a very different way than we are accustomed to in medicine. Product is sampled at regular intervals. The data is plotted on a chart wherein the Y-axis displays the metric of interest against time on the X-axis. With a sufficient number of samples the data should conform to a normal distribution (Fig. 13.2).

Hence 95–99 % of the samples should fall within an upper control line and a lower control line, which represent two or three standard deviations from the mean (Fig. 13.3).

A process that meets this test is said to be "in statistical control." It is important to note that there will be some variation of the products produced by a stable process. Variation that falls within the Control Limits is said to arise from "Common Causes of Variation"—the amount of variation that results from the normal differences within the capabilities of the machines, material, and people that comprise the system.

Common variation is both normal and unavoidable. Just as "no two snowflakes are alike," no two widgets or any other products of a process are identical. Rather they vary within the limits of the ability of the process. Indeed, the normal distribution provides that points residing within upper and lower control limits set at three standard deviations have 997 chances out of a 1000 of not being the result of some "special" factor impacting the process. In the IVF lab "Common Variation" might arise from the lot-to-lot variation in reagents or gas mixtures or the fluctuating ability of incubators to maintain a constant temperature. So long as the data points

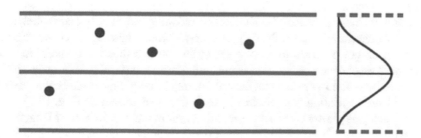

Fig. 13.2 In a stable process products fall within a normal distribution

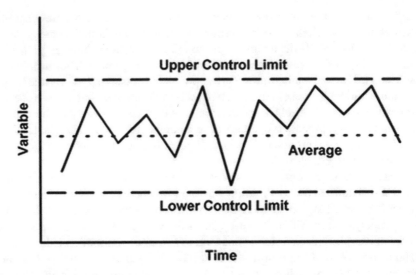

Fig. 13.3 A Shewhart control chart

cluster around the mean in a random fashion and there are not an excessive number (greater than three standard deviations) of defective parts, the production process is said to be stable (Fig. 13.4).

An unstable process will produce a very different control chart. With an unstable process a higher number of samples than expected fall outside the control limits—which is to say that the quality control samples are not normally distributed. Such a process is said to be "out of statistical control." Engineers need to search for "Special" causes of variation such as worn out tools and poorly trained or compromised employees. to address the newly discovered decreased quality of the manufacturing line (Fig. 13.5).

The following image of two collections of curves over time provides a graphic illustration of the difference between a stable and an unstable process (Fig. 13.6).

Other properties of the normal distribution may be used to detect process instability. As noted above, production samples in a stable process are normally distributed. Hence, individual samples should be randomly and equally distributed above and below the sample mean. Prolonged intervals where data cluster above or below the mean do not conform to a normal distribution and thus are unlikely to result from random chance and are consistent with process instability. Likewise sudden increases in variation or data that describe a trend line are most likely the result of Special Cause variation that requires investigation and correction (Fig. 13.7).

SPC analysis allows us to ask a second question: can we do better? Data from a stable process will have a fairly constant mean value and standard variation. While a process may be stable, it may still be inefficient. SPC supports quality improve-

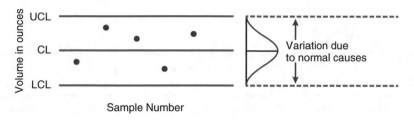

Fig. 13.4 Common variation around the mean and within control limits due to normal causes

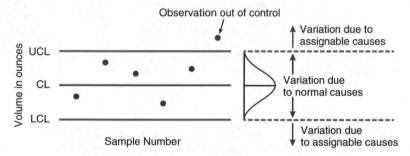

Fig. 13.5 A process that is out of statistical control due to "Special Causes of Variation"

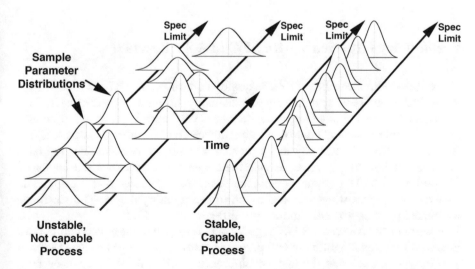

Fig. 13.6 A graphic illustration of the difference between a stable and an unstable process

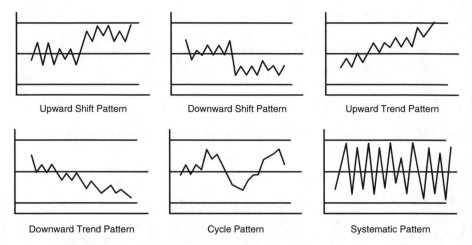

Fig. 13.7 Unstable data patterns that fall with control limits suggest that the process is out of statistical control

ment via "Plan, Do, Assess, Check" (PDAC) cycles, wherein the process supervisor tests quality, makes hypotheses regarding problems, performs and experiment to test an intervention, collects data, and interprets the results. With constant PDAC monitoring we can move to optimize complex systems and gradually decrease process variation and improve quality. This is reflected in tighter control limits and progression towards an optimal value for the finished product (Fig. 13.8).

Preliminary Experience with SPC in ART Practice

To explore the applicability of SPC to quality control in the ART practice setting, we evaluated embryology data from two distinctly different IVF centers. Clinic A is associated with a high volume national-class IVF. This laboratory has been diligent in its environmental control utilizing advanced air handling systems. Clinic B is a low volume center physically located in a surgicenter that does not have advanced air handling systems, leaving the lab environment exposed secondarily exposed to volatile organic compounds used for cleaning and sterilization. Laboratory services were provided by an itinerant embryologist. The mean age for treated patients was not significantly different.

Review of the American SART registry data reveals that these two clinics have produced substantially different IVF pregnancy rates in recent years (Fig. 13.9).

We hypothesized that the marked difference in clinical IVF pregnancy rates between Clinic A and Clinic B might be the result of or at least reflected by differential process variability between the two clinics. To test this hypothesis we

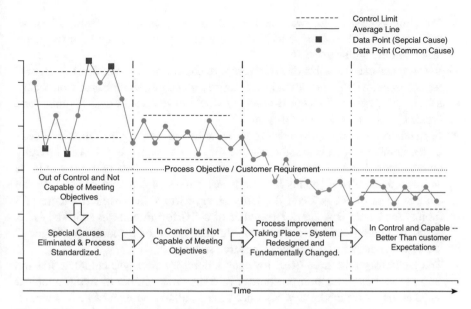

Control Limit
Average Line
Data Point (Sepcial Cause)
Data Point (Common Cause)

Process Objective / Customer Requirement

Out of Control and Not Capable of Meeting Objectives

Special Causes Eliminated & Process Standardized.

In Control but Not Capable of Meeting Objectives

Process Improvement Taking Place -- System Redesigned and Fundamentally Changed.

In Control and Capable -- Better Than customer Expectations

Time

Fig. 13.8 Improved process productivity following iterative PDAC cycles

Fig. 13.9 Delivered pregnancy rates for women aged <35 (Clinic A=*blue bars*, Clinic B=*red bars*)

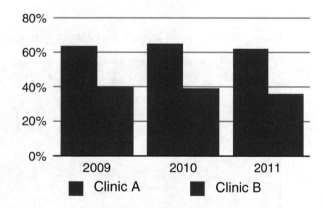

retrospectively collected embryology data for laboratory day one and laboratory day three from each center over an 18-month period. In order to reduce the lab technician's qualitative embryo quality records for statistical analysis, we empirically calculated a laboratory day three "mean embryo score" (MES) for each IVF case. Mean embryo score was calculated as follows:

- Morphology assessment was used to classify embryo quality from "I" = best, "II" = intermediate quality, and "III" = poor quality based on cellular fragmentation and irregularity.
- We assigned each possible day three embryo configuration a Grade of A, B, or C (see chart below). We empirically determined that Grade A embryos would have a factor of 6 "points," Grade B embryos would have a factor of 3 "points," and Grade C embryos a factor of 0 "points."
- Each embryo was assigned a day three score by multiplying the number of cells by the number of points assigned to that Grade. For example, a 10-cell I quality embryo would fall in the group of Grade A embryos. This embryo would be assigned a score of 6 (points for Grade A status) × 10 (number of cells) for an embryo score of 60. A 7-cell II quality embryo would be assigned a score of 3 (points for Grade B status) × 7 (number of cells) for an embryo score of 21. A 4-cell III quality embryo would be assigned a score of 0 (points for Grade C status) × 4 (number of cells) for an embryo score of 0.
- The laboratory day three MES for each laboratory case was calculated as the sum of the individual embryo scores divided by the number of two pronuclear stage embryos on laboratory day one. This results in a range of scores from 0 to 60 (all embryos with greater than 10 cells were classified as 10-cell embryos for calculation purposes) (Fig. 13.10).

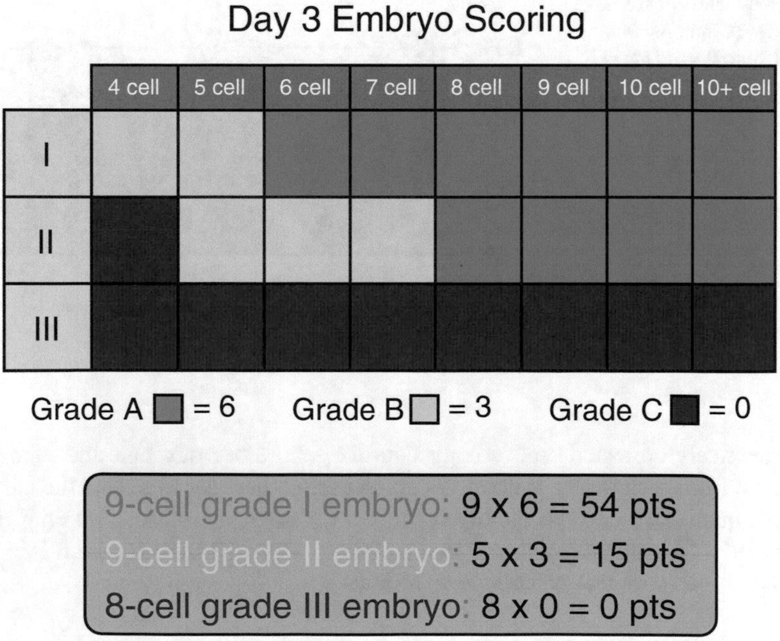

Day 3 Embryo Scoring

	4 cell	5 cell	6 cell	7 cell	8 cell	9 cell	10 cell	10+ cell
I								
II								
III								

Grade A ■ = 6   Grade B □ = 3   Grade C ■ = 0

9-cell grade I embryo: 9 x 6 = 54 pts
9-cell grade II embryo: 5 x 3 = 15 pts
8-cell grade III embryo: 8 x 0 = 0 pts

Fig. 13.10 Day three embryo scoring system

Next we created control charts for SPC analysis. The sequential laboratory day three MES values are plotted on the X-axis while the Y-axis depicts the possible range of MES from 0 to 60.

Review of these data suggests that the two clinics produced significantly different quality control charts that were consistent with their clinical outcomes. Control charting for all patients in Clinic A demonstrated characteristics of a stable process. MES scores were tightly distributed around a high mean. Many of the outlying points were the result of patient characteristics such as poor stimulation or impaired ovarian reserve (Special Cause Variation not attributable to laboratory performance). Of note, control charting demonstrated significant variation due to patient characteristics. Upper and Lower Control Limits (mean± 3 SD) exceeded the range of values for MES (0–60). Hence Control Limits of mean± 1 SD are shown for illustration purposes (Fig. 13.11).

In contrast, control charting for all patients in Clinic B demonstrates significantly more process variation. Average MES was lower than Clinic A with a higher standard deviation. Areas of widely fluctuating values and clusters of values above or below the mean are consistent with a much less stable process than Clinic A (Fig. 13.12).

This superficial control chart analysis suggests that Clinic A has a much more stable "manufacturing" process than Clinic B. It is tempting to speculate that the marked differences in IVF pregnancy rates between the two centers may be attributable in part to process stability. As a consequence, it is possible that Clinic B might improve their results not by "trying harder" with each case, but by analyzing their process and making sequential interventions to improve process stability and quality.

A common refrain from lower performing clinics is "we have tougher patients than everyone else." To explore whether the observed difference in process stability might be a result of patient selection, we performed SPC for a subset of high quality patients from Clinics A and B. Here we limited the analysis to a set of "idealized patients" comprised of women aged <36 that produced eight or more eggs (Fig. 13.13).

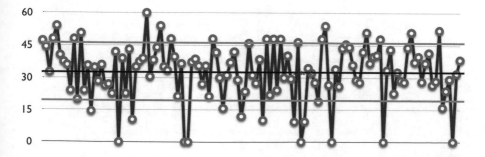

Fig. 13.11 Control chart for Clinic A sequential laboratory day three mean embryo scores

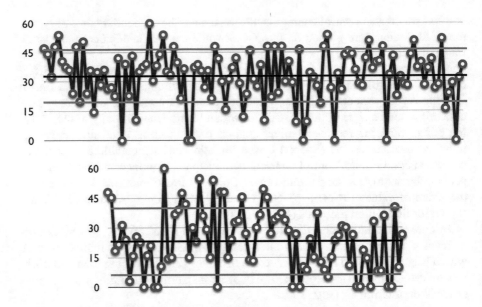

Fig. 13.12 Comparison of laboratory day three control charts for Clinic A (*blue*) vs. Clinic B (*red*)

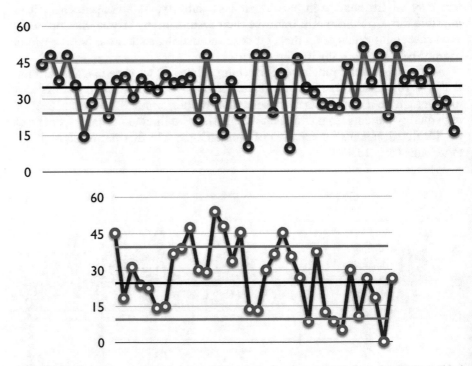

Fig. 13.13 Comparison of "ideal patients" laboratory day three control charts for Clinic A (*blue*) vs. Clinic B (*red*)

SPC analysis for Clinic A demonstrated a higher average MES with a lower standard deviation as compared to the Clinic A unselected patient population. In contrast, even with a selected group of optimal quality patients, Clinic B demonstrated significantly more process variation as compared to clinic A. This suggests that the differential IVF pregnancy success between the two clinics is due to aspects of their clinical or laboratory process and not a function of patient selection.

Given that this early data suggests that SPC analysis of process stability may reflect overall laboratory competence, we sought to explore whether analysis of particular steps in the ART process might differ between high performing and less well performing clinics.

To explore this question control charts were constructed using "idealized patients" for the steps of oocyte aspiration, fertilization, and embryo culture to laboratory day three.

Control charting for numbers of oocytes harvested revealed similar patterns between the two Clinics (Fig. 13.14).

Similarly, the fertilization rate for "idealized patients" was relatively similar between the two centers, although there appears to be a trend toward increased variation in Clinic B (Fig. 13.15).

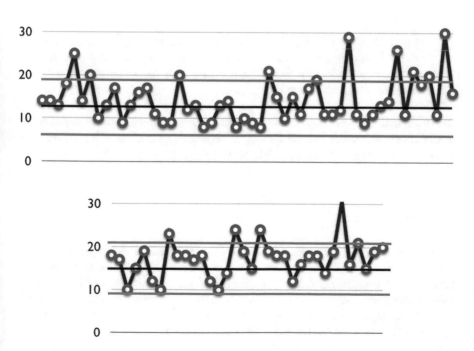

Fig. 13.14 Comparison of control charts for number of oocytes recovered for Clinic A (*blue*) vs. Clinic B (*red*)

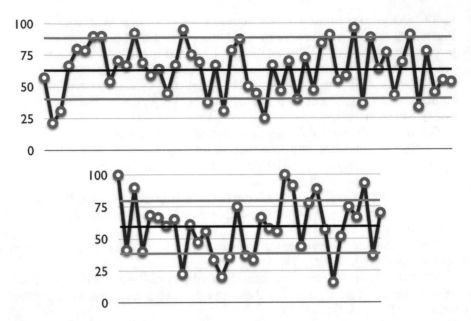

Fig. 13.15 Comparison of control charts for percent fertilization for Clinic A (*blue*) vs. Clinic B (*red*)

In contrast to the similar results for numbers of oocytes aspirated and fertilization rates for Clinic A and Clinic B, the two centers demonstrated considerable difference in day three MES scores. Clinic B displayed markedly greater variation and inconsistency over time (see Fig. 13.13).

This SPC data suggests that the principle difference in performance between the two Clinics lies in the step of embryo culture. Clearly, the next step in process management for Clinic B is to identify Special Causes of Variation in the areas of laboratory environmental control and technician skill in an effort to improve process quality.

Discussion

My interest in applying the principles of SPC to IVF practice dates back to the late 1990s when I read W. Edwards Deming's classic treatise "The New Economics for Industry, Government, Education" [1]. Deming describes a system of both process analysis and personnel management that revolutionized manufacturing in the mid-twentieth century. Utilizing these methods makes obvious sense as a means improving our control over the technologies employed in reproductive medicine.

Surprisingly, no one in our very data driven field has attempted to apply this methodology to the IVF setting. This is due to the fact that SPC requires access to both "big data" to characterize normative trends as well as collections of granular data from individual centers to assess the performance of a given practice's systems. Fortunately, advances in information technology, both at the level of national IVF registries as well as integrated electronic medical records systems finally make it possible to gather the data necessary to employ SPC on clinical level.

The preliminary studies described above offer a glimpse into the potential utility of SPC to assess process variability as a means of objectively assessing IVF laboratory quality. As we have observed, the embryo quality produced by Clinic A is superior to that of Clinic B. Interestingly, Clinic B has a much less stable process, which is to say that Clinic B's laboratory is capable of producing high quality embryos—but it does not do so as consistently as Clinic A. It is tempting to suggest that the difference in process stability is a contributing factor to the substantial difference in pregnancy success rates between the two centers.

The question that arises from this preliminary experience is whether process variability is directly related to IVF clinical success and if there are a number of common process issues that can be uncovered via SPC analysis.

At present we have three investigations underway to this question.

To understand the typical variation in an IVF program we are analyzing a data set of over 4000 procedures performed by twenty physicians in a single high quality laboratory over the course of a 5-year period. The objective of this study is to obtain normative data to characterize the typical variation that results from patient characteristics and from the laboratory process. Our preliminary results suggest that there may be a large degree of inter-patient variation in terms of egg and embryo quality. We suspect that our strategy of creating "idealized" patients will be necessary to eliminate patient-related Special cause variation from the data set in order to examine the impact of laboratory conditions on process variation.

Our second study, working in conjunction with the American SART registry, will analyze over 35,000 IVF cycles performed by clinics reporting success rates across the spectrum from the 10th percentile to the 90th percentile for live birth. We suspect that successful clinics will demonstrate markedly less process variation than that observed in clinics with poorer results.

Lastly, we are sponsoring a prospective study of 100 IVF units worldwide to analyze embryology data from a wide variety of settings. Participating centers will be provided an EMR system to capture IVF laboratory data on a granular basis. It is our hope that this experience will lead to the development of a tool that permits centers to analyze their process in real time and thus utilize a SPC-based PDAC system for quality improvement.

To conclude, it does not matter how hard you try to succeed at a given endeavor. If you have an unstable process, your quality will be poor. ART practitioners are presently handicapped by an inability to assess their process quality and hence make directed interventions to improve outcomes. SPC analytics offer the potential to provide laboratory scientists and clinicians with the objective data they need gain control over their "manufacturing process" and hence optimize quality and patient success.

Reference

1. Deming WE. The new economics for industry, government, education. Massachusetts Institute of Technology Center for Advanced Engineering Study. 1994.

Part III
IVF Units and Society

Chapter 14
Ethics of IVF Treatment: Remember the Patient!

Anne Melton Clark

Introduction

Medical ethics is described as a system of moral principles that apply values and judgements to the practice of medicine. It is based on four basic moral principles [1]:

1. *Respect for autonomy*—the patient has the right to refuse or choose their treatment.
2. *Beneficence*—a practitioner should act in the best interest of the patient.
3. *Non-maleficence*—"first, do no harm."
4. *Justice*—concerns for the distribution of scarce health resources, and the decision of who gets what treatment (fairness and equality).

Unfortunately these will often overlap in a reproductive medicine setting, making it even more difficult to manage how best to assist a couple/individual with fertility issues to achieve the primary aim, a normal, healthy baby.

Respect for Autonomy

In medical ethics this means that the patient has the right to refuse or choose their treatment. In reproductive medicine that is complicated by needing to also act in the best interest of the child, even though the child is technically not the patient, and what the actual patient might desire, a baby, might not be in the best

A.M. Clark, MPS, MBCHB, FRCOG, FRANZCOG, CREI (✉)
Fertility First, 50 Gloucester Road, Hurstville, NSW 2220, Australia
e-mail: anne@fertilityfirst.com.au

© Springer Science+Business Media New York 2016   269
S.D. Fleming, A.C. Varghese (eds.), *Organization and Management of IVF Units*, DOI 10.1007/978-3-319-29373-8_14

interests of that child. For example, a couple who are both carriers of cystic fibrosis, might need IVF treatment to conceive for male factor reasons, but not wish or be unable to afford, to have preimplantation genetic diagnosis (PGD) to avoid delivering a child with cystic fibrosis. So, how best to deal with such situations in managing a fertility unit?

Informed Consent and Counselling

Informed consent, and the counselling that goes into informed consent, is essentially the key. The concept of informed consent has increased in importance since the historical events of the Doctors' Trial of the Nuremburg Trials and the Tuskegee syphilis experiment [2] and thus has been enshrined in law and in the accreditation processes for reproductive medicine units to operate legitimately. A patient must understand the potential risks as well as benefits of their choice of treatment, so the information must be given in a truthful, honest and easy to understand way. It is a rare potential parent who does not want the very best for their child.

The incorporation of professional counsellors and counselling services into fertility clinics has been invaluable in this regard and also allows the patient(s) a safe way to explore their best way forward, particularly when third parties, such as gamete donors or surrogates are involved in the treatment process. Counselling also enables patients to be sure of their motivations prior to conception. It is therefore very important that both the patients, and those involved in the counselling appreciate their role is one of giving information and stimulating thought, so the patient feels safe to express all their hopes and fears.

The counsellor should not be the gate keeper as to who should or should not have treatment. If a patient's treatment is to be delayed or denied, that should be determined by unit policy, an ethics committee and/or the medical director of the Unit.

However, as fertility treatments can be highly technical and involve such high emotions, it is difficult for patients to operate under fully informed consent and understand all the risks and benefits and likelihood of success of any treatment. They are therefore very dependent on the information they receive as to what is the best, simplest, easiest treatment that is likely to work for them. This is a difficult area ethically for individual practitioners as they might have other pressures on them, particularly as increasing corporatisation of fertility treatments globally leads to "IVF being treated more like a commodity and volume becomes paramount to indication" [3].

For example, a Dutch study published in 2015 has demonstrated that stimulated intrauterine insemination (IUI) is as successful in terms of pregnancy for unexplained infertility or mild male factor as an IVF cycle with one embryo transferred; the likelihood of multiple pregnancy was the same [4]. However, Australia and New Zealand data over the past 12 years shows that as an indication for IVF treatment, unexplained infertility alone has risen from 17 % to 23 % of IVF cycles (it is not possible to separate mild male factor from the current data sets). Meanwhile the incidence of IUI cycles as a proportion of combined IVF/IUI cycles has dropped from 30 % to only 17 % in the same time frame [5]. At the same time, in Australia, which has is a high level of Government funding for fertility treatment, there has been a significant rise in commercial fertility units in which IVF is essentially the only option offered to patients irrespective of diagnosis.

The average cost of an IUI cycle, including medications, in Australia is approximately A$1800–A$2000 while the average cost of an IVF cycle, including medications, is approximately A$9000–A$10,000. Would all patients still choose the more complicated, expensive treatment option of IVF if they were aware of this data?

Another example where patients need guidance in relation to informed consent is the decision of at what stage to transfer their embryos. The rapid uptake of blastocyst transfer vs cleavage stage transfer is an example of a treatment being introduced without full evidence of outcome measures compared to shorter in vitro culture. Blastocyst culture has been enthusiastically embraced by most clinics as a way of maintaining good pregnancy rates while reducing the number of embryos transferred, thereby minimising preterm delivery rates [6]. But ironically, a meta-analysis has indicated that the risk of preterm birth in IVF singleton babies is significantly higher following blastocyst transfer compared with cleavage stage transfer; Risk of congenital anomalies may also be higher [7]. Blastocyst transfer, while conveying a higher chance of pregnancy if an embryo transfer cycle occurs, also results in a much higher proportion of embryos being discarded. Analysis of the latest ANZARD database [5] shows that in one year alone, a massive 100,347 embryos were discarded though there is still no foolproof way of knowing which embryos will become babies and which will not. Even if only 1 % of those embryos had resulted in a pregnancy 1000 extra children would have been born in that one year! A 1 % chance of becoming a baby is better than no chance at all if discarded in the bin. That embryo might be a couple's only chance of having their own genetic child.

All units strive for the highest pregnancy rates possible; it is why we come to work, but are we doing that at the expense of our patients? Are we sacrificing the potential of some of their embryos to become babies so our pregnancy rates are better? Certainly we all know of embryos we have felt embarrassed to transfer that have resulted in a healthy baby and other "beautiful" embryos that come to nothing. The literature seems clear that an embryo does not need to be perfect at cleavage stage to result in a healthy pregnancy [8].

The Cochrane database review [6] found that blastocyst transfer results in fewer treatment cycles getting to embryo transfer and a significantly lower chance of frozen embryos for the future. As a result the cumulative pregnancy rate for cleavage stage fresh treatment cycles is actually higher than blastocyst fresh treatment cycles.

However, from a business perspective, blastocyst transfers mean less embryos at the end of a cycle so less embryology time required, less storage and freezing requirements, therefore less paperwork and the need for a more expensive fresh IVF cycle as opposed to a frozen transfer cycle if a pregnancy does not result. Some low cost IVF units say they only aim to collect four to five eggs and/or do not offer embryo freezing but is it ethical and does it comply with the requirements of informed consent?

In an increasingly litigious world it is very important for clinicians to ensure that the unit has documentation of a patient's informed consent to all aspects of treatment prior to proceeding.

Cross Border Reproductive Care (CBRC): The Impact of Restricting or Banning Fertility Treatments Available in Other Jurisdictions

The cross border phenomenon is now well entrenched as a means to an end. The patients' reproductive journeys are designed to deliver them a child that has not been proven possible for them in their home setting. The data show that while many patients travel to evade restrictive legislation in their own country or state, support from their home health providers is variable [9].

Cross border reproductive services are of concern to patients, fertility clinics and policy makers. Patients prefer to obtain care near their home; practitioners often see the complications of treatment abroad returning for care. It is the lack of consistency in types of fertility treatments offered in different jurisdictions that drives reproductive tourism.

Cross border reproductive care occurs within cities, states and countries [8, 9]. As prohibition in America demonstrated, making alcohol illegal did not stop drinking, it just drove it underground, so it was no longer regulated and resulted in those involved being more vulnerable to risk, exploitation and adverse outcomes for both the potential parents [10, 11] and the potential child. An example is a couple undergoing surrogacy in Mexico in which one embryo was destroyed and the documents relating to the transfer of another between clinics were mixed up so they do not know if the surrogate mother received the right embryos [10]. The risks for the third party involved and the potential children is highlighted by the "Baby Gammy" case in Thailand, in which a convicted Australian paedophile and partner left a son with Down syndrome behind with the surrogate but took his sister back to Australia [12].

There will also be inequality in access as only those who are financially able can make use of CBRC treatments [13].

Treatments involving donor gametes, surrogacy, sex selection for family balancing and preimplantation genetic diagnosis (PGD) and screening (PGS) are all treatments that legislators and clinics have restricted access to in different ways and for different patient groups. For example, in Europe, the use of donor gametes is allowed in most countries but in Switzerland, Norway and Germany only donor sperm but not donor eggs is allowed under current legislation. In the Netherlands, PGD is permitted, but in only one centre and then only in the framework of a scientific study [8]. Sex selection for family balancing is not legal in Australia but is for sex linked diseases [14] and surrogacy is only available in some Australian

States. Efforts in Australia to regulate the use of donors and donor sperm, however well intentioned, have led to a dramatic drop in the availability of donor sperm [15] and the rise of websites that offer direct contact between donors and potential recipients without any of the medical, genetic, infection, family limit or counselling oversight offered by fertility clinics. For example, as reported earlier this year, a 67 year old New South Wales man has become the biological father of at least 120 donor conceived children and has no plans to give up. Fertility units in New South Wales are restricted to a maximum of five families accessing the same genetic father with donor conception. The man acknowledges that studies show an increase in the risk of mental, congenital and physical illnesses increase with the age of the father and that two of his children have been born with autism but "on the autism spectrum they're only at the mild end" he says. He is also quoted as saying that with some of the women he donates to "I would find it hard getting an erection because some of them are grossly overweight" [11].

An ESHRE study [9] from 46 ART clinics in six European countries is the first prospective study to present a set of hard data on CBRC. The study found the main reasons for travelling were to circumvent legal restrictions prohibiting the treatment in their own jurisdiction (55 %), followed by an expectation of better quality of treatment (43 %), then difficulties accessing treatment due to patient characteristics such as age, sexual orientation or civil status (7 %). The annual number of cycles was a minimum of 24–30,000 a year.

So, in a clinic setting how best to manage these anomalies? If the service is restricted by legislation in your setting, it is still possible to assist your patients by having knowledge of safe, ethical treatment centres they can go to and assist in counselling before a final decision is made. If your clinic does not offer a service in a timely fashion, for example, donor sperm, but another in your jurisdiction does, ethical guidelines should require the patient be guided to that service, rather than a woman in her late 30s, for example, being put on a several year waiting list until sperm is available at your own clinic.

The ESHRE study [9] reported that 59 % patients received some help from their own doctor, for a drug prescription (17 %), cycle monitoring (17 %) or both (26 %). The amount of help varied from country to country.

Clinicians involved as service providers or service facilitators have an ethical responsibility to ensure appropriate standards of care are provided to all receiving treatment and the third-party providers are not exploited. But that can be easier said than done, particularly if your patient is travelling several continents away and more countries and clinics seek to benefit economically from the expanding market in medical consumerism [16].

The internet has greatly facilitated the spread of CBRC to the extent that in some countries, such as the UK and Australia, more patients access egg donation abroad than do in their home country, despite a permissive legislative environment. Third party exploitation, where treatment can constitute a potential risk to the third party, is a major concern, as it is rare for the movement of patients from areas of low to high technology for assisted reproduction using their own gametes to be questioned.

The clinician may be torn between the desire to support the patient to have a child and their reticence to facilitate medical interventions which may be illegal in their own country. A good example would be sex selection for non-medical reasons.

Should Some Treatments Be Restricted or Banned?

As said above, even if a treatment is banned or restricted, the rise in CBRC has shown if a treatment is available legally somewhere in the world people will try to access it if they are financially able to. Clearly, some treatments, for example, combining of sperm of several men, should be banned but much comes back to the issues of informed consent.

Beneficence

Medical ethics requires that a practitioner should act in the best interest of the patient. In reproductive medicine, of course, that is complicated by also needing to act in the best interest of the child, even though the child is technically not the patient and does not exist at the time of treatment.

Should Anyone Be Able to Treat Patients?

Professional training is essential for the safety and efficacy of any complex operation and reproductive medicine is no exception [17]. There is good evidence that fellowship training and certification in Reproductive Endocrinology and Infertility (REI) has improved clinical outcomes in IVF [18].

So the trend to reduce costs by using general practitioners, for example, who have no formal specialist, let alone subspecialty training, or continuing education requirements, for the assessment, management and treatment of IVF patients might be cheaper, but does not compare with the experience and knowledge of a specialist in treating patients, particularly for complex or unexpected problems. Similarly the use of a unit's nursing staff to do the monitoring ultrasound scans vs the use of a qualified ultrasonographer. Training and appropriate supervision for the task are essential.

How Should Treatments Be Selected?

Patients should be offered the simplest, easiest, cheapest, safest treatment that is likely to work. That can only be done after a full assessment of all factors that can contribute to reduced fertility. Lifestyle factors such as smoking and significantly increased weight, that impact on both male and female fertility should be addressed first.

Essentially the treatment choice will be determined by the woman's fallopian tubes, the man's sperm and the couple's stage in life. The growth of budget clinics that only offer IVF is a worrying trend if the choice of treatment for a couple is based on financial incentives rather than need as discussed above.

Involve the Other Health Professionals Already Treating the Patient

If a person wanting to conceive is already under the care of another health professional, it is always my policy to seek documentation from that person that they are aware their patient is wishing to have a child and they support that decision. Not only is this a matter of courtesy but it ensures I am not proceeding with treatment at a time that is medically inappropriate for other reasons and also ensures that any medication the patient is being prescribed elsewhere is not likely to have detrimental effects on a pregnancy.

Non-maleficence

"First, do no harm" requires that a procedure does not harm the patient(s) involved or others in society. As IVF technologies have limited success rates, uncertain overall outcomes and the emotional state of patients can be impacted negatively if treatment is unsuccessful, it is often difficult for doctors to apply the "do no harm" principle successfully in a reproductive medicine setting. In addition, even the most informed patients are often willing to "try anything" to achieve a baby.

Introduction of New Treatments

Reproductive medicine is such a rapidly evolving field and the drive for success by both the patients and clinics so great, it is easy for tests and therapies to be offered to patients undergoing fertility treatment before their efficacy, and more importantly potential risks to both mother and the resulting baby, have been fully assessed. An example of this has been the proliferation of treatments in relation to uterine natural killer (NK) cells [19].

An industry has grown up to treat women undergoing IVF or attending recurrent miscarriage clinics based on the theory that uterine NK cells need suppressing to prevent damage to the embryo. The function of these uterine NK cells is essentially unknown and despite the lack of scientific rationale and advice from clinical governing bodies, such as the Human Fertilisation and Embryology Authority (HFEA), whole practices have grown up offering, at a not inconsiderable patient cost, financial and otherwise, a range of tests and immunotherapies. Apart from the lack of evidence base for these treatments it is now clear that the potential risks and costs of these therapies outweigh any benefits. As stated by Moffet and Shreeve [19] "It is surely no longer acceptable for licensed medical practitioners to continue to administer and profit from potentially unsafe and unproven treatments based on belief and not scientific rationale."

Keep Up with the Literature: What is Said to Be True Today Might Not Be Tomorrow

The use of anti-Mullerian hormone (AMH) testing is an example. This was a test repeatedly reported in the literature to be a reasonably accurate guide to a woman's fertility, long and short term. For some, including many general practitioners, it has been a first line in assessing then advising a woman on her fertility potential. I have seen women who have been counselled to have fertility treatment immediately, freeze eggs at great cost or told that they would never be able to have children based on a single AMH test result. However, the assay has continued to be less reliable than hoped and women can have AMH levels that are significantly different when tested even weeks apart [20].

In addition, extremely low levels of AMH do not mean a woman cannot get pregnant naturally or on treatment and, therefore, such women deserve the same workup as any other fertility patient [21].

Recent research indicates that AMH levels are not constant as previously hypothesised. So, for example, while a woman is on the oral contraceptive pill her AMH levels will be lower than when she starts cycling again [22].

The recommended treatment of endometriosis has also undergone radical changes in the past decade from treating even small amounts of endometriosis to maximise fertility to the current recommendations that even endometriomas should not be removed for fear of significantly reducing a woman's remaining antral follicle pool [23] and compromising her fertility further.

Epigenetics: What of the Children into the Future?

Pre-pregnancy Assessment and the Male Partner

The often sole focus on the female partner, and her age, in relation to failure to conceive and or recurrent miscarriage ignores the impact of the male's half of the baby, in particular, increased levels of DNA fragmentation, which also result in unsuccessful fertility treatments and increased risk of miscarriage [24, 25]. Increased sperm DNA adversely affects embryo quality starting at Day 2 and continues after embryo transfer, resulting in reduced implantation rates and pregnancy outcomes [26].

With men also delaying fatherhood [25, 27] and the known increase in DNA damage with increasing age [28], testing and treating the male prior to any other fertility treatment is likely to be more effective, less costly, and has the added benefit of reducing the likelihood of birth defects, autism, and childhood cancers such as leukaemia in the resulting child [27, 29].

Adult diseases are also more common with increasing male age and DNA damage, including, achondroplasia, breast cancer and epilepsy.

One could argue that if embryos are less than ideal for couples in their late 30s and 40s, rather than advising the woman to have donor eggs, maybe we should be advising the couple to consider using donor sperm as a much simpler, easier, cheaper option to improve embryo quality and outcomes for the child. Obviously a better alternative is to assess more than just the basics of sperm count, motility and morphology. First, reduce DNA damage if appropriate with lifestyle changes and antioxidants [30] as the first line in any treatment plan.

Pre-pregnancy Nutritional Assessment and the Child in Adulthood

Nutritional deficiencies of some vitamins and minerals can reduce a woman's chance of conceiving, even with fertility treatment, and also increase the likelihood of complications during pregnancy (Table 14.1). Vitamin D, iodine, folate, vitamin B12 and iron are the most important to assess. Table 14.2 contains the recommended levels during pregnancy. To maximise the health of the child and likelihood of pregnancy, these should be assessed and corrected as part of any fertility workup [31].

The World Health Organisation (WHO) now rates acquired diseases, such as diabetes and cardiovascular disease, as the leading cause of death in the world's population. Suboptimal nutrition during pregnancy predisposes to these diseases. The resulting epigenetic changes are also transmitted to, and therefore affect, subsequent generations. Asthma, lung disease, some mental health conditions and forms of cancer have also been reported as increased following inadequate nutrition at the start of life [32]. The association between the intrauterine environment and later health is often referred to as the "Barker Hypothesis" following the finding that lower birthweight was associated with increased coronary mortality [33].

Therefore, assessment and replacement, if necessary, to ensure good nutrition prior to becoming pregnant with fertility treatment is an important, simple method of reducing these risks and increasing the health of all children conceived through IVF into the future.

Designer Babies

Sometimes patients will present wanting a particular type of baby, such as a specific gender, or a match to another child who has specific needs in terms of tissue donation, or a particular ethnicity that is different from their own, for example, a Caucasian couple wanting an Afro Caribbean sperm donor. Where each clinician sits on this will

Table 14.1 Impact of nutritional deficiencies on fertility, pregnancy outcomes and long term health

Women	Iodine deficiency	Vitamin D deficiency	Folate and vitamin B12 deficiency and/or raised homocysteine levels	Iron
% of new patients affected at Fertility First[a]	57 %	45 %	19 %	3 %
Cause of infertility?	Yes	Yes	Yes	Yes
Cause of long term adverse health effects for children and adults?	Yes—irreversible reduction in IQ of up to 13 points, birth defects, linked to autism	Yes—increased risk of rickets, multiple sclerosis, and schizophrenia	Yes—increased risk of neural tube defects, asthma, autism and depression	Yes—increased risk of anaemia when born, reduced IQ and developmental behaviour
Increased miscarriage rate?	Yes	Yes	Yes	
Pregnancy complications increased?	Yes	Yes	Yes	Yes—if deficiency significant
Pregnancy-induced hypertension?	Yes	Yes	Yes	
Placental abruption?	–	–	Yes	
Intra-uterine growth retardation?	–	Yes	Yes	
Prematurity?	–	Yes	Yes	Yes—if deficiency significant
Low birth weight?	Yes	Yes	Yes	Yes—if deficiency significant
Still birth?	Yes	–	Yes	Yes—if deficiency significant

[a]$N = 7368$

Table 14.2 Nutrients essential in pregnancy, recommended levels and supplementation, at risk women

Nutrient	Recommended levels for Australian women	Recommended daily supplementation	Dietary sources	At risk women/pregnancies
Iodine	150 μg/l	150 μg/l	•Dairy products (2– 3 portions per day) •Eggs (1–2 portions per week) •Seafood (1–2 portions per week)	•All pregnant women, particularly •Women with a low dietary iodine intake •Smoking and alcohol consumption
Vitamin D	75 nmol/l	1000–4000 IU	•Seafood (2–3 serves per week) •Eggs (1–2 portions per week) •Mushrooms exposed to sunlight (3–4 per day)	•Women with dark skin •Body Mass Index (BMI) >30 kg/m² •Women who wear sunscreen on a regular basis •Lack of skin exposure to sunlight •Medical conditions or medications affecting Vit D metabolism and storage •Younger maternal age.
Folate (and Vit B12) (Low risk deficiency)	RBC folate 300–1500 nmol/l Vit B12 300–740 pmol/l	Folate— 0.4–0.5 mg/day Vit B12 125–2000 μg daily	•Vegetables (green leafy) •Red meat •Nuts and legumes	•Women in lower socioeconomic groups •Indigenous women •Rural women •Younger women •Multiparous women •Body Mass Index (BMI) >30 kg/m²
Folate (and Vit B12) (High risk deficiency)	RBC folate 300–1500 nmol/l Vit B12 300–740 pmol/l	Folate— 5 mg/day Vit B12 125–2000 μg daily	•Vegetables (green leafy) •Red meat •Nuts and legumes	•Reproductive or family history of NTD •Women who have had pregnancy affected by NTD •Women taking anti-epileptic medication •Women diagnosed with diabetes •Body Mass Index (BMI) >30 kg/m² •Women at risk of folate deficiency, e.g. MTHFR variant •Strict vegans can be low in B12

(continued)

Table 14.2 (continued)

Nutrient	Recommended levels for Australian women	Recommended daily supplementation	Dietary sources	At risk women/pregnancies
Iron	Hb <110 g/l Ferritin >12 µg/l	27–45 mg/day	• Vegetables (green leafy) • Red meat • Foods high in vitamin C to assist in iron absorption	• Vegetarian diet • Multiple pregnancies • Pregnancies close together • Severe morning sickness • Poor diet

NTD neglected tropical disease

be different, but as is the case with the rise of CBRC for other reasons, it is important to decide what the protocol will be for your unit; refer to your Ethics Committee if necessary and refer on to a reputable alternative if you are unable to help.

Justice

Justice concerns the distribution of scarce health resources, and the decision of who gets what treatment (fairness and equality). Reproductive technologies will continue to create ethical dilemmas because treatment is not equally available to all people for both financial and restriction of access reasons. As a rapidly changing field there will always be competing needs and potential conflicts with established legislation.

Therefore, it is important to ensure that when assisting patients both their resources and those of the community are used to their best advantage. To fulfil our ethical responsibilities to our patients, ourselves and our unit we should always be looking for the simplest, easiest, safest, cheapest way to help our patients have a normal healthy child who will grow into a healthy adult. Many times that starts with the fence at the top of the cliff, as above, rather than going straight to the ambulance of IVF at the bottom of the cliff. It is also good business practice. You want your brand be known as a unit that can be trusted and does the right thing for its patients as the best way to survive in this fast moving increasingly commercial world.

Who Should Be a Parent? Can a Patient Be Denied Treatment Ethically?

In some countries and states, some patient groups are denied treatment, hence the rise of CBRC. A unit is not obliged ethically to treat all patients who present for treatment, but they are obliged to be clear as to the true reasons treatment will not be offered and whether treatment would be possible in the future. Patients are most likely to be refused treatment for the following reasons:

Single Sex Couples

There has been a vast amount of research over the decades which shows that children from single sex relationships do well through childhood into adulthood. The biggest disadvantage for children born into single sex relationships seems to be the attitude of others. In terms of health, educational outcomes and sexual orientation they do the same, if not better in some circumstances, than children conceived in heterosexual relationships [34].

Medically Unfit Patients

This is difficult to quantify in some cases as one unit's definition might differ from another. Obesity is the commonest, but with 50 % of women of reproductive age overweight or obese and 70 % of men (Australian Bureau of Statistics figures) [35], defining a cut-off BMI over which treatment will not occur is challenging. It is also more likely, though inconsistent, that a cut-off will be in place for the female patients only, despite evidence that if a man is medically unfit it also impacts on the potential child's future health [36].

Age

Once again there is an inconsistency in that units set limits for female age, when pregnancy is much less likely, but not for male age. Of interest, over the past 12 years in Australia and New Zealand, the woman's age has remained steady at 35.5 years (Fig. 14.1), contrary to male age which has risen slightly. There is now a lot of

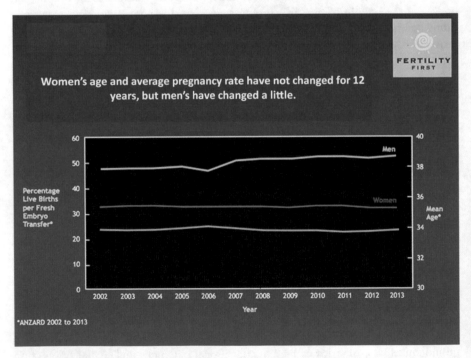

Fig. 14.1 Women's age and average pregnancy rate have not changed for twelve years but men's have changed a little

evidence of the impact of a man's increasing age, particularly from the age of 40, on the couple's chance of not just getting pregnant but staying pregnant. In 38 % of IVF cycles in the latest Australian/New Zealand data the man was aged 40 or older.

Medical Futility

When to say no—it is always difficult to destroy hope but for some patients it is clear that fertility treatment or continued fertility treatment will never result in a pregnancy. But it is also important to ensure that all potential blocks to pregnancy have been eliminated first.

Are League Tables Ethical?

Not according to the HFEA, if patients use them to assess which fertility unit to attend. As Disraeli famously said "There are 3 sorts of lies–lies, damned lies and statistics." To quote the HFEA, it is not meaningful to directly compare clinic's success rates or create "league tables" of clinics performance because:

- Clinics treat patients with different diagnoses and this will affect the average success rates we show for clinics.
- Most clinics carry out too few cycles each year to reliably predict a patient's future chance of success.
- The success rates relate to a period of treatment from about two years ago and may not be a good indication of success rates at the particular clinic today.
- The vast majority of overall success rate data published on our website … is given to us by the clinics themselves!

Patient groups consistently argue against league tables for the same reasons, as "they do not represent an accurate picture of an individual's chance of success and prevents them from making an informed decision about where they choose to undergo treatment" [37].

Is Business Good for Patients?

Sometimes. Economy of scale, sharing of policies and procedures, for example, can all result in easier access and more efficient, safer treatment for patients. However, there is always an ethical danger for clinicians when they have competing obligations to the patient and the shareholder. As stated previously, "When IVF is treated like a commodity and volume is paramount to indication" [3].

Clinical outcomes can be affected by the needs of business to maximise profit by minimising staff costs for example. If a unit is going to use staff who are not trained and supervised appropriately for the task it risks not only its ethical life but its professional life [38, 39]. Short term cost savings can become very expensive long-term in an increasingly litigious world.

The Role of Ethics Committees

Since the 1970s, the growing influence of ethics in contemporary medicine can be seen in the increase in the use and power of Institutional Ethics Committees (IEC) to evaluate experiments, the requirement of ethics committees to oversee public and private medical practice, the expansion of the role of clinician ethicists and the integration of ethics into medical school curricula [38, 40].

However, it is important to remember that the entire IVF industry is not based on a double blind, randomised, placebo controlled trial but a single case report in a letter to Nature, re the birth of Louise Brown in July, 1978 [41] which would have had little chance of being approved by an IEC today. Intracytoplasmic sperm injection (ICSI), one the biggest changes in the way we practise today, was initially reported as occurring by "accident" [42].

New variants of treatments also run well ahead of ethical guidelines. The NHMRC Legislative Guidelines covering ethical regulation of reproductive medicine in Australia, for example, were last revised in 2007 [14].

Conclusion

Ideally, for a medical, and therefore IVF, practice to be considered "ethical", it must respect the principles of autonomy, non-maleficence, beneficence and justice [43].

These values do not give all the answers on how to handle a particular situation, but do provide a framework for understanding and resolving conflicts.

There is a need for professional societies to establish standards for cross border reproductive health. There is also a need for more data as opposed to supposition in some areas and a need for greater focus on what is the simplest, easiest, safest way to maximise the primary aim of a normal, healthy baby who will become a normal, healthy adult.

References

1. Beauchamp T. The "four principles" approach to health care ethics. In: Ashcroft RE, Dawson A, Draper H, McMillan JR, editors. Principles of health care ethics. 2nd ed. Chichester, UK: Wiley; 2006. p. 3–10.
2. Angell M. The ethics of clinical research in the Third World. N Engl J Med. 1997;337:847–8.
3. Cedars MI, Rosenwaks Z. Who are we? A perspective on the reproductive endocrinologist and infertility specialist in the 21st century. Fertil Steril. 2015;104:26–7.
4. Bensdorp AJ, Tjon-Kon-Fat RI, Bossuyt PM, Koks CA, Oosterhuis GJ, Hoek A, Hompes PG, Broekmans FJ, Verhoeve HR, De Bruin JP, Van Golde R, Repping S, Cohlen BJ, Lambers MD, Van Bommel PF, Slappendel E, Perquin D, Smeenk JM, Pelinck MJ, Gianotten J, Hoozemans DA, Maas JW, Eijkemans MJ, Van Der Veen F, Mol BW, Van Wely M. Prevention of multiple pregnancies in couples with unexplained or mild male subfertility: randomised controlled trial of in vitro fertilisation with single embryo transfer or in vitro fertilisation in

modified natural cycle compared with intrauterine insemination with controlled ovarian hyper-stimulation. BMJ. 2015;350:g7771.

5. Macaldowie A, Lee E, Chambers GM. Assisted reproductive technology in Australia and New Zealand 2013. Sydney: National Perinatal Epidemiology and Statistics Unit, The University of New South Wales; 2015.

6. Glujovsky D, Blake D, Farquhar C, Bardach A. Cleavage stage versus blastocyst stage embryo transfer in assisted reproductive technology. Cochrane Database Syst Rev. 2012;7:CD002118.

7. Dar S, Lazer T, Shah PS, Librach CL. Neonatal outcomes among singleton births after blasto-cyst versus cleavage stage embryo transfer: a systematic review and meta-analysis. Hum Reprod Update. 2014;20:439–48.

8. Eshre. Focus on reproduction. 2015;22–23.

9. Shenfield F, De Mouzon J, Pennings G, Ferraretti AP, Andersen AN, De Wert G, Goossens V, Care ETOCBR. Cross border reproductive care in six European countries. Hum Reprod. 2010;25:1361–8.

10. Burlass T, Marriner C. Couple's Mexico surrogacy nightmare with embryos destroyed and mixed up. The Sydney Morning Herald; 2015.

11. Auerbach T. Sydney freelance serial sperm donor John Mayger has fathered at least 18 chil-dren, two with autism. The Daily Telegraph; 2015.

12. Kagi J. Baby Gammy: child protection knew infant was in care of convicted paedophile months before making contact with David Farnell. ABC News; 2014.

13. Pennings G, De Wert G, Shenfield F, Cohen J, Tarlatzis B, Devroey P. ESHRE task force on ethics and law 15: cross-border reproductive care. Hum Reprod. 2008;23:2182–4.

14. NHMRC. Ethical guidelines on the use of assisted reproductive technology in clinical practice and research. National Health and Medical Research Council, Australian Government; 2007.

15. Swanson A. How the biological clock is ticking for men as well as women. The Independent; 2015.

16. Forman R. Cross-border reproductive care: a clinician's perspective. Reprod Biomed Online. 2011;23:808–10.

17. De Ziegler D, De Ziegler N, Sean S, Bajouh O, Meldrum DR. Training in reproductive endo-crinology and infertility and assisted reproductive technologies: options and worldwide needs. Fertil Steril. 2015;104:16–23.

18. Gambone JC, Segars JH, Cedars M, Schlaff WD. Fellowship training and board certification in reproductive endocrinology and infertility. Fertil Steril. 2015;104:3–7.

19. Moffett A, Shreeve N. First do no harm: uterine natural killer (NK) cells in assisted reproduc-tion. Hum Reprod. 2015;30:1519–25.

20. Rustamov O, Smith A, Roberts SA, Yates AP, Fitzgerald C, Krishnan M, Nardo LG, Pemberton PW. Anti-Mullerian hormone: poor assay reproducibility in a large cohort of subjects suggests sample instability. Hum Reprod. 2012;27:3085–91.

21. Yarde F, Voorhuis M, Fauser B, Eijkemans M, Broekmans F. Anti-mullerian hormone as predictor of live birth in imminent ovarian failure. Human Reproduction; 2012. Oxford Univ Press Great Clarendon St, Oxford OX2 6DP, England.

22. Lambalk CB. Anti-Mullerian hormone, the holy grail for fertility counselling in the general population? Hum Reprod. 2015;30:2257–8.

23. Somigliana E, Viganò P, Filippi F, Papaleo E, Benaglia L, Candiani M, Vercellini P. Fertility preser-vation in women with endometriosis: for all, for some, for none? Hum Reprod. 2015;30:1280–6.

24. Leach M, Aitken RJ, Sacks G. Sperm DNA fragmentation abnormalities in men from couples with a history of recurrent miscarriage. Aust N Z J Obstet Gynaecol. 2015;55:379–83.

25. Aitken RJ, De Iuliis GN, Finnie JM, Hedges A, Mclachlan RI. Analysis of the relationships between oxidative stress, DNA damage and sperm vitality in a patient population: develop-ment of diagnostic criteria. Hum Reprod. 2010;25:2415–26.

26. Simon L, Murphy K, Shamsi MB, Liu L, Emery B, Aston KI, Hotaling J, Carrell DT. Paternal influ-ence of sperm DNA integrity on early embryonic development. Hum Reprod. 2014;29:2402–12.

27. Gavriliouk D, Aitken RJ. Damage to sperm DNA mediated by reactive oxygen species: its impact on human reproduction and the health trajectory of offspring. Adv Exp Med Biol. 2015;868:23–47.

28. Stone MP, Huang H, Brown KL, Shanmugam G. Chemistry and structural biology of DNA damage and biological consequences. Chem Biodivers. 2011;8:1571–615.
29. Aitken RJ, Jones KT, Robertson SA. Reactive oxygen species and sperm function—in sickness and in health. J Androl. 2012;33:1096–106.
30. Showell MG, Brown J, Yazdani A, Stankiewicz MT, Hart RJ. Antioxidants for male subfertility. Cochrane Database Syst Rev. 2011;CD007411.
31. Polyzos NP, Anckaert E, Guzman L, Schiettecatte J, Van Landuyt L, Camus M, Smitz J, Tournaye H. Vitamin D deficiency and pregnancy rates in women undergoing single embryo, blastocyst stage, transfer (SET) for IVF/ICSI. Hum Reprod. 2014;29:2032–40.
32. Meher A, Sundrani D, Joshi S. Maternal nutrition influences angiogenesis in the placenta through peroxisome proliferator activated receptors: a novel hypothesis. Mol Reprod Dev. 2015;82:726–34.
33. Barker DJ, Osmond C, Golding J, Kuh D, Wadsworth ME. Growth in utero, blood pressure in childhood and adult life, and mortality from cardiovascular disease. BMJ. 1989;298:564–7.
34. Ilioi EC, Golombok S. Psychological adjustment in adolescents conceived by assisted reproduction techniques: a systematic review. Hum Reprod Update. 2015;21:84–96.
35. Vulliemoz NR, Mcveigh E, Kurinczuk J. In vitro fertilisation: perinatal risks and early childhood outcomes. Hum Fertil (Camb). 2012;15:62–8.
36. Ventimiglia E, Capogrosso P, Boeri L, Serino A, Colicchia M, Ippolito S, Scano R, Papaleo E, Damiano R, Montorsi F, Salonia A. Infertility as a proxy of general male health: results of a cross-sectional survey. Fertil Steril. 2015;104:48–55.
37. Chan JL, Schon SB, O'Neill KE, Masson P. Infertility and the internet: ethical concerns in medical marketing. Fertil Steril. 2014;102:e42.
38. Goldman KN, Moon KS, Yauger BJ, Payson MD, Segars JH, Stegmann BJ. Proficiency in oocyte retrieval: how many procedures are necessary for training? Fertil Steril. 2011;95:2279–82.
39. Petok WD. Infertility counseling (or the lack thereof) of the forgotten male partner. Fertil Steril. 2015;104:260–6.
40. De Ziegler D, Meldrum DR. Introduction: training in reproductive endocrinology and infertility: meeting worldwide needs. Fertil Steril. 2015;104:1–2.
41. Steptoe PC, Edwards RG. Birth after the reimplantation of a human embryo. Lancet. 1978;312:366.
42. Ng SC, Bongso A, Ratnam SS. Microinjection of human oocytes: a technique for severe oligo-asthenoteratozoospermia. Fertil Steril. 1991;56:1117–23.
43. Benward J. Mandatory counseling for gamete donation recipients: ethical dilemmas. Fertil Steril. 2015;104:507–12.

Chapter 15
Implementing and Managing Natural and Modified Natural IVF Cycles

Mara Kotrotsou, Geeta Nargund, and Stuart Campbell

Introduction

The story of the birth of the first IVF baby on 25th July 1978 is well known to all reproductive medicine specialists. It was achieved in a natural cycle for a woman with tubal factor infertility. As means of controlling the Luteinizing Hormone (LH) surge were not available at that time, Patrick Steptoe and Robert Edwards turned to the advantages of a physiological cycle to overcome the problems of an early surge which is associated with stimulated cycles [1].

Nearly four decades after Louise Brown was born, it is now estimated that approximately five million babies have been born worldwide by IVF [2]. Following the advent of Gonadotrophin Releasing Hormone (GnRH) agonist downregulation in the early 1980s protocols were developed where following high Follicular Stimulating Hormone (FSH) stimulation multiple oocytes could be collected for fertilisation with a view to improving the selection potential of embryos [3]. However, iatrogenic complications, high cost of fertility treatment, concerns regarding supraphysiological hormonal levels on both mothers and embryos have led clinicians to rethink their established views on cycle management to seek more physiological approaches to stimulation. This was aided by the development of GnRH antagonists, introduced to the market for the first time in 2001, where patients could be treated within their own natural cycle and milder and more natural protocols could be developed [3]. As a

M. Kotrotsou, MUDr (✉) • G. Nargund, FRCOG
Create Fertility, 3-5 Pepys Road, West Wimbledon, London SW20 8NJ, UK
e-mail: maragys@brinternet.com; geetanargund@googlemail.com

S. Campbell, DSc, FRCPEd, FRCOG
Create Fertility, 150 Cheapside, London EC2V 6ET, UK

34 Corfton Road, London W5 2HT, UK
e-mail: profscampbell@hotmail.com

© Springer Science+Business Media New York 2016
S.D. Fleming, A.C. Varghese (eds.), *Organization and Management of IVF Units*, DOI 10.1007/978-3-319-29373-8_15

result a global trend has emerged over the last few years favouring milder and more natural approaches to ovarian stimulation. The efficiency of these approaches has also been enabled by advances in ultrasound such as Doppler and 3D and by innovative technology in the laboratory such as in vitro maturation (IVM).

In 2006 an international society for implementing mild and natural approaches to stimulation (ISMAAR) was established. Its members advocate that these approaches in IVF treatment are as effective as conventional IVF in achieving comparable pregnancy rates. At the same time they are more patient friendly, resulting in fewer short and long term side effects promoting more natural and physiological conceptions that result in healthier babies [4].

Physiology of Selection of a Dominant Oocyte

In the female, the cells (*oogonia*) that will give rise to the oocytes released during menstrual cycles are formed during foetal life. The oogonia increase rapidly in number and some differentiate into the so-called *primary oocytes* until about the 5th month of foetal life after which some cell degeneration takes place. At birth a female carries 700,000 to 2,000,000 primary oocytes. Cell death or *atresia* continues and at puberty there are only around 400,000 primary oocytes of which fewer than 500 will be ovulated [5, 6].

As oocytes cannot be produced after birth, oocytes released later in life derive from cells that could have been dormant for more than 40 years.

A primary oocyte together with its surrounding flat epithelial cells is known as a *primordial follicle*. Around 1000 primordial follicles start growing every month. Complete follicular development takes over 220 days and can be classified into three phases according to the developmental stage and follicular gonadotrophin dependence. First, the initial recruitment of resting primordial follicles, second the development of pre-antral and early antral follicles and finally cyclic recruitment of a limited cohort of antral follicles followed by the selection of a single dominant follicle during the mid-follicular phase of the menstrual cycle [7, 8].

The very early stages of follicular development, which are also known as "initial recruitment", are possibly under the control of intra-ovarian autocrine and paracrine factors and they are independent of FSH and LH [9]. However, the selection of a dominant follicle from a cohort of antral follicles, also known as "cyclic recruitment", is dependent on FSH [8].

FSH levels increase in the late luteal phase up to the onset of menstruation and the early follicular phase of the following cycle. This inter-cycle rise is also named the "*FSH window*" and stimulates "cyclic recruitment". A cohort of 4–6 healthy follicles start accumulating FSH in their follicular fluid and in the follicle destined to become dominant, this FSH concentrates at a critical threshold [10, 11]. In that follicle FSH stimulates production of estradiol in excess of the production in the non-dominant follicles. Its development becomes a self-supported event through a negative feedback loop where the oestrogen secreted by the dominant follicle suppresses the release of FSH to such levels that the remaining follicles which do not contain adequate numbers of FSH receptors or have not reached a certain stage of maturity (narrowing of FSH window) cannot aromatise androgens to estrogens at a sufficient rate and develop an androgenised environment. It is only the follicles with an estrogenic environment that are rescued for further growth, while those with an androgenic environment become atretic. The above shows that the duration of the FSH window as well as its magnitude is important. The selected dominant follicle continues to grow despite low FSH values. This is partially explained by an increase in the sensitivity of the dominant follicle to FSH. In the midfollicular phase and onwards the follicle becomes dependent on LH.

One needs to realise that in older women or those with low ovarian reserve, high stimulation with FSH will only affect the small number of follicles that are undergoing cyclic recruitment and will not affect follicles undergoing early recruitment. Therefore, in these circumstances downregulation protocols may be counterproductive. In such women natural or modified natural IVF appears to be a more logical treatment.

Definitions

In the nearly four decades since the birth of the first IVF baby several protocols have been developed with nomenclatures often creating a confusion in terminology both among clinicians and among patients.

ISMAAR has published a clarification of the terminology used for ovarian stimulation protocols (The ISMAAR proposal on terminology for ovarian stimulation in IVF, Table 15.1) [12].

Natural Cycle IVF

This refers to IVF performed during a patient's spontaneous cycle without the use of any stimulation medication or medication to trigger final oocyte maturation. The cycle develops spontaneously and oocyte retrieval is timed according to the patient's LH surge. The aim of this treatment is to harvest a naturally selected oocyte at the lowest possible cost.

Table 15.1 ISMAAR definitions (www.ismaar.org)

Terminology	Aim	Methodology
Natural cycle IVF	Single oocyte	No medication
Modified natural cycle IVF	Single oocyte	hCG only antagonist and FSH/hMG add-back
Mild IVF	2–7 Oocytes	Low dose FSH/hMG, oral compounds and antagonist
Conventional IVF	≥8 Oocytes	Agonist or antagonist conventional FSH/hMG dose

Natural cycle IVF usually has higher cancellation rates due to spontaneous ovulation but is valuable in specific circumstances, such as when increased oestradiol levels are to be avoided or because of patient preference for a drug free IVF cycle. The patients should be counselled about cancellation rates. The cycle is monitored with serial ultrasound scans and one or two hormone assays during the cycle. The timing of oocyte collection may be based on an optimum level of serum estradiol (E2) and LH and/or ultrasound measurement of follicular diameter and endometrial thickness [13, 14]. Tests may be carried out to detect urinary LH surge prior to oocyte collection. Follicular flushing may be used during ultrasound-directed follicle aspiration. IVF and embryo transfer techniques are similar to those used in stimulated cycles. Luteal support is not used unless specifically indicated.

No specific protocol template can be applied and both the frequency of monitoring and the timing of the oocyte retrieval are dependent on the woman's cycle.

Modified Natural Cycle IVF

This term should be applied when IVF is being performed during a spontaneous cycle with the use of exogenous hormones or any drugs aiming to collect a naturally selected single oocyte but with a reduction in the chance of cycle cancellation. The drugs used may include:

1. The use of human chorionic gonadotrophin (hCG) to induce final oocyte maturation with or without subsequent luteal support.
2. The administration of GnRH antagonist to block the spontaneous LH surge with or without FSH or human menopausal gonadotrophin (hMG) as add-back therapy.

Luteal support is usually administered.

Standardised template protocols in this type of treatment can include the following:

- *Natural cycles with hCG and indomethacin only*: Monitoring in these cycles is performed via serial ultrasound scans and measurements of serum E2 and LH. The first scan may be performed between day 8–9 of the cycle or as early as day 5 depending on the woman's natural cycle pattern. HCG is used to induce final oocyte maturation when a follicle is ≥16 mm. Indomethacin tablets 50 mg three times a day are administered from the day of the trigger or earlier if there is a spontaneous rise in LH or a spontaneous surge, in order to inhibit ovulation [15].
- *Natural controlled cycles*: Monitoring in these cycles is again performed via serial ultrasound scans and measurements of serum E2 and LH. The first scan can be performed as early as day 5 of the cycle. A GnRH antagonist is administered together with add back FSH (max dose 150 IU) once the leading follicle is 13–14 mm. HCG is used to induce final oocyte maturation when a follicle is >17 mm. Luteal support is administered.

Potential Advantages of a Natural or Natural Based IVF Cycle

As mentioned earlier in the introduction, the recently noted global trend toward natural and milder stimulation approaches to IVF treatment can be attributed to emerging evidence associating certain advantages to these types of treatment. Some of these advantages are summarised below:

- The natural selection process of the dominant follicle is maintained. This ensures recruitment and development of only the best quality follicles and oocytes in each menstrual cycle, a classic example of quality versus quantity.

  The importance of preserving the element of natural selection is associated with the development of better quality gametes, especially in cases of women of advanced age with diminished reserve. In 2001 Wikland et al. compared antagonist protocols with a low starting FSH dose (150 IU) and a high FSH dose (225 IU) and showed that whilst there was a difference in the number of oocytes retrieved in the high dose group, both groups have comparable results in pregnancy rates [16]. Similar results were presented by Yong et al. in a randomised trial comparing cycle outcomes with starting doses of 150 IU r-FSH versus 225 IU [17]. They concluded that higher doses of stimulation could not compensate for the well documented age related decline in numbers of follicles available for stimulation. In conclusion, aiming to develop higher numbers of oocytes does not ensure a better outcome.

- The natural based protocols involve the use of either no stimulation or low dose drugs for a short period of time, hence minimising any potential long-term side effects.

  It is evident that increasingly more women are delaying childbirth, which leads to an increase in the numbers of those who are seeking fertility treatment. As a result the fertility drugs are among the fastest growing group of drugs and it is therefore understandable that they will be attracting studies on potential long-term side effects. Periodically there are epidemiological studies linking fertility drugs to an increased incidence of various cancers. Evidence is already available on the prolonged use of clomiphene citrate for ovulation induction. Use of clomiphene citrate for 12 consecutive months or more has linked this drug to the development of borderline ovarian tumours. The evidence is less clear when it comes to the gonadotrophins used in stimulation and whilst some studies have implicated their use with an increased risk of ovarian cancer, others have failed to show such a relationship [18]. There is similarly conflicting evidence when it comes to any associations between fertility drugs and development of breast cancer but there are studies that have shown an increased risk between use of clomiphene citrate and endometrial cancer [19]. When interpreting the currently available results, we must bear in mind that the fertility drugs were first used in the 1960's and that longer term follow up may reveal new evidence. These limitations are evident to both clinicians and patients seeking milder forms of treatment.

- The risk of ovarian hyper-stimulation syndrome (OHSS) is either eliminated or decreased significantly.

OHSS is an iatrogenic complication that can be very challenging for clinicians and distressing for patients. The prevalence of moderate to severe OHSS in literature varies between 1 % and 10 % [20]. It makes sense that the risk of developing OHSS drops significantly with lower doses of stimulation and that it is completely eliminated in natural cycles and nearly eliminated in modified natural cycles [21].

- The use of no or less drugs decreases the cost of the individual cycle.

When directly comparing the cost of individual cycles, natural and natural modified cycles are cheaper due to the use of no or decreased amounts of drugs [13].

- The discomfort and emotional burden experienced by patients is considered to be less in mild stimulation approaches [22].

The overall discomfort experienced by patients was not higher than that experienced in conventional IVF cycles despite the higher number of IVF cycles undertaken with the mild approach. The cycle drop-out rates were nearly halved in mild stimulation compared to those with standard treatment [22].

- The endometrium maintains its physiological properties.

Embryo implantation is an extremely well controlled process at both cellular and hormonal levels. Therefore, maintaining a receptive endometrium is of paramount importance. There is recent evidence suggesting that conventional IVF protocols using GnRH-agonist may alter the receptivity properties of the endometrium [23]. Horcajadas and his colleagues concluded that endometrial development after a GnRH antagonist mimics the natural endometrium more closely than after a GnRH agonist at both morphological and molecular levels [23]. They showed that no changes were seen in morphology and at the molecular level only 23 genes were dysregulated when high doses of drugs were used. Similar results have been shown earlier by Mirkin and co-workers but they concluded that although ovarian stimulation causes structural and functional changes compared with natural cycles, small changes were found when gene expression patterns were compared, and that ovarian stimulation may therefore not have a major impact on endometrial receptivity [24]. The clinical implications of this need to be evaluated further.

- Lower and more physiological doses of stimulation can result in better quality embryos.

Baart et al. conducted a study where they randomly allocated mild stimulation and conventional stimulation protocols to two groups of patients [4]. One hundred and eleven patients were included in the study, all under the age of 38. The mild stimulation protocol involved stimulation with 150 IU of rFSH commenced on day 5 and the conventional stimulation protocol involved down-regulation with a GnRH agonist and stimulation with 225 IU. A day 3 embryo biopsy was conducted. The study was terminated prematurely after an interim analysis showed lower embryo aneuploidy results in the mild stimulation group. They concluded that reducing the interference with ovarian physiology results in a sufficient number of chromosomally normal embryos [4].

- The success rates of natural cycles are comparable to those of stimulated IVF.

  Early studies on natural cycle IVF have reported live birth rates between 3.8 and 18.8 % per cycle [25]. The lower pregnancy rate per started cycle in natural and modified natural-cycle IVF compared with conventional IVF stimulation is a logical consequence, since only one follicle is available in natural and modified natural IVF cycles. The higher cost effectiveness of stimulated cycles when compared to natural cycles has been the argument that established stimulated IVF as the predominant form of assisted reproduction treatment. Ultimately, a higher number of retrieved oocytes is expected to result in higher pregnancy rates through an improved embryo selection potential compensating for any inefficiencies in the embryology lab.

  Four randomised controlled trials (RCT's) conducted between 1991 and 2004 that compared natural cycles with hCG only to clomid stimulated cycles, hMG and GnRH analogue long protocol cycles and flare stimulation cycles with FSH and GnRH analogues all demonstrated lower success rates for natural cycles [26–29].

  In contrast a study conducted by Nargund et al. in 2001 showed that the overall cost effectiveness of natural cycle IVF may be higher compared to conventional IVF if natural cycles are offered in a series of consecutive cycles [13]. They felt that the lower cost per cycle, the lower stress levels observed during treatment and the ability to have "back to back" treatment in successive cycles made natural cycle IVF a viable option for many women. In their study they looked at 52 women who underwent a total of 181 cycles. The median age of the study group was 34 with a range 24–40. They included women with both primary and secondary infertility and tubal damage and women with primary infertility and poor ovarian reserve. They calculated the cost of natural cycles based on use of hCG and indomethacin including three scans per cycle. They concluded that after four cycles the cumulative probability of pregnancy was 46 % with a live birth rate of 32 % [13, 30].

  The concept of offering a series of natural cycles also attracted Pelinck et al. who conducted a large cohort study in 2006 and looked into the cumulative pregnancy rate after three modified natural IVF cycles in good prognosis patients [31]. A total of 844 treatment cycles in 350 patients of 36 years of age with no previous IVF treatment were included. The ongoing pregnancy rate was 8.3 % with one cycle and 20.8 % after up to three cycles of treatment. A year later Pelink et al. showed that cumulative pregnancy rates reached 44.4 % after nine modified natural cycles [32].

- Performance of transvaginal retrieval under local anaesthetic.

  Since the great majority of natural cycles involve harvesting of only one follicle, the idea of performing the oocyte retrieval under local anaesthetic can be very appealing to both patients and clinicians. The patient avoids exposure to sedation medication, the procedure time and time for recovery in the unit is shortened and the cost of treatment decreases. Selection of patients following assessment of access to the dominant follicle and patient suitability in terms of pain expectations and anxiety levels is important.

- The laboratory procedures are less time consuming due to the low number of oocytes utilised.
  This contributes to a lower cost of the cycles [33].
- Decreased multiple pregnancy rates.
  Clearly multiple pregnancies are the result of the embryo transfer policy and not of ovarian stimulation in itself. The argument for more aggressive stimulation and increased oocyte yield has been the need for an increased number of embryos. In natural cycles single embryo transfer (SET) becomes the default as there is rarely more than one embryo available, there is less embryo wastage and the process appears more efficient.

Challenges and Solutions

Natural cycles require closer monitoring and can be associated with lack of efficacy and overall high cancellation rates (28.9 %) [14]. The high cancellation rates are due to unfavourable cycle events that impact on outcome and occur more frequently than in conventional superovulation IVF cycles. These unfavourable cycle events are inadequate growth of the dominant follicle, premature surge in LH, spontaneous ovulation before oocyte retrieval, failure to collect an oocyte and fertilisation failure or no transferable embryo.

- Use of an antagonist.
  The use of an antagonist in the so-called natural modified cycle has decreased the incidence of premature ovulation from 16.6 % seen in natural cycles to 4.2 %. To avoid follicular developmental arrest, concomitant substitution with rFSH is thought necessary [33]. In natural modified cycles 81 % of started cycles reach oocyte retrieval and 36.5 % reach embryo transfer (or 61.1 % of successful retrievals) as shown by a large cohort study conducted by Pelinck et al. in 2007 [32].
- Use of indomethacin.
  The administration of FSH, albeit for a short period and at low doses, could be considered as an inconvenience for some. The use of indomethacin can be an alternative. Indomethacin is a non-steroidal anti-inflammatory drug (NSAID) and has been shown to effectively delay ovulation [15, 34–36]. It inhibits the production of prostaglandins which are essential for follicle rupture and ovulation. Indomethacin administered before ovulation prevents follicle rupture without apparent effects on menstrual cycle length or FSH, LH, oestradiol and progesterone concentrations [37, 38].
- Use of Clomiphene.
  The continuous use of Clomiphene as another alternative for suppressing the premature LH surge has been described by Teramoto and Kato in a large scale retrospective study [39]. They have successfully used a protocol where clomiphene was used from day 3 of the cycle and continued until the day before triggering oocyte maturation and 83 % of the cycles studied reached oocyte retrieval.

- Use of advanced ultrasound and Doppler images to assess the quality of the developing follicle and optimise the timing of HCG administration for oocyte maturation.

Management of natural IVF cycles requires greater judgement and knowledge of physiological processes. This has led to a greater variability in the success rates and contributed to the initial trend of decreased prevalence of these cycles. The use of colour flow Doppler to assess the perifollicular blood flow can provide additional information about the quality of the developing follicle and contribute to optimising the timing of oocyte retrieval.

Nargund et al. conducted a study assessing the perifollicular flow of stimulated follicles on the day of the trigger injection and immediately before follicular aspiration for oocyte retrieval [40]. They demonstrated a significant relationship between follicular peak systolic velocity (PSV), the ability to recover an oocyte and the subsequent production of morphologically normal embryos. They demonstrated that 72 % of the follicles with PSV ≥ 10 cm/s produced grade 1 or grade 2 preimplantation embryos. Their findings were consistent with previous studies on PSV and pulsatility index (PI) in unstimulated ovaries, at the times of follicular rupture at ovulation, that had demonstrated a rise in the PVS associated with the preovulatory rise in LH [41]. The authors acknowledge the difficulties in accurately assessing the flow velocity in small vessels and the importance of the operator's skills in obtaining accurate findings.

- Use of a series of treatment cycles to improve efficiency.

As shown by Nargund et al. after four cycles the cumulative probability of pregnancy can reach 46 % with a live birth rate of 32 % [13].

Indications

The advantages of natural cycle IVF that we analysed earlier give rise to some of the indications for this type of treatment.

1. Medical contraindications to the use of stimulation drugs and the development of high levels of estradiol.

   Patients with conditions that can be adversely affected by high levels of estradiol, such as hypercoagulable diseases, history of oestrogen dependent carcinomas, etc., can opt to have natural based IVF. In the case of cancer patients awaiting cancer treatment, one should obviously consider the time frame available for IVF treatment and determine whether serial natural cycles or a single mild short stimulation protocol with or without the use of anti-estrogens would be preferable.

2. Women with a history of severe OHSS or those at significant risk of developing severe OHSS.

This group of women can find stimulation very stressful and are challenging to treat. No or low doses of drugs for a short period of time eliminates or decreases the risk of OHSS.

3. IVM cycles.

IVM cycles were initially indicated to eliminate the risk of OHSS in patients with polycystic ovaries.

The increased interest in natural cycle IVF has subsequently led to the evaluation of natural cycle IVM. As we described earlier in a natural cycle, normally only a single follicle develops to the pre-ovulatory stage and ovulates its mature oocyte. Many small follicles also grow in the ovaries during the same follicular phase of the menstrual cycle. These will eventually become atretic following the selection of the dominant follicle but there is a narrow window when they can still be retrieved. Immature oocytes retrieved at this stage have been successfully matured in vitro and fertilised, and they have resulted in several pregnancies and healthy live births [42].

Prevention of ovulation from the dominant follicle in a natural IVM cycle remains important. HCG can be administered 36 h before oocyte retrieval when the size of the leading follicle has reached 12–14 mm in diameter and before atresia takes place in the non-dominant follicles and still result in retrieval of metaphase 2 (MII) oocytes from the majority of leading follicles. It is therefore possible to combine natural cycle IVF with IVM as an alternative to natural cycle IVF, and clinical pregnancy rates of 35 % have been achieved for a selected group of women with various causes of infertility without recourse to ovarian stimulation [42].

Natural IVF with IVM, where in vivo matured oocytes are collected with immature IVM oocytes in the same unstimulated cycles could become a standard approach in assisted reproductive technology (ART) treatments. Lim et al. showed promising results in a study conducted in 2009 that revealed a 40.4 % clinical pregnancy rate from such a combined natural IVF/IVM approach [43].

The applications of IVM have been extended to other groups of patients, such as poor responders and cancer patients. Poor responders to previous gonadotrophin stimulation were found to benefit from immature oocyte collection in an unstimulated natural cycle. In 2001 Child et al. showed that in a group of women with poor ovarian response the number of embryos produced and available for embryo transfer was similar to that for previous IVF treatments [44]. Some of the applications of IVM cycles may be limited by the technical difficulties of oocyte retrieval from follicles less than 7 mm in size.

4. Poor responders and women with poor ovarian reserve.

This group of patients remains difficult to treat and different ovarian stimulation protocols have been tried without a single protocol appearing superior to the other. Natural cycle IVF has been shown to be equally effective as a *"Flare"* protocol with a GnRH agonist in younger poor responders [29]. It has also been shown to produce results comparable to conventional IVF in patients aged between 37 and 43 years old with low ovarian reserve [45]. Natural cycle IVF in poor responders resulted in a higher number of cycles scheduled for oocyte retrieval and thus a higher pregnancy rate per started cycle compared to conventional IVF, where cycles have a higher cancellation rate [46]. Better embryo quality, better endometrium receptivity and the possibility of repeating the cycle monthly can account for the better results seen in this group of patients.

5. Older patients with or without previous poor response to stimulation.

   For these patients who, as a rule, are expected to have a diminished ovarian reserve, the benefits of a natural cycle appear clear. Natural selection of the dominant follicle improves embryo quality. By applying the knowledge we derived from studies on poor responders, the combination of an expected poor response and decreased oocyte quality can justify the use of these protocols as first line treatment in this group of patients [47]. Contrary to these results, Tomasevic et al. in 2007 concluded that age related poor responders rarely benefit from natural IVF cycles [48].

6. Male factor only

   Relatively high pregnancy rates have been reported in young couples with severe male factor infertility as the only fertility-compromising factor. In this category of patients, the success rate per started cycle was 13.3 % and cumulative pregnancy rates of 43.8 % after six successive cycles have been reported [49, 50]. These can be seen as encouraging results that justify offering this type of treatment to such couples while keeping treatment side effects to a minimum. Contrary to these findings Pelinck et al. concluded that natural and modified natural cycles may not be the best choice of treatment protocols in male factor infertility due to the lower fertilisation rate that consequently results in fewer embryo transfers per started cycle [14].

7. Patient preference.

   There is an increased tendency among patients to seek more physiological approaches to fertility treatment. This is understandable considering the possible advantages attributed to these cycles. The simplicity and short duration, the lack or low doses of medication and the fact that natural IVF cycles can fit into patients' spontaneous menstrual cycles are some of the reasons that make these cycles appealing to patients [51, 52].

Conclusions

Natural cycle IVF set the cornerstone upon which ART developed. Conventional IVF once thought as a sophisticated treatment method has been associated with complications such as OHSS, thrombosis, increased multiple pregnancy rates, high treatment cost and increased patient symptomatology including anxiety.

There is now sufficient evidence showing that natural and modified natural IVF cycles are more patient friendly with low complication rates and can be performed at lower cost. Treatment can be given in back to back cycles and there is evidence of similar success rates to conventional IVF treatment in older women and those with low ovarian reserve. Natural cycle IVF is more successful in centres with ultrasound expertise especially in ovarian and uterine Doppler. Natural and Modified natural cycle IVF is valuable in specific circumstances and especially when combined with IVM it will play an increasing role in the treatment options that should be available to couples.

References

1. Edwards RG. IVF, IVM, natural cycle IVF, minimal stimulation IVF-time for a rethink. Reprod BioMed Online. 2007;15(1):106–19.
2. ESHRE ART fact sheet. http://www.eshre.eu/Guidelines-and-Legal/ART-fact-sheet.aspx.
3. Heyden C. GnRH analogues: applications in assisted reproductive techniques. Eur J Endocrinol. 2008;159:S17–25.
4. Baart EB, Martini E, Eijkemans MJ, Van Opstal D, Beckers NG, Verhoeff A, Macklon NS, Fauser BC. Milder ovarian stimulation for in-vitro fertilization reduces aneuploidy in the human preimplantation embryo: a randomized controlled trial. Hum Reprod. 2007;22: 980–8.
5. Sadler TW. Gametogenesis. In: Langman's medical embryology. 6th ed. North Carolina, USA; 1990. p. 3–14. Published by Williams & Wilkins.
6. Sadler TW. Ovulation to implantation. In: Langman's medical embryology. 6th ed. North Carolina, USA; 1990. p. 21–38. Published by Williams & Wilkins.
7. Gougeon A. Regulation of ovarian follicular development in primates: facts and hypotheses. Endocr Rev. 1996;17:121–55.
8. McGee EA, Hsueh AJ. Initial and cyclic recruitment of ovarian follicles. Endocr Rev. 2000;21:200–14.
9. Fortune JE, Cushman RA, Wahl CM, Kito S. The primordial to primary follicle transition. Mol Cell Endocrinol. 2000;163:53–60.
10. McNatty KP, Hunter WM, MacNeilly AS, Sawers RS. Changes in the concentration of pituitary and steroid hormones in the follicular fluid of human graafian follicles throughout the menstrual cycle. J Endocrinol. 1975;64(3):555–71.
11. Brown JB. Pituitary control of ovarian function—concepts derived from gonadotrophin therapy. Aust N Z J Obstet Gynaecol. 1978;18:46–54.
12. Nargund G, Fauser BCJM, Macklon NS, Ombelet W, Nygren K, Frydman R. The ISMAAR proposal on terminology for ovarian stimulation for IVF. Hum Reprod. 2007;22(11):2801–4.
13. Nargund G, Waterstone J, Bland JM, Philips Z, Parsons J, Campbell S. Cumulative conception and live birth rates in natural (unstimulated) IVF cycles. Hum Reprod. 2001;16(2):259–62.
14. Pelinck MJ, Hoek A, Simons AHM, Heineman MJ. Efficacy of natural cycle IVF: a review of the literature. Hum Reprod Update. 2002;8(2):129–39.
15. Nargund G, Wei C. Successful planned delay of ovulation for one week with indomethacin. J Assist Reprod Genet. 1996;13(8):683–4.
16. Wikland M, Bergh C, Borg K, Hillensjo T, Howles CM, Knutsson A, Nilsson L, Wood M. A prospective, randomized comparison of two starting doses of recombinant FSH in combination with cetrorelix in women undergoing ovarian stimulation for IVF/ICSI. Hum Reprod. 2001;16:1676–81.
17. Yong PY, Brett S, Baird DT, Thong KJ. A prospective randomized clinical trial comparing 150 IU and 225 IU of recombinant follicle-stimulating hormone (Gonal-F) in a fixed-dose regimen for controlled ovarian stimulation in in vitro fertilization treatment. Fertil Steril. 2003;79:308–15.
18. Brinton LA, Lamb EJ, Moghissi KS, et al. Ovarian cancer risk associated with varying causes of infertility. Fertil Steril. 2004;82:405–14.
19. Brinton LA. Long-term effects of ovulation-stimulating drugs on cancer risk. Reprod BioMed Online. 2007;15(1):38–44.

20. Serour GI, Rhodes C, Sattar MA, Aboulghar MA, Mansour R. Complications of assisted reproductive techniques: a review. Assist Reprod. 1999;9(4):214–32.
21. Fauser BC, Nargund G, Nyboe Andersen A, Norman R, Tarlatzis B, Boivin J, Ledger W. Mild ovarian stimulation for IVF: 10 years later. Hum Reprod. 2010;25(11):2678–84.
22. Heijnen EMEW, Eijkemans MJC, De Klerk C, Polinder S, Beckers NGM, Klinkert ER, Macklon NS, Fauser BCJM. A mild treatment strategy for in-vitro fertilisation: a randomised non-inferiority study. Lancet. 2007;369:1–8.
23. Martinez-Conejero JF, Simon C, Pellicer A, Horcajadas JA. Is ovarian stimulation detrimental to the endometrium? Reprod BioMed Online. 2007;15(1):45–50.
24. Mirkin S, Nikas G, Hsiu JG, Diaz J, Oehninger S. Gene expression profiles and structural/functional features of the peri-implantation endometrium in natural and gonadotropin-stimulated cycles. J Clin Endocrinol Metabol. 2004;89:5742–52.
25. Daya S, Gunby J, Hughes EG, Collins JA, Sagle MA, YoungLai EV. Natural cycles for in-vitro fertilisation: cost effectiveness analysis and factors influencing outcome. Hum Reprod. 1995;10:1719–24.
26. MacDougall MJ, Tan SL, Hall V, Balen A, Mason BA, Jacobs HS. Comparison of natural with clomiphene citrate-stimulated cycles in in vitro fertilization: a prospective, randomized trial. Fertil Steril. 1994;61:1052–7.
27. Ingerslev HJ, Hojgaard A, Hindkjaer J, Kesmodel U. A randomized study comparing IVF in the unstimulated cycle with IVF following clomiphene citrate. Hum Reprod. 2001;16:696–702.
28. Levy MJ, Gindoff P, Hall J, Stillman RJ. The efficacy of natural versus stimulated cycle IVF-ET. Fertil Steril. 1991;56 Suppl 1:S15.
29. Morgia F, Sbracia M, Schimberni M, Giallonardo A, Piscitelli C, Giannini P, Aragona C. A controlled trial of natural cycle versus microdose gonadotropin-releasing hormone analog flare cycles in poor responders undergoing in vitro fertilization. Fertil Steril. 2004;81:1542–7.
30. Verberg MFG, Macklon NS, Nargund G, Frydman R, Devroey P, Broekmans FJ, Fauser BC. Mild ovarian stimulation for IVF. Hum Reprod Update. 2009;15(1):13–29.
31. Pelinck MJ, Vogel NE, Hoek A, Simons AH, Arts EG, Mochtar MH, Beemsterboer S, Hondelink MN, Heineman MJ. Cumulative pregnancy rates after three cycles of minimal stimulation IVF and results according to subfertility diagnosis: a multicentre cohort study. Hum Reprod. 2006;21:2375–83.
32. Pelinck MJ, Vogel NE, Arts EG, Simons AH, Heineman MJ, Hoek A. Cumulative pregnancy rates after a maximum of nine cycles of modified natural cycle IVF and analysis of patient drop-out: a cohort study. Hum Reprod. 2007;22:2463–70.
33. Pelinck MJ, Vogel NE, Hoek A, Arts EG, Simons AH, Heineman MJ. Minimal stimulation IVF with late follicular phase administration of the GnRH antagonist cetrorelix and concomitant substitution with recombinant FSH: a pilot study. Hum Reprod. 2005;20(3):642–8.
34. Okuda Y, Okamura H, Kanzaki H, Fujii S, Takenaka A, Wallach EE. An ultrastructural study of ovarian perifollicular capillaries in the indomethacin-treated rabbit. Fertil Steril. 1983;39:85–92.
35. Kadoch I, Al-Khaduri M, Phillips S, Lapense L, Couturier B, Hemmings R, Bissonnette F. Spontaneous ovulation rate before oocyte retrieval in modified natural cycle IVF with and without indomethacin. Reprod BioMed Online. 2008;16:245–9.
36. Kawachiya S, Matsumoto T, Bodri D, Kato K, Takehara Y, Kato O. Short-term, low-dose, non-steroidal anti-inflammatory drug application diminishes premature ovulation in natural-cycle IVF. Reprod BioMed Online. 2012;24:308–13.
37. Athanasiou S, Bourne TH, Khalid A, Okokon EV, Crayford TJ, Hagstrom HG, Campbell S, Collins WP. Effects of indomethacin on follicular structure, vascularity, and function over the peri-ovulatory period in women. Fertil Steril. 1996;65:556–60.
38. Hester K, Harper MJK, Duffy D. Oral administration of the cyclooxygenase-2 (COX-2) inhibitor meloxicam blocks ovulation in non-human primates when administered to simulate emergency contraception. Hum Reprod. 2010;25:360–7.
39. Teramoto S, Kato O. Minimal ovarian stimulation with clomiphene citrate: a large-scale retrospective study. Reprod BioMed Online. 2007;15:134–48.
40. Nargund G, Bourne T, Doyle P, Parsons J, Cheng W, Campbell S, Collins W. Association between US indices of follicular blood flow, oocyte recovery and preimplantation embryo quality. Hum Reprod. 1996;11(1):109–13.

41. Campbell S, Bourne TH, Waterstone J, Reynolds KM, Crayford TJ, Jurkovic D, Okokon EV, Collins WP. Transvaginal color blood flow imaging of the periovulatory follicle. Fertil Steril. 1993;60(3):433–8.
42. Lim JH, Yang SH, Chian RC. New alternative to infertility treatment for women without ovarian stimulation. Reprod BioMed Online. 2007;14:547–9.
43. Lim JH, Yang SH, Xu Y, Yoon SH, Chian RC. Selection of patients for natural cycle in vitro fertilization combined with in vitro maturation of immature oocytes. Fertil Steril. 2009;91(4):1050–5.
44. Child TJ, Abdul-Jalil AK, Gulekli B, Tan SL. In vitro maturation and fertilization of oocytes from unstimulated normal ovaries, polycystic ovaries, and women with polycystic ovary syndrome. Fertil Steril. 2001;76(5):936–42.
45. Papaleo E, De Santis L, Fusi F, Doldi N, Brigante C, Marelli G, Persico P, Cino I, Ferrari A. Natural cycle as first approach in aged patients with elevated follicle-stimulating hormone undergoing intracytoplasmic sperm injection: a pilot study. Gynaecol Endocrinol. 2006;22:351–4.
46. Bassil S, Godin PA, Donnez J. Outcome of IVF through natural cycles in poor responders. Hum Reprod. 1999;14:1262–5.
47. Ubaldi FM, Rienzi L, Ferrero S, Baroni E, Sapienza F, Cobellis L, Greco E. Management of poor responders in IVF. Reprod BioMed Online. 2004;10(2):235–46.
48. Tomasevic T, Korosec S, Virant Klun I, Drobnic S, Verdenik I. Age, oestradiol and blastocysts can predict success in natural cycle IVF-embryo transfer. Reprod BioMed Online. 2007;15(2):220–6.
49. Zhioua F, Zhioua A, Chaker A, M'solly S, Meriah S. Efficacy of intracytoplasmic sperm injection in a natural cycle with GnRH antagonists. Hum Reprod. 2004;49 Suppl 1:i105.
50. Vogel NEA, Pelinck MJ, Arts EG, Hoek A, Simons AH, Heineman MJ. Effectiveness of the modified natural cycle ICSI: results of a pilot study. Fertil Steril. 2003;80 Suppl 3:123.
51. Verberg MF, Eijkemans MJ, Heijnen EM, Broekmans FJ, de Klerk C, Fauser BC, Macklon NS. Why do couples drop-out from IVF treatment? A prospective cohort study. Hum Reprod. 2008;23(9):2050–5.
52. Pistorius EN, Adang EM, Stalmeier PF, Braat DD, Kremer JA. Prospective patient and physician preferences for stimulation or no stimulation in IVF. Hum Fertil. 2006;9(4):209–16.

Chapter 16
Public and Low-Cost IVF

Ian D. Cooke

Introduction

Although the first baby from in vitro fertilisation (IVF) was born in 1978, it took some years before IVF became more readily available. The first report covering IVF (and other techniques, and referred to as Assisted Reproductive Technologies, ART) in a number of countries was *presented* in Paris in 1991 [1], and a more detailed report, the 4th, was *published* in 1997 [2]. The latter's Table 16.1 reproduced the original data, which covered 31 countries with 664 clinics and 33,565 treatment cycles, showing how extensively the technology and clinical services were distributed at that time. The most recent data, from 2005, are reported from 53 countries with over a million ART procedures [3]. It was not until 2004 that information became available on whether or not a country had a national health plan covering assisted conception [4]. Those details were included in a discussion of the extent of insurance coverage and showed that 16 of 48 countries had coverage from a national health plan and no available private insurance. The comment was made that (at that time) France had unlimited coverage, and the reason for lack of cover was "mostly economic," but was associated with religious opposition, as "no Latin American country has either public or private insurance coverage" [4].

I.D. Cooke, FRCOG, F Med Sci, FRANZCOG (Hon) (✉)
Academic Unit of Reproductive and Developmental Medicine, The University of Sheffield,
Level 4, The Jessop Wing, Tree Root Walk, Sheffield S10 2SF, UK
e-mail: i.d.cooke@sheffield.ac.uk

© Springer Science+Business Media New York 2016
S.D. Fleming, A.C. Varghese (eds.), *Organization and Management of IVF Units*, DOI 10.1007/978-3-319-29373-8_16

Table 16.1 National plans
for assisted reproductive
technology (ART) coverage
(adapted from Table 3.3, Ory
S and Devroey P, editors,
Surveillance 2013. New
Jersey, IFFS, 2013)

Complete	Partial
Chile	Australia
Denmark	Austria
France	Belgium
Hungary	Bulgaria
Israel	Croatia
Libya	Czech Republic
Russian Federation	Finland
Saudi Arabia	Greece
Slovenia	Hong Kong
Spain	Iceland
	Italy
	Japan
	Kazakhstan
	Latvia
	New Zealand
	Norway
	Philippines
	Portugal
	Singapore
	South Korea
	Sweden
	Tunisia
	Turkey
	UK
	USA

Public Provision

In Surveillance 2010 [5] 30/47 countries were reported as having national health plan coverage and there were 35/60 so described in the 2013 report, although the countries surveyed were not all the same. In 2013, ten countries had complete coverage and 25 had partial coverage (Table 16.1), although the criteria restricting access varied markedly. The criteria could include age, marital state, the number of previous children, a specific number of attempts and type of procedure. The state may cover the cost of the whole procedure or only contribute some or all of the costs of the medication. It may mandate single embryo transfer under particular circumstances; it may only support a specific total number of cycles for the whole country for 1 year. Alternatively a state may only provide reimbursement to patients in government-sponsored programmes; a federal system may delegate the responsibility to states, which vary their provision within a country, or regions may themselves diverge in their criteria, thus limiting patient access. Restrictive criteria may drive patients to the private sector, although of course, more affluent patients often elect to use the private sector in the first instance.

The restrictive criteria, or complete lack of a national plan, may prevent a couple proceeding further in managing their infertility. It may leave them with a feeling of resentment or other psychological trauma, which may or may not have been addressed by offered counselling. Others are driven to invest in further treatment and may not be able to afford it. Catastrophic expenditure on ART treatment has been described by Dyer et al. [6] in a public health system in South Africa, where patient co-payment is required. It is defined as being >40 % of annual non-food expenditure and applied to 22 % of the 135 patients asked. When that patient population was divided into thirds, this applied to >50 % of the poorest third. It cannot be assumed that expensive ART treatment will be denied to poor people in a low resource economy; their determination to have treatment may well drive them into poverty.

An interesting question arises: *what is the cost of ART?*

Outcome data from ART have shown significant improvements, but costs have risen progressively. In the UK, according to the HFEA 2011-2 data, the mean live birth rate has increased from 14 % in 1991 to 25 % in 2011, more embryos are being transferred at the blastocyst stage reducing the multiple birth rate but the embryos are staying longer in culture. de Neubourg et al. [7] analysed the Belgian experience from 2003 to 2010 and the reasons for the reduction in the multiple birth rate while *maintaining* the same pregnancy rate per cycle. They ascribed this improvement to optimisation of laboratory procedures and stimulation protocols, introduction of quality systems and implementation of the EU Tissue Directive [8, 9], all of which add to costs. Laboratory costs have escalated with claims of more expensive quality materials, but each improvement has only been limited and overall is the sum of small gains. The medication cost, particularly when recombinant versions appeared, has been substantial in the developed world (although the cost of urinary products in low resource economies is substantially less) and particularly as the stimulation regimes became more complex.

A call for implementing randomised controlled trials has been made to identify real improvements and to optimise the use of consumables, methods and equipment [10]. Such an approach may also contribute to reduction of costs. Additional costs, however, are generated by screening, by counselling, using intracytoplasmic sperm injection (ICSI) and preimplantation genetic diagnosis (PGD), using donated gametes, as well as implementing quality assurance schemes and by the need to defray the costs of regulation. There has been a major increase in ART units (~3750 reported from 60 countries in Surveillance, 2013; [11]) and in many countries this has been predominantly in the private sector, suggesting that there is an opportunity to be commercially successful, as private enterprise has moved to counter the lack of public provision. In health provision in general, the cost of private provision is greater than that which the state would pay for a comparable service.

Other questions arise: *what impact does cost have on governments considering whether to include ART in public health provision; what determines whether the state pays all costs or whether co-payment (out of pocket expenses) is required?*

    The criteria that determine answers to these questions are not readily accessible, but some facts are available. In France a national plan offers four cycles of treatment, and in Israel pays until there have been two live births. In Germany the national plan covers 50 % of the cost of three cycles, although when the 50 % co-payment was introduced in 2004, as the government was concerned at rising health-care costs, there was a significant reduction in the use of ART as shown in the combined data from the public and private sectors [12, 13]. In Australia in 2010 restrictions were placed on the amount that Medicare paid in benefits for ART treatments and in the subsequent 15 months there was a significant reduction in the number of fresh ART cycles [14], experienced across all socioeconomic groups as a similar percentage reduction [15]. In New Zealand publicly funded procedures are controlled using Clinical Priority Access Criteria (CPAC), obtained using earlier clinical outcome data, perhaps a more justifiable approach [16].

    In the Netherlands there is mandatory private insurance. If insurance is mandated, cost is spread much more widely, so is much cheaper. In Belgium it was decided to reduce expenditure on neonatal intensive care for the markedly increased number of multiple births and transfer the money saved to pay for more ART, provided that multiple births were avoided. This led to specific requirements for Single Embryo Transfer (SET) in patients <36 years old having their first cycle of treatment. So at least in Western Europe the more affluent governments have accepted that modern and appropriate infertility treatment should be funded by the state, although there are various restrictions largely to reduce the total state expenditure, which throws a greater economic burden on those requiring treatment and promotes further stress. The support for state funding may be driven by a pronatalist approach, as in Denmark where there is a falling population or in Israel simply to increase the population. On the other hand, the Rand Corporation [17] has suggested that ART alone will not address the problem of population decline in Western Europe. In a review of European countries' public financing Berg Brigham et al. [18] stated that countries with the most generous schemes tended to restrict access to covered IVF to a greater degree.

    In 2012, in the UK there were 47, 422 women treated by ART [19]. The population was 63.23 million. If one assumes that the women of reproductive age comprise 20 % of the population, then that represents 3.7 % of the eligible population. If one assumes also that the rate of infertility in the population is 16 %, then only 23 % of the eligible population has been treated with ART, which is a gross under-provision. Recent estimates of the prevalence of infertility have suggested that previous estimates using demographic methods have been too low. Using different methodology of "time to pregnancy," Thoma et al. [20] in the USA estimate that the number of women in the population suffering infertility is 15.5 %, not the traditional 7.0 % and that for nulliparous women it is 24.3 % rather than 13.2 % with similarly high figures in France [21]. Thus the 23 % stated above, the proportion of the eligible population treated by ART, may be a gross *overestimate*.

    In low resource economies the provision is much less and the general health problems and financial constraints are even greater. Lu et al. [22] reported that government expenditure on health in many developing world countries increased by about 100 % from 1995 to 2006, although it reduced in sub-Saharan Africa. With problems such as HIV, malaria and TB the claim of infertility for funds lacked advocacy and urgency, so there was no additional allocation for ART. Murage et al. [23] from Kenya call for a simplified, less costly and more accessible ART to deal with the undoubted demand. Makuch et al. [24] aver that charges for ART have been incompatible with the financial possibilities of the majority of low-income Brazilians, so treatment should be offered at no cost to low-income populations as part of public health policy.

Rationale for Public Provision

The International Covenant on Economic, Social and Cultural Rights [25] enshrines access to basic social services as a fundamental human right. Governments have an obligation to provide those services for their people and so committed themselves to the UN Millennium Declaration and UN Millennium Development Goals (MDG) [26] as a reflection of this, to achieve by 2015 universal access to reproductive health (MDG5B; see UN MDG goals 5A and B) [27]. Nevertheless, if a country's institutions are weak and there is poor accountability for the use of public resources, as is often seen in developing countries, public provision may not be the best use of resources [28]. However, simply allowing the management to pass to the private sector may not be the best use of resources either; rather the government should contract the private sector to *deliver services* (not manage them). For equitable access to services, especially for the poor, there needs to be state sponsored universal provision. These general principles also apply to health. Infertility has been defined as a disease [29] and ART is now a major treatment, so it should be included in health provision. The critical points are the cost and the adequacy of regulation that ensures that both the public and private sectors are seen to adhere to the same high standards. Murphy [30], writing from the USA, posits that if society is required to accept ART as a basic right, it has the right to regulate access for its physical, social and economic wellbeing.

When ICMART and WHO defined infertility (the clinical definition, as opposed to the demographic definition) in 2009 as "a *disease* of the reproductive system defined by the failure to achieve a clinical pregnancy after 12 months or more of regular unprotected intercourse" [29], the potential health benefit case was significantly advanced as a health issue. The argument was made more persuasive when the World Report on Disability [31] was published by the WHO and reported that the fifth most prevalent disability in the world from the ages of 0–60 years was infertility. The category only included cases due to abortion and maternal sepsis and those categories alone had a prevalence of 32.5 % in the population of low and middle-income countries. This frequency was about the same as unintentional injuries, coming below hearing and visual problems and depression, and clearly affecting those of potential working age. The fact that the WHO refers to this as the "burden of disease" is informative.

So infertility is being recognised as a major problem for society and civil government, particularly in low resource economies and especially in sub-Saharan Africa where the problem is greater, the resources more scarce and the funding allocation even more limited. It is said (personal communications) that 70 % of patients in gynaecological clinics in Africa present with infertility, often initially undisclosed. Treating infertility has become a major issue and given the context, so has its cost. As at least 50 % of infertility is best treated by ART, so there is a great need to provide a relevant service at an appropriate, but low cost. Habbema [32] has considered factors influencing cost in low resource economies and calculated that a cycle would need to cost US \$50–75 to have a chance of being included in state health provision in those economies. He went on to conclude that greater emphasis would need to be given to infertility for it to be supported at greater cost. That low a cost seems unrealistic, so perhaps ART, that has limited provision, will fail to cater for all members of a society that need it. So the alternatives may be either to recognise the burden infertility places on individuals, families and the economic state of the country or to try and minimise the cost of ART or more likely, both. If Connolly et al. [12, 13] can calculate that the economic benefit of ART (at least in the UK) is by producing another individual who has long term economic benefit to the state, then, taking the longer term view, there is a powerful argument to support the provision of ART. However, a more recent calculation of the cost to the state in the Netherlands suggests that the state continues to support both naturally conceived and ART-conceived individuals if only fiscal considerations are taken into account and wider benefits need to be evaluated [33]. Habbema went on to consider what trade-offs could be made, so that more affluent societies could consider supporting state provision to a greater extent. Thus the affordable maximum for low-income countries could be a total cost of \$100 per cycle, if it is to be sustainable, and for middle-income countries it could be \$200. For higher middle-income countries it may be \$3–400. Co-payments seem always to reduce uptake of a service.

A further dimension also needs to be considered. The physical and psychological impact of ART on an individual is substantial and there have been moves to make ART more "patient friendly" [34, 35]. The emphasis is on reducing the degree of stimulation (see The International Society for Mild Approaches to Assisted Reproduction [ISMAAR] classification of mild stimulation for IVF) [36] to obtain fewer, better quality eggs [37] and avoid the possibility of ovarian hyper-stimulation. It will also reduce the costs of stimulation and lab consumables, as well as reducing the ovarian enlargement and accompanying discomfort and distress. It should also reduce the time and cost of monitoring.

However, the problem with using a minimal stimulation regime and SET is that the outcome is perceived as being poorer than using a conventional, greater stimulatory regime. The false analogy, of course, is simply to compare the mild regime with the conventional one. A fairer comparison would be the cost of a singleton, term, live baby per cycle started, not per embryo transfer (ET), as many cycles are cancelled for suboptimal response. That juxtaposition would suggest that a comparable cost would be the cumulative cost of a series of the lower cost cycles against a single higher cost treatment. Moragianni and Penzias [38] advocated use of cumulative live birth rates (CLBR) and claimed that they provide a more realistic estimate of outcome for individual couples. They state that elective SET and natural cycle IVF do not affect CLBR while achieving a significant reduction in the rates of multiples (and hence the neonatal care costs).

The reason for this continuing comparison to the perceived detriment of the milder stimulatory regime is that there are few data available. Many of the data have been obtained in ideal situations and there are hardly any data obtained under field conditions in low resource economies. There is a great need to obtain those data to make valid comparisons. Further, adding a degree of sophistication to a simple form of ART, by vitrification of embryos supernumerary after SET, could lead to greater gains, but also greater costs and the relative benefits need to be calculated. Groen et al. [39], using actual data, modelled three scenarios changing the number of cycles, single or double ET and using cryopreservation, compared the minimal stimulation of modified natural cycle and controlled ovarian stimulation ART. They suggested that minimising medication may be cost-effective if a strict SET policy is accepted. There would need to be a willingness to trade off effectiveness as live birth rate against the benefits of the milder stimulation regime, which would include a very low rate of multiple pregnancy and ovarian hyper-stimulation syndrome and the resulting lower costs per birth. A Cochrane analysis [40] concluded that further data from well conducted, large trials on natural and modified natural cycle IVF against standard IVF are required. They should include cumulative live birth and pregnancy rates, the number of cycles required to reach live birth, treatment costs and adverse effects.

In addition, if a country wishes to address the issue of infertility provision, it will need to improve its infrastructure to provide access to quality basic investigation and management [41]. It will need to generate a system that uses evidence based medicine principles to treat those that can be treated by simpler means and identify those that should be treated using ART. Such principles should apply equally in the private sector and should be exercised by regulation, ideally voluntarily through professional societies using agreed Guidelines, such as the Reports of The Practice Committee of the American Society for Reproductive Medicine or more comprehensively, as in the UK, through the National Institute for Health and Clinical Excellence [42]. Such recommendations, as important for well-based practice as they are, also have an economic edge, in that they should steer practitioners away from ineffectual, suboptimal or cost-inefficient practices and prevent exploitation. There is little point in having patients with limited means spending all their resources before they even arrive at the point of having ART, because inappropriate drug therapy or surgery has exhausted their financial means in a wholly private system or in a state system requiring additional out-of-pocket payments (co-payments). Chambers et al. [43] from Australia assert that the higher the cost paid by consumers, the greater the likelihood of having an increased number of embryos transferred. They show that a decrease in the cost of a cycle predicts increased usage. The uptake of ART is highly influenced by income, but having private insurance did not lead to greater utilisation of infertility services when reviewed in 1995 [44]. Presumably those that could afford insurance come from the small stratum of society that could afford ART in any case. On the other hand Hammoud et al. [45] reviewed 2005 US Census data to show in some of the 50 states that lower rates of IVF utilisation were correlated with a *lack* of insurance cover and a reduced availability of physicians providing this service. Perhaps the difference reflects a decade's better public recognition of IVF treatment and greater preparedness for its costs in an affluent society.

Low-Cost IVF

Another option, with or without attempting universal access, is to provide ART at the lowest possible cost. That involves rethinking the current standard approach. Heng [46] has described the reluctance of medical professionals to adopt minimal ovarian stimulation protocols, as they perceive maximising their "success" as giving them a competitive edge and economic advantage, particularly when regulatory authorities produce comparisons. Balic [47], in starting a programme in Bosnia and Herzegovina with a standard regime observed that the delivery rates were not acceptable and the twin rate was too high. It was concluded that a low-cost programme would make IVF affordable to a larger number of infertile couples.

If benefit can be justified and the economics of minimal cost can be validated, then possible technical and therapeutic options must be examined carefully. The early regimes of minimal stimulation from 1999, particularly with comparisons against natural cycles, have previously been reviewed in detail [48]. A more recent regime is that of Aanesen et al. [49] who compared the use of hCG to trigger ovulation ($n = 43$) with 100 mg clomiphene (days 3–7)/hCG, termed mild IVF, in 145 patients. In the latter group a mean of 1.9 oocytes were retrieved (range 1–10), but 40 % of patients failed to reach ET. The ongoing pregnancy rate/embryo transfer (SET) was 17.5 % in those <38 years; there were no pregnancies in older women. In historical controls using a conventional regime the cancellation rate was 14 % and the pregnancy rate per embryo transfer was 34 %. However, the costs were 96 % lower than the conventional regime, the risks of complications were dramatically reduced and the treatment may have been psychologically more acceptable. This reflects the earlier findings of Hojgaard et al. [50], who reported that 93 % of patients would undergo a mild regime again whereas only 53 % who had experienced a long protocol of down-regulation would do so. Hammoud et al. [51] also felt that this approach would leave fewer embryos unused. It was being used for younger, good prognosis patients and also for older women and poor responders.

Gianaroli et al. [52] described preliminary data from an ongoing study in SISMeR, Bologna, Italy using clomiphene 100 mg daily from days 3–7 and FSH 150 IU on days 5, 7 and 9 of the cycle with hCG on day 12 (IVF-Lite). There was a mean of 5.6 oocytes retrieved per cycle. Of 204 patients starting treatment, 50 dropped out at the first cycle, but others remained in until they were pregnant or had had a third cycle. The cumulative ongoing pregnancy rate for them was 58 % compared with a conventional IVF result of 37 %, which included both fresh and frozen/thawed transfers.

A very detailed analysis of retrospective data was published by Zhang et al. [53] covering a wide age range and segregating the data according to FSH levels being below or above 15 IU/l. They used 50 mg Clomiphene and 150 IU hMG every 48 h with occasional use of Indomethacin to delay ovulation or used an antagonist and later an agonist to trigger ovulation. They did SET if a good embryo was available or two if not, and vitrified supernumerary embryos with later transfer. Although there was only an ET in half the cases, the live birth rate/ET was 8.9 % with a multiple pregnancy rate of 1/247 on fresh transfer and live birth rate/ET of 13.5 % for vitrified/thawed embryos with a multiple pregnancy rate of 7/250. These data clearly show the result of meticulous management, based on Teramoto and Kato's [54] approach.

Zarek and Muasher [55] refer to "minimal stimulation" as being Clomiphene and low-dose gonadotrophins with a GnRH antagonist, whereas they use the term "mild" to apply to a regime of low-dose gonadotrophins and GnRH antagonist without the Clomiphene. They emphasise the advantages of cost and tolerability, but also the merit of using these routines for patients with a history of high or low response. They point out that even in resource rich economies, not all patients would choose to use a conventional regime and would opt for a mild/minimal stimulation regime. Even so, Gleicher et al. [56] and Baker [57] fail to see any role for these approaches in the USA.

An alternative approach could be the use of Letrozole. In India Mukherjee et al. [58] used Letrozole 5 mg daily from days 3–7 and recombinant FSH 75 IU from day 5 until the 10,000 IU hCG trigger at a follicle size of 18 mm. An antagonist, Ganirelix 125 µg, was given daily from 14 mm follicular size. The patients were normal 25–35 year old women with azoospermic partners treated by testicular sperm aspiration and intracytoplasmic sperm injection. There was a mean of 6 follicles developed and 5 oocytes aspirated. No patients dropped out and a pregnancy rate of 36 % was achieved from a mean of 3.5 transferable embryos from which 2 were transferred. There was no hyper-stimulation and the cost was reduced by 34 % in comparison with a continuous FSH only group. The live birth and the multiple pregnancy rates were not reported. Nevertheless, using an alternate day cheaper urinary product, hMG, would bring the costs down further.

Recently, van Blerkom et al. [59] reported the first seven live births using a method in which the CO_2 for the embryo culture environment was generated in a bicarbonate solution by citric acid and connected to the culture medium by a U-tube, the whole being kept in a heated block. This is a simple method that has the potential for much wider use in resource poor environments.

The need for low resource economies to develop a simpler, inexpensive approach to infertility treatment was raised at WHO in 2001 [60] and elaborated by Hovatta and Cooke [61]. The importance of the social impact of infertility in resource poor environments was recently emphasised by Hammarberg and Kirkman [62]. Yet public understanding of reproductive biology and medicine, infertility and ART is limited in many communities [63]. WHO [60] had already emphasised the important role of governments in public education and the important advocacy role of patient organisations.

Yet it has been difficult to establish low-cost ART units. The Low Cost IVF Foundation attempted to start such programmes and realised that they would need continuous external financial support, an unsustainable situation. Attempts to establish programmes in university environments should have had a better outlook, but required political support, which was withdrawn. Providing a programme in the private sector [64] risks adding physicians' fees to the basic cost. So the commitment needs to come at government level with a recognition that the net benefit can be argued in the face of alternative health spending and that the benefit to members in that society can provide the justification, an approach that is currently being pursued in Zambia.

There needs to be separate space for the clinic, the staff need training in clinical selection of patients, so that initially women of <38 years with tubal occlusion and males with normal or nearly normal semen data are chosen and screened for HIV. The staff should be trained in the use of pelvic ultrasound and education and counselling are important obligations. Embryological training needs to be developed, perhaps in a local university, so that those externally trained do not rapidly leave for the private sector. A quality service could be a significant counterweight. There needs to be use made of the ICMART Minimum Data Set [65] and in due course the data should be reported to national and international data registries. Later, ICSI and cryopreservation need to be added to the repertoire, and these will require reappraisal of the economics. A patient support group can add another dimension [66] and provide additional advocacy. Of course, it should be possible, given the motivation, to add a low-cost programme to an existing one and serve an entirely different and supplementary population. Perhaps this will be a singular way to draw attention to the health needs of the local population and create the political climate for wider adoption and ultimately state support.

Conclusion

The whole area of ART provided at low cost has had a slow trajectory. There are now sufficient data to support a concerted effort to apply the examples that are available, to establish programmes and accumulate significant data. There is a need to conduct randomised studies against conventional IVF and that will always be difficult in low resource environments. Perhaps the establishment of low-cost programmes that are able to offer prospects of appropriate treatment to infertile couples in low resource economies will be justification enough. With good quality data there should then be a compelling case to promote this approach in the *developed* world for the large number of patients currently denied access to conventional ART.

References

1. Cohen J, de Mouzon J, Lancaster P. International Working Group for Registers on Assisted Reproduction, World collaborative report on in vitro fertilization, 1989. Presented at the 7th World Congress on In Vitro Fertilization and Assisted Reproduction. Paris, France.1991, as quoted in World Collaborative Report on in vitro fertilization, 2000. International Committee for Monitoring Assisted Reproductive Technology (ICMART), Fertil Steril. 2006;85:1586–622. doi: 10.1016/j.fertnstert.2006.01.011.
2. de Mouzon J, Lancaster P, International Working Group for Registers on Assisted Reproduction. World Collaborative Report on in vitro fertilisation: preliminary data for 1995. J Asst Reprod Genet. 1997;14:S251–65.
3. Zegers-Hochschild F, Mansour R, Ishihara O, Adamson GD, de Mouzon J, Nygren KG, et al. International Committee for Monitoring Assisted Reproductive Technology: world report on assisted reproductive technology, 2005. Fertil Steril. 2014;101:366–78. doi:10.1016/j.fertnstert.2013.10.005.
4. Insurance coverage. In: Jones HW Jr, Cohen J, editors. IFFS Surveillance 04. Fertil Steril. 2004;81:S17–8.
5. Jones HW Jr, Cooke I, Kempers R, Brinsden P, Saunders D. International Federation of Fertility Societies (IFFS) Surveillance: preface 2010. Fertil Steril. 2011;95:491. doi: 10.1016/j.fertnstert.2010.08.011, https://c.ymcdn.com/sites/iffs.siteym.com/resource/resmgr/newsletters/iffs_surveillance_2010.pdf.
6. Dyer SJ, Sherwood KM, Ataguba JE. Catastrophic payment for assisted reproduction techniques with conventional ovarian stimulation in the public health sector of South Africa: frequency and coping strategies. Hum Reprod. 2013;28:2755–64. doi:10.1093/humrep/det290.
7. de Neuborg D, Boghaerts K, Wyns C, Albert A, Camus M, Candeur M, et al. The history of Belgian assisted reproduction technology cycle registration and control: a case study in reducing the incidence of multiple pregnancy. Hum Reprod. 2013;28:2709–19. doi:10.1093/humrep/det269.
8. Commission Directive 2006/17/EC of 8 February, 2006 implementing Directive 2004/23/EC of the European Parliament and of the Council as regards certain technical requirements for the donation, procurement and testing of human tissues and cells. http://eur-lex.europa.eu/LexUriServ/LexUriServ.do?uri=OJ:L:2006:038:0040:0052:EN:PDF.
9. Commission Directive 2006/86/E of 24 October 2006 implementing Directive 2004/23/EC of the European Parliament and of the Council as regards traceability requirements, notification of serious adverse reactions and events and certain technical requirements for the coding, processing, preservation, storage and distribution of human tissues and cells. http://pharma.be/assets/files/859/859_128902168074519980.pdf.
10. Sunde A, Balaban B. The assisted reproductive technology laboratory: toward evidence-based practice? Fertil Steril. 2013;100:31–8. doi:10.1016/j.fertstert.2013.06.032.
11. Ory SJ, Devroey P, editors. IFFS Surveillance 2013. IFFS, New Jersey 2013. p. 21–9, https://c.ymcdn.com/sites/iffs.site-ym.com/resource/resmgr/iffs_surveillance_09-19-13.pdf.
12. Connolly M, Gallo F, Hoorens S, Ledger W. Assessing long-run economic benefits attributed to an IVF-conceived singleton based on projected lifetime net tax contributions in the UK. Hum Reprod. 2009;24:626–32. doi:10.1093/humrep/den435.
13. Connolly MP, Griesinger G, Ledger W, Postma MJ. The impact of introducing patient co-payments in Germany on the use of IVF and ICSI: a price-elasticity of demand assessment. Hum Reprod. 2009;24:2796–800. doi:10.1093/humrep/dep260.
14. Chambers GM, Hoang VP, Zhu R, Illingworth PJ. A reduction in public funding for fertility treatment—an econometric analysis of access to treatment and savings to government. BMC Health Serv Res. 2012;12:art. no. 142. doi: 10.1186/1472-6963-12-142.
15. Chambers GM, Hoang VP, Illingworth P. Socioeconomic disparities in access to ART treatment and the differential impact of a policy that increases consumer costs. Hum Reprod. 2013;28:3111–7. doi:10.1093/humrep/det302.
16. Gillett WR, Peek JC, Herbison GP. Development of clinical priority access criteria for assisted reproduction and its evaluation on 1386 infertile couples in New Zealand. Hum Reprod. 2012;27:131–41. doi:10.1093/humrep/der372.

17. Grant J, Hoorens S, Gallo F, Cave J. Should ART be part of a population policy mix? A preliminary assessment of the demographic and economic impact of Assisted Reproductive Technologies. 2006. www.rand.org/pubs/documented_briefings/DB507.html.
18. Berg Brigham K, Cadier B, Chevreul K. The diversity of regulation and public financing of IVF in Europe and its impact on utilization. Hum Reprod. 2013;28:666–75. doi:10.1093/humrep/des418.
19. Human Fertilisation and Embryology Authority. Fertility treatment in 2012: trends and figures. http://www.hfea.gov.uk/docs/FertilityTreatment2012TrendsFigures.PDF.
20. Thoma ME, McLain AC, Louis JF, King RB, Trumble AC, Sundaram R, et al. Prevalence of infertility in the United States as estimated by the current duration approach and a traditional constructed approach. Fertil Steril. 2013;99:1324–31. doi:10.1016/j.fertnstert.2012.11.037.
21. Slama R, Hansen OKH, Ducot B, Bohet A, Sorensen D, Georgis Allemand L, et al. Estimation of the frequency of involuntary infertility on a nation-wide basis. Hum Reprod. 2012;27:1489–98. doi:10.1093/humrep/des070.
22. Lu C, Schneider MT, Gubbins P, Leach-Kemon K, Jamison D, Murray CJ. Public financing of health in developing countries: a cross-sectional analysis. Lancet. 2010;375:1375–87. doi:10.1016/S0140-6736(10)60233-4.
23. Murage A, Muteshi MC, Githae F. Assisted reproduction services provision in a developing country: time to act? Fertil Steril. 2011;96:966–8. doi:10.1016/j.fertnstert.2011.07.1109.
24. Makuch MY, Simonia de Padua K, Petta CA, Duarte Osis MJ, Bahamondes L. Inequitable access to assisted reproductive technology for the low-income Brazilian population: a qualitative study. Hum Reprod. 2011;26:2054–60. doi:10.1093/humrep/der158.
25. International Covenant on Economic, Social and Cultural Rights. 1966. www.ohchr.org/EN/ProfessionalInterest/Pages/CESCR.aspx.
26. United Nations Millennium Development Goals: Goal 5B. http://www.un.org/millenniumgoals/maternal.shtml.
27. UNFPA. How universal is access to reproductive health? A review of the evidence. 2010. https://www.unfpa.org/webdav/site/global/shared/documents/publications/2010/universal_rh.pdf.
28. Human Development Report. Millennium development goals: a compact among nations to end human poverty. New York: United Nations Development Programme (UNDP); 2003. www.unic.un.org.pl/hdr/hdr2003/hdr03_complete.pdf.
29. Zegers-Hochschild F, Adamson GD, de Mouzon J, Ishihara O, Mansour R, Nygren K, et al. The International Committee for Monitoring Assisted Reproductive Technology (ICMART) and the World Health Organisation (WHO) Revised Glossary on ART. Hum Reprod. 2009;24:2683–7. doi:10.1093/humrep/dep343.
30. Murphy JB. Access to in vitro fertilization deserves increased regulation in the United States. J Sex Marital Ther. 2013;39:85–92. doi:10.1080/0092623X.2011.632072.
31. World Report on Disability. WHO, World Bank. Geneva: WHO; 2011. Table D1, p. 297.
32. Habbema JDF. Is affordable and cost-effective assisted reproductive technology in low-income countries possible? What should we know to answer the question? Human Reprod. 2008;Sp Iss 21–4.
33. Moolenaar LM, Connolly M, Huisman B, Postma MJ, Hompes PGA, van der Veen F, et al. Costs and benefits of individuals conceived after IVF: a net tax evaluation in The Netherlands. Reprod BioMed Online. 2014;28:239–45. doi:10.1016/j.rbmo.2013.10.002.
34. Pennings G, Ombelet W. Coming soon to your clinic: patient-friendly ART. Hum Reprod. 2007;22:2075–9. doi:10.1093/humrep/dem158.
35. van Empel IWH, Nelen WLDM, Hermens PMG, Kremer JAM. Coming soon to your clinic: high-quality ART. Hum Reprod. 2008;23:1242–5. doi:10.1093/humrep/den094.
36. Nargund G, Fauser BC, Macklon NS, Ombelet W, Nygren K, Frydman R, Rotterdam ISMAAR Consensus Group on Terminology for Ovarian Stimulation for IVF. The ISMAAR proposal on terminology for ovarian stimulation for IVF. Hum Reprod. 2007;22:2801–4. doi:10.1093/humrep/dem285.
37. Verberg MFG, Eijkemans MJC, Macklon NS, Heijnen EMEW, Baart EB, Hohmann FP, et al. The clinical significance of the retrieval of a low number of oocytes following mild ovarian stimulation for IVF: a meta-analysis. Hum Reprod Update. 2009;15:5–12. doi:10.1093/humupd/dmn053.

38. Moragianni VA, Penzias AS. Cumulative live births after assisted reproductive technology. Curr Opin Obstet Gynec. 2010;22:189–92. doi:10.1097/GCO.0b013e328338493f.
39. Groen H, Tonch N, Simons AHM, van der Veen F, Hoek A, Land JA. Modified natural cycle versus controlled ovarian hyperstimulation IVF: a cost-effectiveness evaluation of three simulated treatment scenarios. Hum Reprod. 2013;28:3236–46. doi:10.1093/humrep/det386.
40. Allersma T, Farquhar C, Cantineau AEP. Natural cycle in vitro fertilisation (IVF) for subfertile couples. Cochrane Database Syst Rev. 2013;8:CD010550.
41. Widge A, Cleland J. The public sector's role in infertility management in India. Health Policy Plan. 2009;24:108–15. doi:10.1093/heapol/czn053.
42. National Institute for Health and Clinical Excellence. Fertility: assessment and treatment for people with fertility problems. 2013. http://guidance.nice.org.uk/CG156/NICEGuidance/pdf/English.
43. Chambers GM, Hoang VP, Sullivan EA, Chapman MG, Ishihara O, Zegers-Hochschild F, et al. The impact of consumer affordability on access to assisted reproductive technologies and embryo transfer practices: an international analysis. Fertil Steril. 2014;101:191–8. doi:10.1016/j.fertnstert.2013.09.005.
44. Staniec JFO, Webb NJ. Utilization of infertility services: how much does money matter? Health Serv Res. 2007;42:971–89. doi:10.1111/j.1475-6773.2006.00640.x.
45. Hammoud AO, Gibson M, Stanford J, White G, Carrell DT, Peterson M. In vitro fertilization availability and utilization in the United States: a study of demographic, social and economic factors. Fertil Steril. 2009;91:1630–5. doi:10.1016/j.fertnstert.2007.10.038.
46. Heng BC. Reluctance of medical professionals in adopting natural-cycle and minimal ovarian stimulation protocols in human clinical assisted reproduction. Reprod Biomed Online. 2007;15:9–11.
47. Balic D. How to make assisted reproductive technologies (ART) affordable in Bosnia and Herzegovina: experience after the first 105 cycles. Med Arhiv. 2011;65:119–21.
48. Cooke ID. Mild stimulation. In: Hedon B, Mettler L, Tinneberg H-R, editors. Proceedings of the IFFS world congress on fertility and sterility, September 12–16, 2010. Munchen: Lukon Verlagsgesellschaft; 2010. p. 187–93.
49. Aanesen A, Nygren K-G, Nylund L. Modified natural cycle IVF and mild IVF: a 10 year Swedish experience. Reprod Biomed Online. 2010;20:156–62. doi:10.1016/jrbmo.2009.10.017.
50. Hojgaard A, Ingerslev HJ, Dinesen J. Friendly IVF: patient opinions. Hum Reprod. 2001; 16:1391–6.
51. Hammoud AO, Gibson MBE. Minimal stimulation IVF. In: Infertil BR, Racowsky C, Schlegel PN, Fauser BC, Carrell DT, editors. Vol. 2, 2011. p. 11–8. doi: 10.1007/978-1-4419-8456-2_2.
52. Gianaroli L, Ferraretti AP, Magli MC. Minimal stimulation. In: Training people in low-cost infertility and ART treatment, postgraduate course 23, American Society of Reproductive Medicine, Boston. Accessed 13 Oct 2013.
53. Zhang J, Chang L, Sone Y, Silber S. Minimal ovarian stimulation (mini-IVF) for IVF utilizing vitrification and cryopreserved embryo transfer. Reprod Biomed Online. 2010;21:485–95. doi:10.1016/j.rbmo.2010.06.033.
54. Teramoto S, Kato O. Minimal ovarian stimulation with clomiphene citrate: a large scale retrospective study. Reprod Biomed Online. 2007;15:134–48.
55. Zarek SM, Muasher SJ. Mild/minimal stimulation for in vitro fertilization: an old idea that needs to be revisited. Fertil Steril. 2011;95:2449–55. doi:10.1016/ferttnstert.2011.094.041.
56. Gleicher NW, Weghofer A, Barad DH. A case-control pilot study of low-intensity IVF in good-prognosis patients. Reprod Biomed Online. 2012;24:396–402. doi:10.1016/j.rbmo.2011.12.011.
57. Baker VL. Mild ovarian stimulation for in vitro fertilization: one perspective from the USA. J Assist Reprod Genet. 2013;30:197–202. doi:10.1007/s10815-013-9946-8.
58. Mukherjee S, Sharma S, Chakravarty BN. Letrozole in a low-cost in vitro fertilization protocol in intracytoplasmic sperm injection cycles for male factor infertility: a randomized controlled trial. J Hum Reprod Sci. 2012;5:170–4. doi:10.4103/0974-1208.101014.

59. van Blerkom J, Ombelet W, Klerkx E, Janssen M, Dhont N, Nargund G, et al. First births with a simplified culture system for clinical IVF and embryo transfer. Reprod Biomed Online. 2014;28:310–20. doi:10.1016/j.rbmo.2013.11.012.
60. World Health Organisation (WHO). In: Vayena E, Rowe PJ, Griffin PD, editors. Current practices and controversies in assisted reproduction, Report of a WHO meeting on "Medical, Ethical and Social aspects of Assisted Reproduction" (2002) held at WHO Headquarters in Geneva, Switzerland, 17–21 September, 2001. Geneva: WHO.
61. Hovatta O, Cooke I. Cost-effective approaches to in vitro fertilization: means to improve access. Int J Gyn Obstet. 2006;94:287–91.
62. Hammarberg K, Kirkman M. Infertility in resource-constrained settings: moving towards amelioration. Reprod Biomed Online. 2013;26:189–95. doi:10.1016/j.rbmo.2012.11.009.
63. Fabamwo AO, Akinola OI. The understanding and acceptability of assisted reproductive technology (ART) among infertile women in urban Lagos. Nigeria J Obstet Gyn. 2013;33:71–4. doi:10.3109/01443615.2012.730077.
64. Aleyamma TK, Kamath MS, Muthukumar K, Mangalaraj AM, George K. Affordable ART: a different perspective. Hum Reprod. 2011;26:3312–8. doi:10.1093/humrep/der323.
65. The ICMART Toolbox for ART data collection, Version 1.0, April, 2011. http://www.icmartivf.org/toolbox/toolbox-main.html.
66. Ombelet W, Cooke I, Dyer S, Serour G, Devroey P. Infertility and the provision of infertility medical services in developing countries. Hum Reprod Update. 2008;14:605–21. doi:10.1093/humupd/dmn042.

Chapter 17
Private and Corporate IVF Units

Amparo Ruiz and Luis Saurat

Determining Factors of Health Services

One of the most common definitions in economics refers to the study of how societies use scarce resources to produce goods or services and distribute them among individuals. Two ideas underlie this definition: resources are scarce and should therefore be used efficiently [1].

From the point of view of the producers of these goods or the providers of these services, the consequences are clear. As both material and human resources are limited, you cannot do or cover everything. You will have to choose an option, a path. But whatever option you choose, you will always have to abide by the rules of the game set by the need to use these scarce resources in the best possible way, as efficiently as possible. If it is a private company, this is due to the fact that the market will demand it; if it is public, because it is the responsibility of all good managers, and in respect for taxpayers' money.

In the case of organizations that provide health care, we must bear in mind that these services are not only useful for the individuals who receive them but also for society in general, they have a social nature regardless of whether the provider is public or private. Sometimes, the determining factors of this social service may clash with the purely economic factors [2], making the whole situation more complex. But, apart from this peculiarity, every organization, whether medical or not, be it a Reproduction Unit or otherwise, must have a certain strategy and this strategy will influence the way the organization relates to its stakeholders.

A. Ruiz, MD, PhD (✉)
IVI Valencia, Valencia, Spain
e-mail: amparo.ruiz@ivi.es

L. Saurat, MD (Economics), MD (Law)
IVI Group, Valencia, Spain
e-mail: luis.saurat@ivi.es

© Springer Science+Business Media New York 2016
S.D. Fleming, A.C. Varghese (eds.), *Organization and Management of IVF Units*, DOI 10.1007/978-3-319-29373-8_17

The above applies to any organization operating in any market with the clarification that we have made above as regards healthcare organizations. However, below we focus on the case of what may arise at strategic levels and of relations with their stakeholders in a Reproduction Unit operating in the private sphere independently, as this is the case of IVI and, therefore, the area we know best.

Many of the comments that we make below, and, particularly, in the case of how the strategy affects relations with stakeholders, are applicable to other types of organizations. Therefore, if it were a Reproduction Unit integrated in a larger private organization the main clarification would be that the Unit's strategy should be set within a broader strategy, the organization's global strategy. If we were dealing with a Reproduction Unit integrated in a public organization, the main clarification would be that the sustained creation of value over time should be reflected more strongly in stakeholders, taxpayers, and society in general.

In other words, as we see it, the stakeholders of a public practice are not exactly the same as those of a private practice and their relations have a different approach. To begin with, although we understand that a private practice should also be highly focused on providing the best care possible to patients, because there are people who have invested a given capital (whether these are the physicians or not) from which they logically demand a certain return, profitability that should be sufficient to repay this capital and to ensure the continuity of the business over time, which is not apparent in public practice although this comparison becomes more complicated by introducing efficiency factors that we do not discuss now. On the other hand, there is a need to attract patients in private practice that is not the case in public practice, meaning we will need to take into account the importance of marketing in its broadest sense as a closely related aspect to the strategy, both regarding the market positioning of the actual clinic and the specific actions to attract patients.

The Strategy and Its Impact on Relations with Stakeholders. Our View

From the business point of view, the strategy describes how a company intends to achieve its objectives with the ultimate aim of creating sustained value over time for its shareholders, clients and citizens [3]. Because, in the final analysis, the aim is to create valuable relations with the different stakeholders and only if value is provided will the company's existence continue over time.

Thus, any organization that offers a product or service to the market has a particular competitive strategy, is positioned in a certain way before its potential clients and its competitors, and all of this irrespective of whether the organization is aware of it or not.

There are numerous advantages in having a clear strategy, developed through an adequate process for planning, deployment and control, particularly because it implies that the actions of the organization's different departments act in a coordinated way in order to complete a series of targets set, allowing us to monitor how close we are to achieving these goals. This process is called strategic planning.

Although there are many diagrams that can guide us in this respect, the most typical and common way to present the aforementioned strategic planning process is through a circular diagram of five stages [4], which are as follows:

1. Initial or strategic thinking phase. In this phase the aim is to reflect on the key concepts of the organization, particularly the mission, vision, and values.
2. Internal and external analysis. This is the longest phase of the process. It involves studying the fundamental parts of the company and its environment, aiming to link them to each other. Therefore, firstly, we look around us to see where we are and, secondly, we analyze internally to see, according to our capabilities and our limitations, where we could be.
3. Strategic formulation. From the above analysis we will have to decide the strategy to follow and formulate the main objectives. The result of this formulation will be the strategic plan.
4. Implementation of the strategy. Once formulated, the strategy must be deployed. It will seek to identify actions to develop and align the organization's different objectives with the strategy.
5. Evaluation and control. This will consist of defining management indicators and monitoring compliance with the objectives set, so its effectiveness will depend on the management control systems available to the organization. According to the analysis of the data and the deviations produced, feedback can be generated for future reformulations of the strategy and organizational change. For this reason, the strategic planning process is presented as a circular diagram, because this evaluation and control phase provides feedback to the process again.

From the point of view of the strategy's impact on relations with the different stakeholders, we focus, firstly, on briefly analyzing the first two phases and what approaches we have made from IVI. Subsequently, the third phase will be the object of greater development, insofar as the strategic option chosen will totally condition the allocation of resources and market positioning and, ultimately, the operation of the organization and relations with the various stakeholders.

Strategic Thinking. Key Concepts

Any planning process must begin with a reflection on the starting position of each organization. The first thing to do is to know ourselves well and be sure of our starting point. Therefore, the main thing in this phase will be to reflect on each organization's so-called key strategic concepts.

(a) The values.
   In the same way that people have values and beliefs that shape the way we act in life, from a strategic point of view we say that organizations have certain values that determine how they want to act and behave. In some way they resume the beliefs about what is desirable, valuable and fair for that organization.

Values are usually understood and shared by the organization (anyone who does not share them does not fit in) and they are not easy to change because they somehow shape the personality of the entity.

In short, the values of an organization define its character. This way, the values determine how a given business project develops and how decisions are made within it, even if the organization is not completely aware of it. It is therefore very important, before carrying out any strategic planning process, to be clear about the values of the organization to which we belong.

Normally the values are set by the promoters or founders of the organization and they determine how it will behave and develop its relations with stakeholders. IVI's values are:

- Freedom of initiative and innovation.
- Desire for self-improvement.
- Satisfaction for a job well done.
- Team work.
- Honesty.
- Loyalty.

(b) The mission.

The mission defines what an organization does, the business of a company. We cannot reflect on what strategy we will follow if we are not reasonably sure what we are doing.

When defining our business we must be able to answer three fundamental questions:

- What do we do (what client needs do we satisfy)?
- For whom (for which market segment)?
- How we do it (with what technology or know-how)?

At any given time, an organization may decide on a new strategy, for example offering products that meet other needs of our clients, but for this we must be very sure of the starting point, i.e., the mission, and therefore, what we are currently doing, what and who our clients are. If we are not very sure who our clients are and what they want it hardly makes sense to consider a strategy based on meeting their needs.

IVI defines its mission as follows: *We are a team of qualified professionals working on a common project: carrying out reproductive medicine of the highest order and fostering research, education and professional excellence.*

(c) Vision.

Lastly, the third key strategic concept is vision. It is no longer a question of defining what we do, what we are, but rather to reflect on what we want to be that we are not yet. In short, the vision determines where we want to be in the future, where our organization is going.

To ensure the vision has a meaning it should be challenging. It must motivate and guide the everyday actions towards that great future ahead. It must define what the company wants to be, what goals it wants to achieve and how it will stand out from other organizations. But it should not be a utopia or an empty statement of intention, because if it is not believable or achievable we are generating the opposite effect to that desired. It would not be a challenge or have a motivating effect. In that case, it would be best to change the view as soon as possible. Depending on the vision, relations with stakeholders will go one way or another. IVI defines its vision as follows:

To be a world-leading team in the field of reproductive medicine, becoming the most widespread group with the best clinical results. To be an international reference point in quality care, research and teaching. Prioritizing the development of people and team sprit as the pillars of our project.

Internal and External Analysis

Once we are sure of the key factors that influence our strategic choice we must analyze the environment around us as well as our own internal capabilities in order to conclude on what we could do, depending on the environment, and what we can do, based on our own means and possibilities.

We now look at this in more detail.

(a) Internal analysis.

The aim of the internal analysis is to identify the organization's strengths and weaknesses. What we do well and what we do not do so well. It is very important to be as critical and as honest with yourself as possible for this exercise to be positive. Because the idea is to reflect on how we can maintain and enhance, if possible, our strengths and how to correct, as best and as soon as possible, our weaknesses. In short, the aim is to answer the question: in line with the circumstances, what can we do?

In this context, it is very important to reflect on what we do better than our competitors and what we do not do so well. In relation to what we do best, the fundamental objective will be to take advantage of that fact as much as we can and to try and make it sustainable over time. This is the concept of competitive advantage [5].

A competitive advantage will allow us to survive over time. In the case of the Reproduction Unit we reflect on what is relevant and what is not when it comes to providing an excellent service to our patients (who are also clients). To do this we focus on the activities that are most closely related to the critical success factors of our business. What are these factors? It depends on each situation and how they are focusing on service, as well as their own resources and capabilities.

It is important to identify which activities are critical and which are not within the service provided by our Unit. It is recommended that critical activities are directly made by our unit and their implementation closely monitored by those responsible. Activities not critical to its success can be outsourced if the criteria of timeliness and efficiency recommend it; For example, the performance of certain laboratory tests.

(b) External analysis.

In this part of the reflection we focus on the analysis of what is outside. We do not look inside our organization but rather beyond it, in order to conclude on what is happening in our environment in general, what is happening in the area of those who demand our services, of our potential clients (demand analysis) and in the environment of our sector (supply analysis).

As regards the general environment, the aim is to identify what advantages or opportunities may arise from changes that may occur in the environment and what threats, or in other words, what changes could be to our advantage if we know how to utilize them, and which will not. Evidently, the idea is to identify opportunities to try to take advantage of them and threats to try to tackle them with the least possible negative impact, even, if feasible, turning them round and converting them into opportunities.

Regarding the demand analysis, we must focus on the best possible understanding of our clients (patients). It is essential to understand what they want, what is valuable to them. It is the critical factor for success and even more so in an activity where we cannot ensure that the client gets what they want because a percentage of cases will not get pregnant at the first attempt.

Here it is essential to be sure of what the client values and what our organization offers in order to meet their expectations and for them to be sufficiently satisfied to repeat the treatment if they do not get pregnant in the previous attempt.

We must be aware that we exist because there is a need to cover and a market in which to offer our services. In short, we exist because there are clients interested in our services; we exist because of our clients.

More often than we would like, we commit the error of investing efforts and resources in virtues or qualities of products or services that clients do not value or consider relevant. We may think that we are the best providers of medical services in the world but if we do not respond to what our clients expect from us, and we do not know how to convey our supposed excellence and the client does not perceive it, all these efforts will be of little use. Client satisfaction depends on their perception of what the service offers and their expectations [6].

Therefore, it is equally ill advised to invest efforts in exceeding client expectations as it is to create expectations that cannot be met or promises that will not be fulfilled.

When calculating our clients' expectations and measuring their level of satisfaction with the services provided it is advisable to conduct market research. It is not always necessary to invest great resources in these matters. A simple well-designed survey conducted on a well-defined sample of our clients can give us a lot of relevant information.

After analyzing our market and our clients we must reflect on our sector and the supply that exists in it. Firstly, because our sector will be totally different to others (e.g., reproductive medicine versus the automotive sector) and we have to be sure about what aspects are relevant in it. And secondly, because we will not be lucky enough to be the only ones offering our services to the market, but rather we must compete with other suppliers and other options that will be offered to our clients and we must be sure about what sets our organization apart from its competitors.

Strategic Formulation

From the above analysis we have to decide the strategy and formulate the main objectives. The result of this formulation will be the Strategic Plan.

Although each company will design its own strategy it is interesting to note that, from a competitive point of view, there are three major options or generic strategies [7].

Thus, we can talk about:

Differentiation strategies.
Low-cost strategies.
Specialization, or niche strategies.

Companies that follow a differentiation strategy tend to emphasize aspects such as quality, service, design, technology, brand, and innovation, and they invest a lot of resources and efforts into them.

Companies that follow cost leadership strategies seek to offer customers a good product or service at a low price, which does not mean in any way that because the price is low they give a bad product or service. But to achieve this they emphasize aspects such as large-scale production, efficiency in assembly and design of the product or service, sharing activities with other companies; the company stops providing part of the service and the individual takes over.

In the case of IVI we have clearly opted for a differentiation strategy based on achieving maximum patient satisfaction, a strategy which contains the following fundamental aspects.

Implementation of the Strategy: The Management Model Based on Patient's Satisfaction

Taking into account what has been said, it is not difficult to conclude that a management system that takes into account the company as a whole, that has global reach, and that also takes into account non-financial elements at the time of decision-making, will be much more effective. Obviously, in a private organization there will always be the objective of increasing profitability, which is even necessary to guarantee the continuity of the organization and, therefore, of the service it provides and its continuous improvement through the necessary investments. Nevertheless, the ways to achieve it can be very diverse and that is precisely what the management model consists of: the set of decisions and actions carried out by the leadership to implement the strategic directions. Said management will be based on the fundamental strategic principle of each organization, which in our case is differentiation through patient satisfaction.

Management, in being always subjected to strategy, is dynamic; and its development, evolution, and optimization are performed through management control.

According to Serra and colleagues [8], management control is the direction technique that basically consists of:

– Establishing objectives at all responsibility levels in the company.
– Quantifying said objectives through a budget.
– Periodically controlling and evaluating the degree of their fulfillment.
– Taking the appropriate corrective decisions.

We believe this definition to be the most accurate, since it considers the institution of objectives as part of the strategic plan, not as something isolated that is decided "de novo".

According to this reasoning, the first thing to do is to find out what really satisfies patients and not to assume it due to its apparent obviousness: achieving gestation. To know what satisfies patients and what does not—and act accordingly—all that is needed is to ask them. Logically it will be asked in an organized manner, with questions involving the degree of satisfaction in all the aspects that the patients have experienced, from the waiting time to be assisted by phone, obtain an appointment, or enter the office, to the kindness and professionalism of each of the collectives and departments, as well as the amount and quality of received information, and many other details.

Furthermore, the collection of data must be simple and it must be registered in a way as to permit its later measurement and the production of statistical reports.

It is surprising to discover that some patients—even having achieved pregnancy on their first attempt—can be found to be dissatisfied because they had a feeling of insecurity after receiving seemingly contradictory sets of information, or due to having been taken care of by a physician they did not expect without previously being informed. It is possible that these patients will not recommend our clinic or may not speak well of it. On the other hand, on numerous occasions, even if gestation is delayed or is never obtained, patients reveal very positive opinions when they perceive the true implication of the entire team in achieving their goal and they feel that they have been very exclusively and personally treated.

Once we have the patients' opinions, we know what satisfies them the most and what they believe needs improvement; but we will have also asked them to score— and we can now measure—the degree of importance that they place on each of the consulted areas. Thus, it may be that a high percentage of patients convey themselves as dissatisfied by the waiting times to enter the office or the operating room, but that they do not consider this such an important aspect; however, a particular percentage of patients may be dissatisfied because they were not allowed to participate in decision making regarding their treatment, and also mark this aspect as one of great importance. Therefore, at the time of deciding improvement actions to achieve the patient's satisfaction goal, those areas that combine the lowest satisfaction index with the greatest importance will be prioritized, postponing other aspects that may be even significantly dissatisfying, but that are not deemed as important by patients, for further assessment.

Surveys can be designed internally or an external, specialized company can provide the service, but it is necessary not only to carry them out: they must be well designed and offer useful statistical reports.

The management designed for the fulfillment of the company's strategic plan and the patient's satisfaction will begin by defining objectives, which must be few and challenging—but achievable—and the management tool to attain those goals is clinic organization, which will differ depending on whether the practice is public, private, corporate, etc. and on the company's philosophy.

Therefore, on a day-to-day basis, the management of the unit, clinic, or company is really how it is organized, and it comprises:

- Organization of the activity: departments and sections.
- Organization of the employees: charts and roles.
- Organization of time: schedules and timetables, work hours, etc.

(a) Organization of the activity.

In the majority of clinics, there are many activities and services around the patient:

- Patient attention services such as general information, telephone assistance, front desk, and appointment management.
- Office visits: gynecology, psychology, genetics, andrology, endocrinology, etc.
- Laboratory procedures: hormones, serology, semen analysis and preparation, in vitro fertilization (IVF), preimplantation genetic diagnosis (PGD), etc.
- Surgery: oocyte retrieval procedures, embryo transfers, testicular biopsies, endoscopies.
- Administrative services: financial office, price information, insurance agreements.

All these activities must be distributed in departments in a logical way, and this entire distribution must be fit into a larger design that includes other activities that are not provided directly to patients, but that are equally important, such as management, research, teaching, or relationships with other doctors and institutions (Fig. 17.1).

On the other hand, the different activities of the unit not only have to do with the service they provide, but they must also be grouped according to the types of professionals or collectives that perform them, the treatment to which they belong, or the department that carries them out, as is observed in the example in Fig. 17.2.

Once the activities have been organized in groups according to the different criteria, the personnel performing said activities must be well dimensioned and organized.

(b) Organization of the employees.

The size of the clinic's staff is a topic of capital importance. If it is scarce, it can result in bad attention to patients and duties, as well as unrest and a bad work environment, which can equally impact productivity and quality. But the staff's dimension is not the topic of this chapter, its organization is.

We have devised a complete organization chart—even for small IVI clinics—that could be easily adapted to growth and increasing complexity in the

Services for patients
Consultation
Admin. Services
Labs
Surgery
Pat. Att. Services.
PATIENT
Research and Education
Managem ent
Services for patients

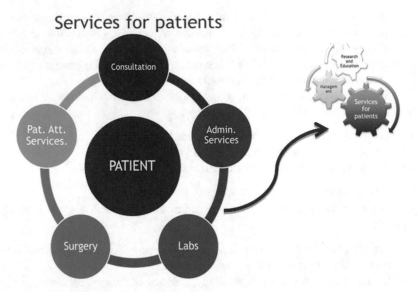

Fig. 17.1 Services for patients

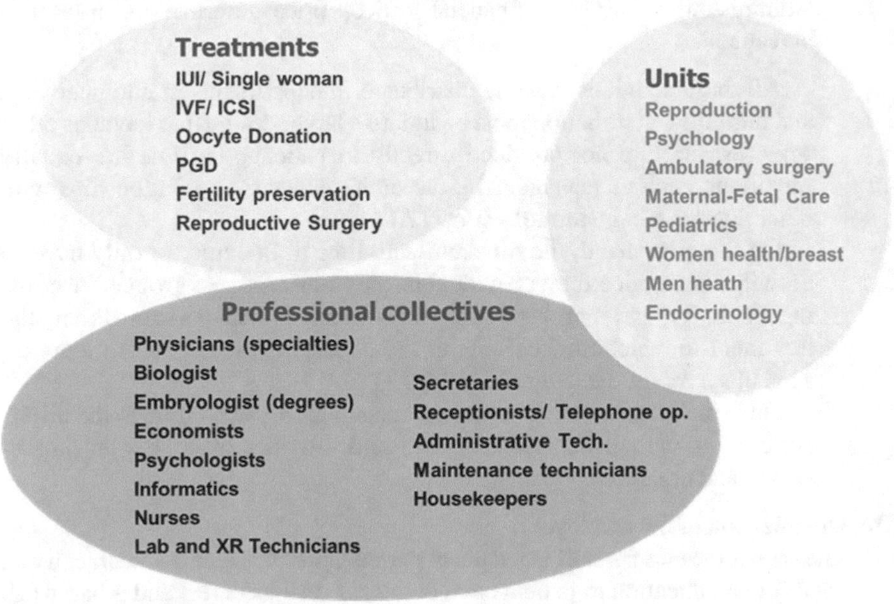

Treatments
IUI/ Single woman
IVF/ ICSI
Oocyte Donation
PGD
Fertility preservation
Reproductive Surgery
Units
Reproduction
Psychology
Ambulatory surgery
Maternal-Fetal Care
Pediatrics
Women health/breast
Men heath
Endocrinology
Professional collectives
Physicians (specialties)
Biologist
Embryologist (degrees)
Economists
Psychologists
Informatics
Nurses
Lab and XR Technicians
Secretaries
Receptionists/ Telephone op.
Administrative Tech.
Maintenance technicians
Housekeepers

Fig. 17.2 Unit activities

future. In new or small IVI clinics, one person assumes several roles in the chart and—as the volume and complexity increase—there is already a plan on how to allocate new professionals.

Regarding the hierarchical pyramid, we prefer it to be as flat as possible, since this facilitates internal communication and teamwork. We only have three hierarchical levels:

- Direction level: clinic and medical director, administrative responsible, clinic supervisor, etc.
- Mid-level management: one manager for each functional unit or department (e.g., IVF Lab, Andrology Lab, Egg Donation), and one coordinator for each professional collective, even if they belong to different departments (e.g., nurses, technicians, front desk—patient services, international department).
- Rest of the employees: every single person in the clinic has a representative in the mid-level management.

This structure allows effective communication and rapid diffusion of novelties or changes, since it facilitates internal communications and teamwork.

(c) Organization of time.

Most clinics organize patient flow according to their doctors' schedules, and very few establish their doctors' and departments' schedules based on patient preferences.

Visiting reproduction units and clinics in general all over the world, I have been able to observe that in most of them, time organization begins by taking into account the different activities, needs, and preferences of the doctors and other collaborators, to then try to fit the patients around that. For instance, doctors may have other parallel activities which make them only available at certain hours, or the laboratory requires that all blood samples for the determinations must be in by a particular time of the day, or the follicular development ultrasounds are only performed by one person and must all be grouped into a few-hours shift, or the entire team directly wants to have free afternoons… and taking into consideration all these variables, patient flow, office appointments, and operating room schedules are organized.

In an organization based, for example, on cost control, the mentioned system may make sense, although other factors would have to be considered as well. Certainly, however, if our strategy is differentiation based on patient satisfaction, this approach is frontally opposed to what we need.

Following our plan to manage through clinic organization and placing our focus on time organization, in addition to the regulations and habits of each country, it is important to analyze the preferences and needs of the patients to optimize each activity's efficiency. In this line, we define the number of hours per day for patient attention, the patient distribution or density along the day, whether it will be convenient to see patients until the late hours because that is what they request in some places (such as Spain) to avoid giving explanations at work, or whether appointments for first visits should be offered on Saturdays (e.g., in Japan).

All the working hours of our laboratories, of our personnel, the establishment of the different shifts, etc. will be based upon this information in order to facilitate a complete service to the patient, at the hour that the patient prefers, and with enough staff to be seen without waiting lists or delays at the clinic.

We also measure precisely the mean duration of each type of procedure to assign it the appropriate time in the schedule. These calculations allow us to design the appointments, since it is necessary to minimize the waiting time for the patients and the bad work distribution for the professionals: the objective is that they do not have to wait for us and we do not have to wait for them.

Finally, although we have focused on the term 'patient' because we are devoted to a medical activity, private and corporate IVF units must be viewed as service companies. Therefore, in terms of management, when we speak of patient satisfaction, we should really see it in the more ample sense of client satisfaction, which includes both the external client (the patient) and the internal one (the staff).

The organization and the concepts described are applicable, therefore, to the satisfaction of all the people who integrate the team and to the relationships with providers, affiliated institutions, and societies in which we play a part, in the sense that satisfying relationships—in the long run—help to achieve goals and to be coherent with our strategic plan.

Last but not least, no matter how deeply rooted an IVF unit's organization is, it must be a totally dynamic thing, always remembering that what we do not ask or we do not measure, we do not know. And what we do not know, we cannot improve.

References

1. Samuelson PA, Nordhaus WD. Economía. México: McGraw-Hill; 2010.
2. Stevens RE, Loudon DL, Migliore RH, Williamson S. Fundamentals of strategic planning for health care organizations. New York: The Haworth Press Inc; 1997.
3. Kaplan RS, Norton DP. Mapas estratégicos. Barcelona: Ediciones Gestión 2000; 2004. p. 31.
4. Gimbert X. El enfoque Estratégico de la Empresa. Bilbao: Deusto; 2003. p. 24–6.
5. Porter ME. Competitive advantage. New York: The Free Press; 1985.
6. Kotler P. Dirección de Marketing. Madrid: Prentice Hall; 2000.
7. Porter ME. Competitive strategy. New York: The Free Press; 1985.
8. Serra V, Vercher S, Zamorano V. Sistemas de control de gestión, metodología para su diseño. Barcelona: Ediciones Deusto; 2007. p. 32.

Part IV
Advertising and Marketing IVF Units

Chapter 18
Marketing of IVF Units and Agencies

Veronica Montgomery

Case Study: Barbados Fertility Centre (BFC)

Background

I have had the privilege of marketing the services of BFC for the last 10 years, from a new start-up clinic in 2002 to a world-class center of excellence for IVF that is now listed in the elite category for their latest Joint Commission International (JCI) accreditation in early 2014.

When the clinic opened in 2002, located on the Caribbean island of Barbados, the medical team led by Dr. Juliet Skinner and Anna Hosford, RGN, knew that this tiny dot in the Caribbean Sea was not big enough to sustain a full time IVF unit. Their vision was to become an international IVF clinic offering patients a 2-week holiday to destress, unwind and receive fertility treatment.

Their success story makes compelling reading when looking for a role model of how to market yourselves successfully and they have a sound sales story with well-documented evidence from previous patients.

Year on year, BFC have exceeded success rates from first world countries such as the UK and the USA (Table 18.1).

The national average live birth rate per treatment cycle started for all ages in the UK is just 25.6 % [1], while the USA national average is just 46.9 % for women under 35 years of age [2].

V. Montgomery (✉)
Department of Marketing, Barbados Fertility Centre, Hastings, Barbados
e-mail: ladymonty@me.com; ronnie@madmonty.com

© Springer Science+Business Media New York 2016
S.D. Fleming, A.C. Varghese (eds.), *Organization and Management of IVF Units*, DOI 10.1007/978-3-319-29373-8_18

Table 18.1 BFC 2013 success rates

IVF using own eggs	Success rates per ET (%)
<35-year-olds CPR/ET	80
ICSI using own eggs + blastocyst transfer	
<35-year-olds PR/ET	77.3
35–39-year-olds PR/ET	53.3
40–42-year-olds PR/ET	50
>42-year-olds PR/ET	11.1
CPR—Clinical pregnancy rate	
PR—Pregnancy rate	
ET—Embryo transfer	

BFC also offers low cost treatment, $5750USD for an IVF cycle, which they have not increased since 2007. This is very competitive for USA and UK patients who are being quoted double that figure for treatment in their home country; add to that the location and the on site spa to ensure patients are at their optimum of relaxation and the sales story is complete.

How a Medical Facility Can Employ Commercial Marketing Methods

It is a fine line to balance being a medical practitioner and having to drive the sales to make your facility a viable business, but with the right staff on hand throughout the patient journey, this transition should be seamless. The patient should never feel that they have been sold or committed to procedures that they cannot afford.

In this section I look at all the marketing elements that you should have in place to reach prospective patients, but the key to your marketing efforts being successful is having a good team to handle the enquiries. The receptionist who gives the first impression of your facility should be friendly and open; a patient is nervous making this call and needs to be reassured. Next the patient will speak to an IVF Nurse Coordinator, and this is where the balance of being a medical professional and sales driver really comes in to play. The patient needs to give a full medical history and the nurse needs to advise them on their next course of action, but also at this stage needs to win the patient's confidence and assure them that your facility is where they will find the help that they need. The patient may then be scheduled to speak with the leading clinician and this call is ultimately when the patient will make the decision to have treatment at your facility. If a patient decides on treatment with you then they should then have all the nonmedical aspects of their treatment handled by a patient liaison officer, who can arrange their flights, accommodation and any nonmedical procedures, such as holistic therapies.

Setting Your Marketing Budget

All of the activities outlined in the coming paragraphs require a decent marketing budget, and as a rule of thumb this should be anything between 2–10 % of your annual sales revenue. To get the right mix of marketing methods and to reach patients through as many channels as possible with your budget, I generally favor a spend at the top end of this bracket. It is important to target this spend and get an even spread between all the methods outlined below. Also allocate your spend on a monthly basis, remember that infertility patients are an ever replenishing market and you need a constant presence in the market to reach them and the more they hear your name and read articles about you, the more comfortable they feel to get in contact with you.

Websites

The first port of call for most patients is your website and you need to ensure that this is clean and easy to navigate. Remember this is the first impression that a patient has of your facility, so make sure it has good quality photographs of your clinic and has good information. IVF patients have spent years researching infertility on the Internet and will quickly dismiss you if information on success rates and costs are not found quickly. Employ a Web specialist to ensure your site is optimized to rank highly in the search engines and make sure your text is not too technical. Remember they could have recently been diagnosed and need to understand why they are not conceiving, so use basic descriptions of medical conditions. Language can be a big problem for clinics when attracting overseas patients. For example, if you are targeting patients in the UK, have your text written by someone who speaks English as a first language. Patients can easily feel alienated if your website has spelling mistakes or incorrect use of grammar.

Always make sure contact details are available on every page of your site, including your social media links and make it easy for prospective patients to get in touch. Have a simple contact form for patients to complete and on this form ensure you ask how the patient heard of you; this is essential in monitoring response from your marketing efforts.

Think about what makes you different from your competitors; what do you offer that they do not? Maybe you offer surrogacy or gender selection; if you do make sure this is highlighted on your home page of the website.

Finally, make sure that your site has Google Analytics installed so you can track where your visitors have come from, how many you have on a monthly basis and also geographically where your patients are coming from; this data is so important when planning your marketing activities.

Print Advertising

You must always check with your governing medical council on advertising guidelines as these can vary with location. For instance, it may be that you are allowed to advertise to patients internationally but you may not be allowed to place advertisements in your local area.

There are many forms of media in which you can reach potential IVF patients and the nature of our market means it is ever replenishing with one in six couples worldwide suffering with infertility. Mainstream media, such as national newspapers, will use up a huge chunk of your advertising budget and are not targeted enough. Generally, I would advise against mainstream advertising and only consider it if there is an editorial opportunity to support the advertisement.

There are many specialist publications dedicated to the subject of infertility and print advertising in these is far more cost effective and generally you see a better response.

When placing print advertisements it is important to just have one key message that you wish to get across to the audience via the advert. Think about the audience that will be reading that publication and tailor your advert to appeal to that audience. Do not try to list every procedure that you offer. Just have a good visual, that is eye catching and just a couple of paragraphs about your facility; highlight your unique selling point. Please see the example print advert (Fig. 18.1).

Website Banner Advertising

It is really important to include advertising on other websites as part of your marketing strategy, as these adverts link back to your site and is another way to drive traffic to your site. Again there are many specialist sites that focus on the subject of infertility that you can use to get your message across. The cost of advertising on these sites is very low for the year and the more you are on the better chance you have of reaching patients. Space on these banner adverts is limited, so again you just need a strong visual image and only a few key words about why a patient should click on your advert for more information. Please see the example banner advertising (Fig. 18.2).

Website Profiles

There are many other websites that you can advertise on to drive traffic to your own clinic's site. You may wish to advertise on a tourism website for your country, as this is a good way of raising your profile and reaching potential patients. If someone is already planning a trip to your country then it is good idea to make them aware of your facility. They may just want to call in and check out your clinic while they are there and then return for treatment, or they may even combine their vacation with

Fig. 18.1 An example of a print advertisement

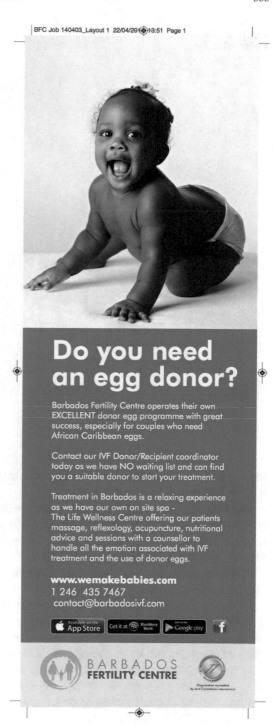

Fig. 18.2 An example of
banner advertising

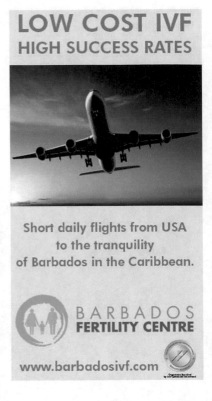

treatment; either way make sure you catch their attention while they are investigating your country.

Medical tourism in on the increase and there are a number of sites that specialize in the subject and it is important that you look at all of these sites; they cover all medical procedures so make sure IVF is in their options and also check that they also have your country on their map as well.

There are also a number of websites dedicated to infertility and again you should also have a presence on these as well.

You may choose to have a profile page and actual banner advertisements. Most websites offer a package for the year, which can include a social media outreach to promote you on their site. They may also offer to publish your patient success stories and can often offer you the option of blogging on their site as well. I would suggest you go for a package that gives you maximum exposure for the best price. Remember to always negotiate on their rate card; you are providing content for their site and the arrangement should be beneficial to both parties.

Billboard and Screen Advertising

It is important that you choose your billboard or screen advertising in prominent places. A static billboard at your airport can be a good investment if you are able to catch people in the arrivals hall while they queue for immigration. Another prominent place is the port if your country has one; while ports attract the cruise line passenger who may be older than your target market, never rule out the potential grandparents, who quite often will fund IVF treatment to get the much-desired grandchild. But always check first with your local medical council to ensure you are allowed to advertise.

In terms of screen advertising, you can normally source a good package deal that offers combined print advertising with screen promotion as well. Popular spots include Times Square in New York and The Path—the underground walkway in the financial district in Toronto, Canada.

When placing screen adverts, a 5 s spot is all that you need, which is run on rotation, you need a clear image to catch people's attention and a memorable way to get in touch. For example, for USA advertising we have bought the domain name www. wemakebabies.com, primarily because people often confuse Barbados, Bahamas and Bermuda; so if you are in a country that people might not remember or you have competitors' clinics near you, then just choose a domain that people can remember; this then redirects to your main site.

Radio Advertising

Placing short radio commercials locally is a good way to reach potential patients. Adverts need to be short, around 30 s and I would suggest a series of different adverts to run in rotation highlighting different areas of treatment offered. Do not try to get too much information in to 30 s; you should be able to read your script without rushing in the time allocated. Less is more with radio, one clear message and a method of contact is all that you need. Start the script with who you are, what you do and then repeat who you are again at the end once you have their attention and end with the contact information. Developing a good relationship with your local radio stations is essential to your business and often they are very interested in women's health issues and have regular programs dedicated to their female audience. Working closely with your local radio station means that you can offer your head clinician to take part in phone in programs and gives you a really good stage to promote your work in an educational way.

TV and Video

Actual TV advertising can be very expensive and like other forms of mainstream media, there is a lot of wastage. But like radio, there may be specific health programs on your local TV station that you can offer content for; you can use this to highlight various issues surrounding infertility or even have your successful patients being interviewed with their child to highlight your work. Patient videos are a really good tool for promoting your clinic, and in the age of social media it is great how quickly potential patients can view these.

You will be approached by a lot of TV production companies who are interested in making documentaries on the subject of IVF, however proceed with caution; a lot of the companies are looking for you to fund the production cost which can vary from US$20,000–US$50,000. If a program has actually been commissioned by a broadcaster then the broadcaster usually funds this as well so there should not be any outlay from your clinic. You may be able to offer them flights to your location if you have special rates in place with airlines or offer them accommodation while they are with you.

In Flight Infomercials and Print Adverts

Take a look at the nearest airport to you and see which airlines fly to your country. Also look at where there are direct flights from. This gives you a good idea of where to target your advertising in other countries or cities. Then find out what the advertising options are on board these flights. This is a great place to get patient stories published or videos shown. Some airlines just have communal screens for watching safety demonstrations, and as you have a captive audience for the duration of the flight, an infomercial about infertility can be very effective. You may have business people travelling who have focused on their career and left starting a family until later in life. If the airline has their own magazine then allocated some budget for advertising and asking if you can run an editorial is also very effective.

Publicity

People believe what they read in an editorial far more than what they see in an advertisement, and every single patient you treat has an individual story to tell. Encourage patients to raise awareness about their own infertility journey and everybody loves to read a happy ending that results in a newborn baby. There are many different angles you can use for stories; usually cost for patients in their home country is a popular topic along with patients that have had many unsuccessful attempts at other clinics before finding success with you. Make sure you have regular stories that come out of your clinic, and subscribe to a good news service for your target market; this way your stories will be published and this is another way to drive potential patients to your website through story-back links. Also develop good relationships with your national newspapers; again women health issues are popular topics and most national newspapers will have a specific health editor. It is worth investing time and money with these publications so that when they do a special feature on infertility then you will feature in it. Always make your head clinician available for consultations with editorial staff when they are writing a feature and make yourselves very accessible for reference material.

Exhibitions

Deciding to exhibit can be very costly and you need to ensure that the outlay will be recouped through patient numbers. Only exhibit at events that are targeted to the patient; exhibiting at other industry events will not prove lucrative to get actual patient enquiries.

When you have found a show that offers the right audience and is specifically targeting IVF patients, the first cost to consider is the price of the exhibition space. Usually there will be different rates for charitable organizations but as an IVF unit you will be charged the highest rate.

Then you have to consider your actual display; do you have an exhibition stand, either pop-up graphics or a full pop-up stand? These can be hired for the event but as this is something you will do at least once a year it is more cost effective to buy your own.

Then you need to have the exhibition panels designed to go on the stand itself.

What else will you need on your stand? Probably furniture, which again can be hired, usually through contractors who are supplying this particular event.

Will you want to have actual patient consultations on the stand? If so, then you may want to think about partitioning to make these private or at least some seating to talk to your patients away from the thick of the traffic passing your stand.

Make sure you have booked a big enough space to fit in your own display stand and the furniture that you order.

You will also need somewhere to display your marketing material; either a display cabinet or shelving so people can help themselves.

Also make sure you have experienced staff to man the stand; they must have good knowledge of your treatment procedures and be able to answer any question thrown at them.

Exhibitions are hard work on the team; they are long days, standing for many hours on hard floors so make sure you have enough cover to allow breaks and remember you could potentially speak to over 1000 patients in a day!

So think really hard before deciding to exhibit as to whether you can afford all the extra costs such as content on the stand, staff, and all the extra marketing material that needs to be printed and all the promotion and advertising expenditure to make people aware that your team are there to talk to throughout the event.

Conferences

Attending conferences is one of the best ways to keep abreast of new developments in the area of both IVF techniques and also the development of medical tourism. Before you register for an event, always find out the deadline for submitting abstracts. Conferences are much easier to network at if you are a speaker as people will always come and find you after you have spoken with further questions and further develop relationships with you and your organization. Do not be afraid to share your best practices; even competitors can work with you. When submitting a call for papers choose a subject that you think will be unique to the conference and offer content that the organizers may not be already covering. Try to add value to the event with your contribution. If you are selected to speak then registration fees for the conference are normally waived. If your paper is not selected then it is still worth going out in to the market place and networking and making contacts for future development of your clinic. When speaking to your competitors establish what services they offer in comparison to yours. If you have something to offer that they do not and vice versa then find a way to work together, referring patients between your two facilities.

Social Networking

There are around 50 social network sites out there that you can have a presence on and are a great method of speaking directly with patients on a daily basis with no costs associated with the site itself. It is really important to have somebody manage the content of your pages and profiles on these sites and answer direct messages and questions on a daily basis. The main two social networks to focus on are a Facebook page and a Twitter account. Make sure you create a page and do not create yourself as a person; you can do a lot more as a page than you can as a person. Also be aware that this is a public domain so if a patient has had a good or bad experience with you, they will write about it on one of these social networking sites. It is really important that you respond to these posts; if someone has a bad experience with you then respond publicly; this can be turned in to a positive experience and how you handle this negative publicity can make a good impression on potential patients. Use these pages to post useful and educational material for patients and as a link to news stories that might interest them. This is a less formal environment, so speak in a more casual manner and talk to the patients as real people. Post your success stories, ask your patients to post their baby photographs and write about their own struggles with infertility. You can also use these sites to post videos about your clinic. Always make sure you have your contact details on these pages and your website address.

Advertising: Facebook

The beauty of these social networking sites is that advertising on them has got very advanced and you can target patients by gender, age, location and relationship status. Adverts are limited in words for your headline and text. So you just need an attention-grabbing headline, and get your point across so that they click on your advert for more information. You only pay when someone clicks on your advert so essentially you only pay for a response. You can pause your advertising at any time and it is a great way for keeping control of your budget. It is better to run multiple adverts and direct some of these to your website, and some to your Facebook page encouraging them to like you, so that your posts come up in their news feed and you can also promote posts or events that you are holding. You may like to consider employing a specialist agency to run your social media advertising as getting the most from your advertising dollars can be done quickly and effectively with the right expertise.

Advertising: Google

Again the beauty of Google adwords is that you can target your advertising by country, gender, and age, but here you can also sponsor specific search terms that a user might key in to the Google search engine. Also this is pay per click advertising and you only pay once somebody clicks on your link. You will see these adverts come up in the top three of sponsored links and also appear in the side bar. Depending on your location you can also link your advertising to Google places and link to your Google + page. This type of advertising can reach hundreds of thousands of potential patients per month with a good click through rate. You can expect to see an actual enquiry rate of about 2 % from the total number of people who saw your advert, which is again a great return on investment. These adverts can also be paused at any time and give you better control of your budget. Again you might consider a specialist agency to handle both your Facebook and Google Adwords advertising to ensure you get the best response.

Educational Seminars

It is really essential to provide patients with good educational material as infertility has so many aspects. Often the patient does not take in what has been discussed at their original diagnosis, then they go away and scour the Internet for information on their specific problems. Therefore educational seminars on specific medical conditions such as polycystic ovarian syndrome (PCOS) or endometriosis can be really useful for potential patients and makes you the authority on the subject matter.

You can go about educational seminars in a number of ways.

Firstly, you might like to rent a conference room in a local hotel and have your medical team present on various subject matters; these can be very popular and you will be surprised at the number of people who will take time out at the weekend to attend.

Apps

Developing an app for your clinic can be quite costly; however you have to look at the app's long-term shelf life and how it puts your clinic on the international stage via the Apple app store, Blackberry World and Google Play for android devices.

Your app needs to be content rich with lots of educational and useful advice for patients on managing their IVF journey. BFC developed *The Fertility App* in 2012; this has a calendar that syncs with the user's device to remind them of ovulation dates and when to take medications. There is a full medical glossary outlining all medical terms associated with infertility and this includes an explanation of all medications and their effects on the body. It also has helpful tips on preparing the body for IVF treatment. Patients can also ask questions within the app and talk directly to the medical team.

Material Sent to Prospective Patients

When you are creating marketing material to send out to prospective patients you have to think of where your audience are located and write in a language that is familiar to them and preferably have it written by someone who speaks that language as their first language. Your brochure needs to demonstrate the quality of your facility and explain all aspects of treatment to patients. This is one of the only publications that you can fill with lots of information as prospective patients need to know as much as possible about you before they make their final decision. Also work with other publishers to have pieces written about you that you can also send out to prospective patients. A third party recommendation is a good endorsement. Your material should also match your corporate branding of all other material that is in the public domain so that patients can easily recognize that this is the same clinic they have seen or heard of previously.

The Treatment Experience

From the moment the patient makes their initial enquiry with you, your goal is to make their experience with as positive as possible.

As I outlined in the beginning this must start with your receptionist and the continuity of their care must continue all the way through their treatment process. If your patients are travelling from overseas then ensure they are met at the airport and transported to their hotel. Have the patient liaison officer meet them at their hotel and ensure that they are happy with their room and outline their full itinerary throughout their stay.

Make sure they know when they have to attend your facility for medical procedures and also advise them where and when their treatments are. Make sure transport is provided to collect them and bring them to your clinic.

If you are treating patients from the local vicinity then just go the extra mile to ensure their treatment experience is one they want to shout about. Despite all of the marketing methods used to reach potential patients, the strongest and best method is still word of mouth, and so many patients quote that other IVF units they have been to have treated them like a number, not as an individual. As we continue to strive to offer the best possible patient experience, just think what can your unit offer that none other does?

Patient Follow-Up for Strategic Marketing

Always follow up with your patients; obviously the whole medical team are keen to know whether or not the pregnancy test is positive but do not let your contact end there. Work closely with the patient; each and every patient has a unique and individual story to tell and encourage them to share their story. Have your marketing department call them and ask them if they will be filmed, ask if they will speak to journalists and ask them if they will blog about you on infertility networking sites. The majority of patients will be happy to do this if they had a good experience of treatment at your clinic regardless of the result. There are no guarantees with IVF but you do control your patient experience and just strive to do your job to best of your ability and patients will do the selling for you.

Good luck!

References

1. Human Fertilisation & Embryology Authority. Fertility treatment in 2012: trends and figures. (http://www.hfea.gov.uk/104.html)
2. Centers for Disease Control and Prevention, American Society for Reproductive Medicine, Society for Assisted Reproductive Technology. 2012 Assisted Reproductive Technology Fertility Clinic Success Rates Report. Atlanta (GA): US Dept of Health and Human Services; 2014.

Chapter 19
Websites for IVF Clinics

James D. Stanger

Static or Interactive Web Sites

Website functionality can range between static and interactive and the cost of development and maintenance reflects what the clinic may want from it. The cost of developing a basic website remains very low for the activity it generates and the function it performs, and most clinics will have commissioned one. In its basic form, a clinic's basic website will provide details of the clinic, the staff, list of services and contact details. They are largely static displays that may or may not require regular maintenance. Changes such as new technology or clinical programmes, changes in staff, patient education evenings and, above all else, the current success rates all require regular updating. Patients are quickly aware if the clinic's website is static or out of date. The cost of maintaining a static format is another issue for most clinics. While the initial costs for static websites are low, these can become significant over time both monetarily and in staff time. This is because each change requires the website developer to make the changes to text or content (images, videos, etc) and each page needs to be approved before it should be loaded on to the sites' provider. While not prohibitive, repeated changes can be an impediment to keeping the site current and has the effect that the website will stagnate. Static sites do record the activity for each page when displayed and service providers can or should provide this information to clinics. Depending on the structure of the website, some information say, on the number of clicks/page, can give the clinic some measure of the impact of any change or client's interest.

J.D. Stanger, PhD (✉)
FertAid Pty Ltd., Newcastle, NSW, Australia
e-mail: office@fertaid.com

© Springer Science+Business Media New York 2016
S.D. Fleming, A.C. Varghese (eds.), *Organization and Management of IVF Units*, DOI 10.1007/978-3-319-29373-8_19

Given that most IVF staff have no computing or Internet skills, the cost of commissioning a more dynamic website will be significantly greater than for developing a static site but the rewards will be significantly greater. While a static website will consist of a number of web pages written in html (the standard web language), a more interactive one will need a database attached to it to record not only requests for information but more importantly, the information stored on each page.

Most dynamic web pages display information stored in tables. The developer may then prepare for the clinic staff, the tools to actively manage the content in the tables and therefore what is displayed on the website. By adding new rows, deleting redundant rows to a table, one can then add or remove content as required. Each page will display information from different tables that can be dynamically maintained. Further, if the tables are arranged correctly, the same page may display vastly different information in a seamless manner. Each request for information may be tagged to identify what information is displayed and statistics could be shown on the clinic's administrative pages. For instance, a page showing the staff groupings (clinical, nursing, laboratory, counselling etc) could lead to individuals that could show a list of skills, publications or experience. Each selection will lead to different information and the statistics data could show which staff groupings, individuals, experience, skills etc. The information may show one clinician who has an interest in endometriosis or polycystic ovarian syndrome (PCOS) even though the website is for IVF. A clinic may in response to this hold information on this subject or dedicate a clinic to it. Since most clients will ultimately attempt IVF, this may provide a valuable conduit for a specific class of client. So while the initial costs may be considerable, there should be significant downstream savings or increases in activity.

Key Performance Indicators and Statistics

Information contained in tables can be easily searched and displayed upon a search request. The clinic can then record what terms are being searched as an indication of items that are of interest to consumers. Key performance indicator (KPI) statistics could be developed to track the changed content. It is acknowledged that IVF is a medical process and not a sales programme and if an IVF clinic is the only clinic in town, none of this is applicable. However, increasingly more clinics will continue to seek new clients as long as demand is unmet. Further, it is likely that IVF clinics may service only about one third of potential clients. The application of integrative websites is a subtle but powerful tool to explore competition and unmet demand.

One limitation of this approach is that search engines use programs to search and record the content on each page and the activity on any page will then be a reflection of the activity of both clients and search programmes. Therefore a database system can interrogate the internet service provider (ISP) identification of each browser and create a list of genuine private requests by clients as distinct to searches by web bots. The "spiders" used by search engines return regularly to all websites following and recording links on the page both to other pages on the same website and to links to other websites. The search engines use this information and well as content plus other unknown details to decide on how to rank each page and each website. A clinic may also enhance their ranking by paying for advertising that will promote them in the order of relevance in a list shown in response to a browser's request. This is a field that some clinics may need professional advice on how to manage their advertising budget. The activity of spiders is a two edged sword since on one hand it is good that a search engine can monitor your site while on the other, their activity creates a false illusion of activity and may in some cases slow down the activity of the site. There are commands that can be placed upon web pages to ask "bots" to move on but no one can enforce it. However, the database can track such search engine views if desired. It should be noted that if a clinic is subscribing to Google advertising, such page statistics can be obtained but this is only for requests that flow from a Google advertisement selection.

One last comment about search engines is that one never knows how a browser may chance upon their website and, therefore, content is key. One may request "oocyte activation in Timbuktu", "overseas surrogacy" or "IVF Clinics" in their local area. Each search engine may deliver different rankings but that can only find your site if the words are mentioned in the search request (or their algorithm). Each page has a script that can contain key words that may help but more recently content and links have become important, so consideration should be to develop a process on your website that mentions key words in several places and make links to the pages that have the primary content. There is a skill to providing links to enhance a browsers experience while not making it confusing.

Honesty

There is a requirement for honesty in both the medical and the success information, with an appraisal of the clinic's website now part of some accreditation surveillance. Data shown for success rates needs to be validated and current. Of course, where there is little or no accreditation process in place, the content of a clinic's website can be largely unregulated. This has the potential to mislead potential clients.

There are several not-for-profit organisations that can certify if the information on a website meets minimal standards for honesty. One such body is the Health on the web Foundation [2].

The principles of the Health on the Net Foundation code of conduct (HONcode) are:

1. Authority—information and advice given only by medical professionals with credentials of author/s, or a clear statement if this is not the case
2. Complementarity—information and help are to support, not replace, patient-healthcare professional relationships which is the desired means of contact

3. Confidentiality—how the site treats personal and non-personal information of readers
4. Attribution—references to source of information (URL if available) and when it was last updated
5. Justifiability—any treatment, product or service must be supported by balanced, well-referenced scientific information
6. Transparency of authorship—contact information, preferably including email addresses, of authors should be available
7. Transparency of sponsorship—sources of funding for the site
8. Honesty in advertising and editorial policy—details about advertising on the site and clear distinction between advertised and editorial material (ref http://en. wikipedia.org/wiki/Health_On_the_Net_Foundation)

These general rules do not reflect the potential for a clinic's website to mislead and misinform. There are very few clinics that display a declaration or a certification (such as from HON) that their websites meet these principles. Adherence to the principles probably is not a major issue since prospective clients are largely younger and more Internet savvy than the medical practitioners who operate the site and any discordant information will quickly become apparent and the clinic's reputation tarnished. In some circumstances, an accreditation review may explore the content of a clinic's website to also check for honest content.

Referral

The purpose of a clinic's website has historically been promotion. Only a short time ago, all referrals to a clinic would have been via a client's general practitioner (GP), newspaper advertising or by word of mouth. Increasingly, clients can now browse the results of a search request and preview the information on a clinic's web page. Their impression can then influence how they request a referral. Since infertile couples are often busy and in a hurry, this decision is an important one. They usually do not have many years to try for conception and while some couples move between clinics, most are relatively loyal and therefore the first choice is often their only choice. It is important for a clinic to portray confidence, compassion, skill and the likelihood of success via their promotional activity that includes their website. There is little information or published reports on how clients find a clinic [3] and in reality, the historical referral process of clinical allegiances between GPs and specialists, location, local news stories and gossip most likely continues to reflect the recruitment pathway for the majority of new clients. In this argument, the role of the website is a secondary one to provide confidence that the referral by one's GP is appropriate.

Couples rarely have the money and time to pursue IVF outside their hometown or region. Newer clinical services such as medical tourism (where cost, and a conjoined holiday, is the main driver), oocyte donation, gender selection and surrogacy have a different clientele and do not reflect the majority of clinics' clients. In fact, patients from outside a clinic's locality often consume more resources and are more demanding unless the clinic is geared to accommodate them. Therefore, the primary purpose of a clinic's website is directed to local competition.

Changing Role of Providing Information

Before the Internet gained traction, most clinics provided clinical information to clients prior to gaining their consent for treatment. Early on, there were concerns that clinics were vulnerable to litigation if they failed to provide sufficient information that allowed the giving of informed consent. In the early 1980s, our clinic provided a 100+ page book that combined all our information sheets. As IVF was changing very rapidly, the time and cost of maintaining such a plethora of information sheets was considerable. It was not surprising therefore that very quickly, clinics rapidly started to move much of this activity to the Internet environment. One problem with this is that if information can be quickly modified, how then a clinic records what changes have been made becomes critical. In response to litigation for services performed several years prior, a clinic may need to be able to reconstruct the information provided at the time of treatment. Written information can have a degree of traceability (version number, etc) while changes to Internet content runs the risk of loss of traceability. Therefore, it may be in a clinic's best interest and as a quality activity, that all changes are logged and retained. Extinct static web pages may be retained on the website with archival file names in archive folders and never accessible by the public but able to be printed on special request.

Recording Activity

One thing the Internet is very efficient at is recording of activity. It is unclear whether clinics trace the activity on their websites but recording the number of page requests and the IP address from where the request originated can provide a clinic with considerable information of what words are of interest to the potential clients. The design of the website then needs to be able to allow the browser the opportunity to explore the various treatments offered by the clinic.

Public and Private

Another approach would be to provide a vehicle whereby a clinic's website may prompt for browsers to register with name and email to receive regular reminders of information nights or clinic activities. A clinic may also provide a regular review of recent publications on topics or procedures they have recently started doing or introduced. For instance, many clinics are now using some form of embryo video imaging to fine-tune the embryo selection process. An email circulation summary of one recent publication explaining the finding and pointing out the clinic now has this capability is a very passive way to inform future clients of the clinic's attitude to new technology. As discussed above, a website with such capability may be more expensive to initially develop but once established will require considerably less cost to operate.

In essence, by providing a private portal for private information accessed by a client joining a private area, you provide the clinic with an address for future contact. Furthermore, depending on what information is asked at the time of joining a mail group/private portal, a clinic may then discriminate on what information is given to which client. For example, if the client's age as asked, then you may provide different success rate data to older than to younger women.

One further advantage of creating a mail group is that you can ask them to nominate for a list of items of interest. For example, male-factors, endometriosis etc and potentially fine-tune information to them but at the same time collect some patient information outside of their protected medical history. Other data that can be collected may include, how did they find a clinic's website or whether they would like the clinic to contact them. This is in effect a dynamic online survey.

Extending this communication concept, by registering the email address of each new patient, and using an e-newsletter to current and past clients allows a clinic to "keep in touch". If a clinic is operating an Internet savvy database to manage clinical history, the database may have the capability to provide such follow-up independently of the website but since this is unlikely, the website with an attached database is another alternative. The essence of this concept is that prior to the Internet, maintaining patient contact was both time-consuming and expensive. Printing and posting of a written newsletter made everyone feel proactive but the number of mail returned was always disheartening. While many clients move frequently, using their email (better still the emails of both partners and alternative contacts) is a better mechanism for communication. One aspect of this is that a returned email is a warning that the patient contact may have been lost. This has other implications with, for instance, the management of couples with frozen embryos in storage where loss of mail contact creates many headaches. Actively managing the couple's email via regular updates will, in some way, warn the laboratory staff of problems and provide an alternative route for correspondence.

Of course the issue of privacy is important and any mailing list may be regarded as exploitable but, unlike medical information, a website email address would constitute a very low risk given the ubiquitous use of using emails to contact individuals. As long as the database did not contain personal details and consent was given to receive electronic news, the issue of privacy is addressed.

Website Design

Online advertising such as GOOGLE is increasingly popular since such delivery can be localised and tracked with online statistics. However, the design of a website can be important in how a website may appear on the ranking of search engines. For instance, having all the staff and their skills on the website may allow browsers to fine-tune searches, especially for the clinical staff with all the skills outside of IVF (e.g. tubal surgery, endometriosis, andrology) and may capture search requests for specific medical conditions by directing them to the clinic's website. Sites with all their staff listed with photos can be expensive and time consuming but it defines the personal nature of a clinic, allows clients to identify individuals and create intimacy between clinic staff and patients, which is often the heart of good IVF practice.

Some clinics are actively involved in research and regularly present findings at scientific meetings. Listing these presentations and research the clinic is currently (or has been) involved in is another way for a clinic to use its website to promote an image of itself that is progressive with new technology.

Listing all the procedures and new activities can be important since most clinicians like to offer alternative procedures, stimulation regimes and techniques for each new stimulation cycle. Couples often feel that since the last cycle was unsuccessful, just repeating the same thing is a waste of time. Being able to offer alternatives can sometimes be the difference in returning for another attempt. Being able to highlight the new options from the website means the clinician can reduce the consultation time and allows the client to return to the page afterwards. It also is a tool for search engines to identify and link a browser's request to a clinic's website.

However, there is a price to pay for too much information—confusion. Early websites tended to throw all their information sheets on their websites, but, more recently, many sites are becoming more frugal with content and navigation around the site. Following new trends in web design and standardisation, websites are more professionally presented with softer colours and images and better browser experience. In some ways, a clinic's website will often be a future client's first contact and this experience must be positive, informative and inviting. By all means have as much information as possible on as many pages as possible but the first initial links should be inviting. It will be expected that as bandwidth increases and technology improves, more information will be provided by video content and text and, depending on what is done, may be very effective at establishing contact, or may be just very expensive. There are probably many traps in using videos but it is a powerful tool to transfer information. An example here is the changing platform for viewing websites. Tablets are replacing home computers and some tablets limit video formats. Apple iPads for instance do not show videos in Flash format, so the website needs to know the platform and show different formats accordingly or provide different formats online.

Some basic initial information could include:

- A welcome statement often with rotating images of 4–5 key pieces of information.

- A list of key services.
- A list of key clinical staff containing an image, a very short resume and key clinical interests.
- Your location; often, including an image of the clinic and a map creates a sense of identity and permanence.
- An invitation to contact the clinic by completion of a form that includes their email and sometimes a box asking if they could receive your future information.

If the clinic's language is not primarily English, having an English page is also a good idea since it allows foreign browsers to have some idea of your clinic. From each of these pages, you can develop cascading pages of more information. If you can add a search button, this can provide an alternative tool for browsers to locate information. As stated above, a dynamic web format can deliver increased functionality such as a search bow or textual suggestions. For example, a page discussing stimulation may also suggest pages discussing hyper-stimulation, oocytes or cryopreservation.

A clinic may wish to display general public information and retain some information for private browsers. In order to view say success rates or costs, you may need a browser to register with name, location and email address. Not many clinics actively manage email content but being able to post regular information content will be an important clinic activity in the future. Additionally, by restricting access to some pages, a clinic can control what pages are seen by a search spider and what pages remain hidden.

Client Interaction

Finally, the difficult subject of interaction concerning a client's patient treatment needs to be discussed, since in the future activity at this level will become very busy. There are a number of IVF databases that are used to manage a couple's treatment. By and large, these databases are not existing live on the Internet but running on a local server protected from prying eyes. Some of these databases have or are developing capability to export information to clients about treatment via email. Such interaction may include instructions about future treatment. The databases can effectively post emails or SMS messages to clients and obtain responses from clients but this acts over the Internet via secure server access rather than over the open Internet.

Currently there are few databases operating live over the Internet and to my knowledge, there are no multi-clinic online services. One can see in the future with better security that such services may arise. While the disadvantages may be self-evident, there are some advantages that could drive it. These include both cost and the capacity to develop an on-line community for data comparisons and KPIs of performance. It may also allow clients to move between clinics for specific services. For example, a clinic may request sex-selection to be performed in another clinic in another country but still retain management of pregnancy or other treatment. This, while far-fetched, may allow clinics to specialise in some services, e.g. PGD. Currently, movement of clients between clinics creates difficulties in continuity of care.

Back to reality, despite desires to implement online health services, the risk to hacking remains real. Clients will need to provide consent to have their data linked to an external portal and all data needs to be encrypted. An example of how a patient specific portal may work can be found at the Pacific Fertility Centre in USA [4] or Boston IVF [5]. Their websites have many of the interactive features discussed above. They do however use a separate portal developed by Pacific Highway [6] to provide a patient logon specific to their clients [7]. While the clinic use the database (SQL Server) to manage its own data management, the client portal provides tools for surveys, appointment reminders, medication instructions, laboratory results consent forms and instructions, accounts and payments. Each clinic has its own database and portal. There will undoubtedly be more competition in this area as the clients themselves become more Internet savvy and demanding. The past times of couples spending a lot to time visiting the clinic for trivial information may well be replaced with a virtual information portal by clients who no longer have the time or are living outside the clinics range. An example, of how this interaction may follow is the Institut Marques in Spain providing a portal for clients to see their embryos from videos generated using the EmbryoScope time-lapse system [8]. They, as do other clinics, also allow couples to book an online information consultation via Skype.

There are rules for managing client's medical records over the Internet [9] that govern privacy, security, transactions, identity and enforcement. How this will develop is uncertain but clinics will explore ways to interact with clients to improve productivity and ensure contact is maintained. The productivity issue is an interesting one since in its earliest days, IVF has always been a team activity. Clients will interact with many clinic staff at various staff during a treatment cycle all of which can be time consuming. Moving to a semi-digital process will probably be appreciated by clients who no longer have to wait to see staff but it also has elements of traceability and checking. This may have the effect of reducing staff loads and even staff.

Finally, there are several other areas where the Internet is impacting on IVF clinics. These include online data submission for national statistics, quality assurance such as www.QAPonline.com, education and training, news groups such as embryomail or IVFDaily and access to online reference material. The large number of consumer websites and patient friendly sites with links to finding clinics and spreading news and information has made client management increasing difficult. It requires the clinical and contact staff to be more aware of new developments and ideas. The consequences of the mass of information in the digital age are that the first point of contact for many clients will be their web interface. Clinics will need to be aware of how their clinic is being discussed over the chat rooms and blogs and ensure that criticism is addressed. Actually any clinic seeking to follow best practice should regularly survey their clients and the internet is a powerful tool with which to do this.

References

1. http://en.wikipedia.org/wiki/History_of_the_Internet
2. https://www.hon.ch/HONcode/
3. Haagen EC, Tuil W, Hendriks J, de Bruijn RPJ, Braat DDM, Kremer JAM. Current internet use and preferences of IVF and ICSI patients. Hum Reprod. 2003;18(10):2073–8.
4. http://www.pacificfertilitycenter.com/
5. http://www.bostonivf.com/
6. http://www.practicehwy.com/
7. https://connect.pacificfertilitycenter.com/patient/
8. http://www.institutmarques.com/advances-assisted-reproduction.html
9. http://www.hipaa-101.com/

Chapter 20
IVF Units and Social Media

Jonathan Pollinger

Definitions

Social Media

There are numerous definitions of "social media" and the term is often used interchangeably with "social networks". For me, social media refers to the whole picture and the definition I like the best, is from Marta Kagan's What the f*** is social media (2008) [1]. "Social media is an umbrella term that defines the various activities that integrate technology, social interaction, and the construction of words, pictures, videos and audio." I like this holistic definition and the specific inclusion of pictures, video and audio as well as text. Posts and tweets that include multimedia tend to receive the most interaction.

Social Networks

Social networks refers to the actual channels, for example Facebook, and my definition is "a digital channel where users interact and share".

The defining characteristics of a social network are the ability to interact and share. For a clinic this means that as well as the ability for a message to be published, the patient can also respond. Social networks facilitate two-way communication. For example, a clinic can post a question on Facebook that can generate answers from one or more patients. This is what makes social media different from more traditional marketing practices such as newspaper adverts and billboards as well as more recent channels such as television adverts and websites.

J. Pollinger (✉)
Intranet Future – Social Media Consultancy, Cheltenham, UK
e-mail: jonathan.pollinger@intranetfuture.com

© Springer Science+Business Media New York 2016
S.D. Fleming, A.C. Varghese (eds.), *Organization and Management of IVF Units*, DOI 10.1007/978-3-319-29373-8_20

The key to success with social media is to provide engaging content that creates conversations and encourages readers to share across their own social networks. This helps raise awareness of the clinic and will encourage prospective patients to find out more.

Benefits

There are many benefits that an IVF clinic can obtain from social media.

Effective and Powerful

First and foremost, social networks can be a very effective and powerful form of marketing. Effective because it is digital word of mouth but unlike face-to-face word of mouth, there are no physical barriers to communication. A message can travel right across the globe reaching huge numbers of people. To use the jargon, it can "go viral". For a clinic, awareness can be spread in the local area but to a large number of prospective patients.

Real Time

Social networks allow communication in real time that helps conversation flow and facilitates promotion of events and campaigns. If a patient asks a question on Facebook or Twitter, a notification is immediate and a reply can be the start of a conversation. Twitter works particularly well for conversations given the short nature, 140 characters, of tweets.

Real time communication allows promotion of events and campaigns right up to the start of the event or end of a campaign, e.g. promotion or competition. Furthermore, conversation around the event can take place whilst the event is going on and after it has finished.

Low Cost

Facebook and Twitter accounts are currently free to set up and Social Media is often described as "free" but this is not quite right. It is worthwhile incorporating professionally taken photos and/or designed images to make your Profile/Page attractive and to ensure it stands out from the competition. Furthermore, it takes a lot of resources and time to manage and run social networks and of course there is cost attached to this.

How to Make Social Media Work for Your Clinic

Listen

Demonstrate to your Fans and Followers that you are available for them by responding promptly to comments and interacting with them. Whether you are having a conversation face to face or on a social network it is important to listen. Make your audience feel that their concerns are important to you.

Provide Value

The single most important characteristic of any posts onto social network is value. Your post or tweet must be of use to your reader. For example, providing advice and tips around health and well-being would be of interest and use to a clinic's audience.

If your posts are enjoyable or useful then it is more likely that members of your audience will share your posts on Facebook and retweet on Twitter, thereby increasing awareness.

Be Human

As social media is all about conversation it is important to be human, as people prefer to talk to another person rather than a clinic. It is worth investing the time to tag people (use the @ symbol) and refer to people by first name only which along with politeness, can help build relationships.

Ask Questions

Start conversations with questions. You can then get to know your audience better. Seek opinions on what content you are providing. If you are not sure of what type of content your audience is looking for, then why not ask?

Provide Answers

Good customer service means answering questions from customers with complete answers. Providing full answers means that others may come across your reply that they could find useful.

Publish Photos and Videos

Facebook is more likely to publish a post including an image or video in News Feeds of your Fans and such posts have a higher engagement rate too. Furthermore, according to Hubspot (2012) [2], photos get 53 % more likes, 104 % more comments and 84 % more click-throughs on links than text-based posts. Plus according to Twitter #TweetAcademy webinar (2014) [3], Tweets with images have a 200 % higher engagement rate than those without. This is not surprising as Twitter has really improved the way that photos and videos are displayed, with thumbnails for images and videos automatically displayed. Most mobile Twitter apps now display photos and videos in this way too.

"Don'ts"

There are also some "Don'ts":

- Do not post photos without permission and/or crediting the photographer—you could be infringing copyright laws.
- Do not automate your posts and tweets—social media should be personal and conversational.
- Do not link Facebook with Twitter—they are different channels, e.g. tweets are limited to 140 characters but there is no limit on Facebook posts.
- Do not send the same update to Facebook and Twitter at the same time—if someone is following you on both networks this can be irritating.

Strategy and Planning

The goals you have for your use of social media should reflect your business objectives. Give some thought about what you want to achieve. Asking yourself the following questions should help:

- Do I want to raise awareness of my clinic?
- Do I want to increase the number of patients?
- Do I want to improve communications with my existing patients?
- Do I want to provide customer services via social media?
- Do I want to increase the traffic to my website or blog?

The main thing is having business objectives for your use of social media. There is little point in setting up a Twitter account and tweeting if you do not know why you are doing it. Once you have decided on what is important then you will need to consider, plan and create content. You can do this by putting together a content plan that should include the following:

The source of your content—is this going to be your blog, medical articles or news websites?

The type of content—are you posting and tweeting articles, links, tools, tips, photos or videos?

Channels—which social networks are you going to use for which types of content. For example, Facebook works better for longer posts when you need to explain how to do something, perhaps accompanied by a photo, whereas on Twitter there might only be space for a sentence with a link. Twitter is better for conversations such as answering queries and responding to patients.

There is plenty of good content around IVF on the Web so it is important that your content is not just good but great. It needs to provide value, and be meaningful to your audience and help achieve your objectives.

How to Make Facebook Work for Your Clinic

Encourage Interaction on Facebook

Crafting your posts in a way that engages readers and creates a response is very important. This response can be measured in Likes, Commenting or Sharing of posts. Good interaction on posts increases the visibility of your brand as they will feature more in your reader's newsfeeds. This interaction, also known as engagement, is about creating feelings and establishing an emotional response with your fans. As Jason Falls states—"Engagement is communicating well enough that the audience pays attention"—www.socialmediaexaminer.com (2011) [4].

Ask Questions

It is a simple but effective technique to encourage interaction and engagement. Fans like answering questions and can use Comments to reply with their answers. A good tactic is to make a statement, for example offer an opinion, and then ask your fans what they think.

Keep Your Posts Concise

Keeping posts concise creates more engagement. Research has shown, published in the Buddy Media Report (2011) [5], that posts made up of 80 characters or less have 27 % higher engagement rates.

Ask People to Engage

"Calls to action" and action words result in higher engagement. Action words such as Visit and phrases such as Sign Up, Tell Us and Ask Us work well in posts and they are worth adding to the About section of your profile too.

Post After 5 pm or at the Weekend

Facebook is visited most after 5 pm on weekdays and perhaps surprisingly, most post sharing occurs on Saturday; Buddy Media Report (2011) [5].

Use Facebook Apps

Facebook Apps (also known as Tabs) have become an attractive feature for owners of Facebook Pages, even though they are slightly less visible following the redesign of Pages in Spring 2014.

Apps provide an opportunity to have your own customised space on Facebook (see Fig. 20.1—Example of a Facebook App).

Effectively, it is your own web page on which to provide any content or features that you wish. With a width of 810 px and no ads or sidebars you can provide engaging content that the reader is focussed on. You should customise your App Thumbnail Image with an eye-catching image that should be 110×74 pixels. Then, add a call to action that encourages visitors to click, e.g. "Sign Up" or "Go To".

If you have a budget for advertising, you can drive traffic directly to your App with Facebook Ads. This can really help increase engagement if your App invites participation, such as with a competition or a poll.

Your Facebook App can reinforce the purpose of your page. Here are some ideas:

- Sell your services—set up a shop for your services
- Newsletter sign-up—add a sign-up form to increase subscribers
- Showcase your videos—display a video
- Run a competition—setup a competition or draw
- Ask for patient feedback—set up a poll or feedback form

For design and setup of Facebook Apps, speak to your web developer about using a third party site. I would recommend Shortstack (www.shortstack.com) as they provide some great templates, Apps are easy to design and install and they display on mobile devices.

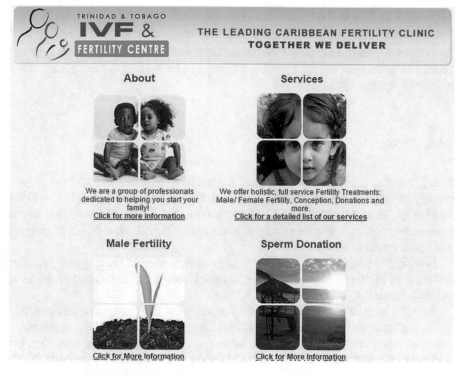

Fig. 20.1 Example of a Facebook App

Add Milestones to Your Facebook Timeline

Timelines allow you to tell the story of your clinic as you can provide the history of your clinic by including key events, known as Milestones. For example, details around when and how the clinic was founded, moves to new premises, numbers of pregnancies achieved and so on. Each milestone is displayed across the Page and can be accompanied with a photo or a video, which I would strongly encourage.

Enhance Your Cover Photos

Cover Photos take up more than a third of most screens so make sure you choose a high-resolution image that has a powerful impact. The size of the image should be 851×351 px although if you upload a larger image it will be resized. Professionally taken photos of employees and patients would work well. You can also add text to an image so if you are having a marketing campaign or wish to promote an event, you could add some wording to an image to reinforce your message.

How to Highlight Posts

You can ensure that important posts standout more with a star banner by "highlighting" them. Hover over the top right corner of the story you want to star and click ˅. Then select the star symbol to highlight.

How to Tag

A tag is a hyperlink that makes it easy for readers to click and visit the entity— usually a Profile or Page that you have tagged. It is displayed onto your Wall and the Wall of the Friend or Page that you have tagged. So it is a great way to mention someone as well as raising awareness of you or your Page. Be careful not to over tag and spam Profiles or Pages.

Ensure that your are using Facebook as your Page then to start tagging just type the name of Profile or Page or use the @ symbol, then select the correct entity from the drop down list.

Tagging is great for cross promotion—work with your suppliers, advisers and contacts to promote each other's service. So for example you could tag an advisers' event on your Wall and a few weeks later they could do the same for a seminar. On each occasion your Page and that of your advisers will be promoted on both Pages.

Tagging is a great way to acknowledge and thank the author of content that you have Shared. So if you find an interesting article that you share on Facebook, you can credit the originator alongside the link.

Enable Messages Button

Your patients might want to message you privately, so make sure that you Enable the Message button under Settings/General/Messages (see Fig. 20.2—Enable Messages).

Get Mobile

The best way to update your Facebook Page when on the move is to use the Facebook Pages Manager App on your smartphone or tablet. This app is totally dedicated to Pages so you can fully focus on your clinic and not be distracted by the personal side of Facebook. You will need this app if you want to take photos and upload them to your Page, which I would recommend you do frequently. It is also very good at providing notifications when Fans interact with your Page.

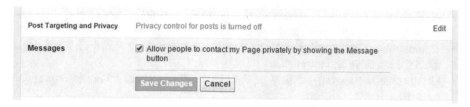

Fig. 20.2 Enable messages

Setup Your Own Facebook Page Web Address

You can have your own web address for your Facebook Business Page, for example www.facebook.com/intranetfuture. If you do not yet have a customised address, you can check to see if the address of your choice is available by going to Settings/Page Info/Facebook Web Address. The best option for your Page's web address is facebook.com followed by your clinic's name.

Once created, you should publish this address on your website, in your email auto signature and on all your marketing collateral such as business cards and brochures as well as mentioning it alongside publication of your phone number or website address. Your own Facebook Page address can have a number of benefits; it is easier to remember so can help increase visitors to you Facebook Page and your Page is more likely to show up in Facebook's Search and Google Search.

It can be difficult to change your Page more than once so make sure you have the address you want and that it is spelled correctly, before you confirm.

How to Use Facebook Groups

Facebook Groups have great features, despite not being as popular as Personal Profiles and Pages. Groups are ideal when you have a set number of people with the same objective or shared interest; for example, consultants working on a project or patients wishing to discuss IVF and pregnancy. The emphasis is on discussion, collaboration and sharing of ideas. Groups are flexible and easy to use and are straightforward and easy to set up at www.facebook.com/groups.

There are three types of Facebook Groups:

1. Open—Anyone can see the group, who is in it and what members post.
2. Closed—Anyone can see the group and who is in it. Only members see posts.
3. Secret—Only members see the group, who is in it and what members post.

Useful features include:

- Easy wall updates—no need to select a Share button; just tap the enter key.
- Page rendering—the latest Wall Posts rise to the top of the Page.

- Navigation/menu—easy access to all the main actions at top of page—Posts, Photos, Videos, Questions and Docs.
- Documents—Create notes and short text docs or upload Word and pdf docs; ideal for agendas and minutes.
- Group chat messaging—ability to chat with all members of the Group at the same time.
- Update via email—send and receive updates using the Group email address.
- For more advice on using Facebook for your clinic, I recommend you visit Facebook's own business guide at www.facebook.com/business.

How to Make Twitter Work for Your Clinic

It is All About Conversation

Due to the limit of 140 characters per tweet (including spaces), Twitter lends itself to discussion and conversation. It is easy to communicate quickly and easily, particularly via smartphone and tablet. It is great for obtaining information and communicating real time. For example, a clinic could provide the latest news on IVF and live updates from seminars.

Listen

In order to make Twitter successful for your clinic you need to "listen". Finding and reading content that is relevant to your area of expertise and the types of service you offer is essential. In order to listen to the conversations relevant to your business, try using the Advanced Search tool, which you can find at twitter.com/search-advanced. The various filters allow you to fine tune your search. For example, you can find prospective patients local to you by searching for tweets within a certain area of your clinic.

You can also use a tool like TweetDeck (www.tweetdeck.com) to listen on an ongoing basis using columns to monitor mentions of your clinic, services and topics like IVF and pregnancy. You can monitor conversations and join into conversations in real time as each column is updated as tweets are posted. Another option is to use a tool like Twilert (www.twilert.com) that works by emailing you tweets containing certain key words or hashtags (see below) that you have specified.

Use Twitter Hashtags

Twitter Hashtags group conversation around a topic, theme or event, e.g. #pregnancy, #ivf or #IVFLive. You can view the entire conversation in a single stream.

You can use to follow a conversation and find out useful information or join into the discussion—simply click on a hashtag or enter into Search.

You can also use hashtags to raise awareness of your clinic and services and build your audience.

Hashtags are also great for promoting events, running competitions and campaigns. In this case your hashtag should be unique so the focus is on your conversation only rather than one that is mixed up with another event or campaign.

You should also ensure your hashtag is concise (maximum of 15 characters) but that it also conveys meaning and is easily understandable. There is little point in including your business or brand name as your account name will reflect that.

It is a good idea to use capital letters within Hashtags to separate words—known as "camel case". This also prevents problems of misunderstanding.

If you are using a hashtag for an event, then ensure that all attendees are aware of the hashtag via joining instructions and delegate packs as well as displaying on event notices, signage and TV/display screens using a tool like twitterfall.com. Encourage attendees to tweet about the event at all times, e.g. before, during and after the event.

You can view the conversation around any hashtag by using the following web address:—www://twitter.com/<#Hashtag>

How to Grow Your Audience

On Twitter it is important to have an audience of quality followers; people who are genuinely interested in your tweets. Ideally, your audience should be made up of potential and existing patients, suppliers, advisers, contacts, fellow professionals and perhaps local people.

Your audience should provide access to a large group of people who can discuss your business and interests and help grow awareness through retweeting. Of course, your tweets are public and can be found via Twitter Search and search engines like Google, but your followers are the most likely people to see your tweets as they will appear on their home page.

If you have a budget you can attract quality followers with Twitter's Promoted Accounts. You pay for each new follower with prices starting at 1 US cent; the more you pay the more followers you will acquire. Once you have set up a campaign, Twitter will display your account name on relevant profiles at the top of the "Who to follow" box and in the timelines of mobile Twitter users. You can even target the followers of other clinics.

But there is plenty you can do to get noticed by other tweeters using the following tips and you do not need a budget.

Add twitter ID as a hyperlink to other marketing channels—For example, a hyperlink on Facebook raises awareness to Friends, Followers and visitors to your Profile or Page. Select About on your Timeline then Contact and Basic Info, then Screen Names under Contact Information.

You should add your twitter ID to your YouTube channel—select the pencil symbol then Edit links and add your Twitter and other social network web addresses under Social Links. The links are then displayed as icons to your YouTube viewers, which makes it easy for them to visit your profile and follow you.

Even if you do no have a budget for Promoted Accounts, you can still reach the followers of other clinics. Their followers are likely to be interested in what you tweet about and you may provide them with a better value and quality of service. You can find and then follow your competitors using Twitter's Advanced Search tool or ManageFlitter (www.manageflitter.com) Paid subscription is required for the latter.

Engage with people who are not yet following you but who have noticed you send @messages to people who have favourited one of your tweets or retweeted you. Even a simple "Thank you" or "Hi" gets your presence on Twitter noticed.

Include key words in tweets—include key words relating to topical issues around IVF, fertility and pregnancy. This will help you show up more in search results.

Optimise your profile—Use your Bio to give people reasons to follow you. Tell people what you tweet about and stress the benefits of following you, e.g. Follow for tips on increasing the chances of getting pregnant.

Mention popular accounts in your tweets—by tagging influential users your tweets will become more visible as such accounts are more likely to show up in search results.

Most importantly of all your tweets should provide value—Tweets that are valued are more likely to get noticed and they will be retweeted which will bring you more followers. So make sure you entertain, inform and engage. Try and generate an emotional response. Look for topical events or news stories around IVF and pregnancy that you can tweet links to or comment about.

Scheduling Tweets

The practice of scheduling tweets allows you to set aside a defined period of time for updating Twitter and other social networks as well as helping you reach as many people as possible with your tweets. Scheduling helps organisation; setting aside a dedicated time, say a 30 min window every morning, makes it more likely that your updating will happen. It also has the advantage of providing a steady stream of tweets throughout the day thus giving more people an opportunity to view your updates.

Scheduling tweets has its dangers though and it is important to keep an eye on Twitter to ensure that questions are answered and comments replied to. Do not forget that Twitter is about conversation; not just broadcasting your own message.

How to Create and Use Twitter Lists

Twitter lists help you organise people and their tweets into groups, thus creating your own customised Timelines. Lists can either be public or private which means they can only be viewed by the creator of the list. Viewing the Timeline of a list will show you a stream of tweets from the users on that list.

It is really straightforward to add someone to a Twitter list:

1. Select the cog symbol that represents the profile of the person you wish to add.
2. Then select "Add or remove from lists".
3. You can then create a new list or select a tick box to add the person to one of your existing Twitter Lists.

You can view existing Lists and create new ones from your Lists page, which you can access via Lists on your Profile page. See Fig. 20.3—"How to create Twitter lists". Twitter lists can be used in a number of ways:

- Segment people into useful groups—create Lists for suppliers, prospects, clients or people that tweet about a particular subject, e.g. fertility. This helps you focus on a particular type of person and their tweets.
- Group people you are not following—you do not have to be following someone in order to add them to a List. For example, if might be useful to have a list of your competitors or local people.
- Research—you do not always need to create your own lists as you can subscribe and follow public lists.

How to Use Twitter Favourites

Twitter Favourites have limited functionality; you cannot create folders by category or subject like you can for Internet browser bookmarks, as they are all stored together. Nevertheless, here is a couple of ways they can be useful:

Use the favouriting feature as a "read later" function—simply save your tweets that you want to read another time. Handy if you are busy and do not have the time to click the link and read a useful article that has been posted.

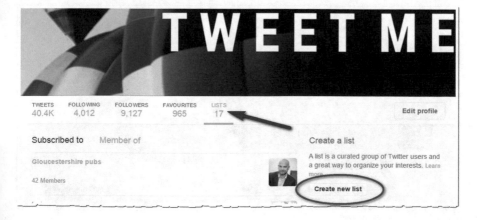

Fig. 20.3 How to create Twitter lists

- Use to record testimonial tweets—you can build up an authentic record of testimonials tweets that recommend your clinic. If patients are tweeting positively about your clinic and its services, why not use their tweets to help promote your business?

How to Embed Tweets

Twitter makes it easy to embed tweets on your website or blog. By embedding a tweet you retain the full functionality that users have on Twitter. For example, readers can retweet, reply or favourite the embedded tweet direct from your website.

To embed a tweet you need to copy and paste the HTML code of the tweet you wish to display into your website or blog. On Twitter.com, hover over the tweet you wish to embed and select …, then Embed Tweet. See Fig. 20.4—"How to embed a tweet".

The code for you to copy and paste into your website or blog will then be displayed. You can choose how the tweet is aligned on the page, e.g. Left, Right or Centre.

Here are some ideas on using embedded tweets:

- Use embedded tweets containing quotes as an alternative to a text quote.
- Instead of quoting opinions, you can display original tweets—far more authentic than putting text in quotation marks.
- Embedded tweets can help promote awareness of events and gain feedback about events.
- Use embedded tweets when you receive positive feedback or testimonials.

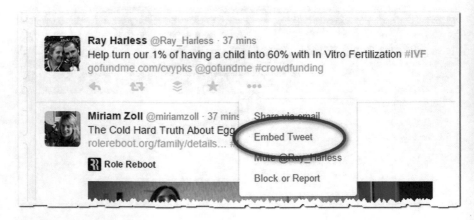

Fig. 20.4 How to embed a Tweet

For more advice on using Twitter for your clinic, I recommend you visit Twitter's own business guide at www.business.twitter.com.

Social Advertising

You can set up your own adverts or "promotions" on Facebook and Twitter. On Facebook, you can use Ads in a number of ways including; to increase Page Likes, to increase clicks to your website and to boost engagement on Posts on your Page.

Facebook Adverts

Advertising to increase Page Likes can be an effective way to boost the audience for your Page. All Facebook Ads should be set up to target and reach your appropriate audience. Criteria includes age, gender, location and interests.

You can display your website or blog on an Ad to encourage visitors to your website. This can be effective if there is content such as a new blog post or a video that you wish to promote.

With only around 6 % of Page Posts now appearing in Facebook News Feeds [6] Social@Ogilvy (2014), advertising is required if you want your posts to reach a meaningful sized audience. You can promote or boost Posts so that they reach not only all your Fans but other people on Facebook too. Targeting can be very precise, reach large numbers of people and when compared with other types of advertising are good value. You can boost a page directly from your Page or using the Ads Manager, which is recommended as this gives you more options.

Each Facebook Ad includes a title, thumbnail image and body copy which is limited to 90 characters. Ads can be displayed on the right hand side and in the News Feed both on desktop and on mobile.

Twitter: Promoted Accounts and Tweets

On Twitter you can promote tweets as well as your account.

With Promoted Tweets you can extend the reach of your tweets. You can select which tweets you wish to promote or create a specific tweet for your campaign.

With a Promoted Account, in return for payment of anything from 1 US cent upwards, Twitter will add your Account to the top of the "Who to follow" section and mark it as "Promoted".

With both Promoted Accounts and Tweets you can target your audience by interest as well as followers of any Twitter accounts. This means that you can target Twitter followers of other IVF clinics.

Recommended Social Media App/Tool

Buffer

There are plenty of Social Media Apps and Tools available but if I had to recommend just one, it would be Buffer (www.bufferapp.com). It is a web based tool and mobile App that provides a smart way to share your posts to your social networks. It enables you to schedule your favourite articles, photos, videos and links so that they are posted out across your social networks at a schedule of your choosing. You can also set a specific time for publication of a post or tweet.

So for example, you could share four or five articles early in the morning that would be published onto Twitter at different times throughout the day. This approach has the advantage of helping you both organise your time and maximise the visibility of your posts. You can also post to Facebook (both your Profile and Page), LinkedIn (Profiles, Pages and Groups and Google + (Pages only).

If you use Chrome, you can add the Buffer extension, which makes it easy to post and tweet content you find around the web.

Measurement

To make sure that your social media efforts are worthwhile you need to measure the results of your activity. To measure the effectiveness of your use of social networks, as stated in the Strategy and Planning section, it is vital that you are clear on your business objectives. To be able to measure you will need to have clearly defined goals and a timeframe for each. For example, "increase website visitors from Twitter from 200 to 500 in 3 months".

You can apply this approach to each of your objectives, although some are harder to accurately measure than others, e.g. increase in patients resulting from social media use. To help with measurement I would recommend the following three tools:

1. Google Analytics—use for measuring origin of website visitors
2. Facebook Insights—use for general measurement of Facebook activity
3. Tweet Analytics—use to measure reach on Twitter

You need to have a Google Account to access and use Google Analytics. As a Facebook Admin you can access and use Insights once you have more than 30 Likes and Twitter Analytics is part of Twitter's Advertising platform. If you are not going to use Twitter Ads, then Tweet Binder (www.tweetbinder.com) is a good alternative.

Measurement should be carried out regularly and your efforts should be tailored accordingly. You should aim to repeat and build on Facebook posts that are providing results and reduce posts that are less successful.

Following the advice in this chapter and taking this approach to measurement will help to ensure that your use of social media in achieving your clinic's business objectives is effective. Good luck!

References

1. Kagan M.: What the f*** is social media. www.slideshare.net/mzkagan/what-the-fk-social-media. 2008.
2. Hubspot   Study.   www.blog.hubspot.com/blog/tabid/6307/bid/33800/Photos-on-Facebook-Generate-53-More-Likes-Than-the-Average-Post-NEW-DATA.aspx. Accessed Oct 2012.
3. Twitter for Business #TwitterAcademy webinar. www.webcaster4.com/Webcast/ListenPage? companyId=214&webcastId=3892. Accessed 16 Apr 2014.
4. Falls J. www.socialmediaexaminer.com. 2011.
5. Buddy Media Report (now salesforce.com). 2011.
6. Social@Ogilvy Survey (2014)

Index

© Springer Science+Business Media New York 2016
S.D. Fleming, A.C. Varghese (eds.), *Organization and Management of IVF
Units*, DOI 10.1007/978-3-319-29373-8

Printed in the United States
By Bookmasters